T0214794

# Modern Management of Perinatal Psychiatric Disorders

For James and Richard
*Carol Henshaw*


For Karin, our three daughters Christina, Ann-Marie and
Susanne, granddaughter Suzannah and grandson Joshua
*John Cox*


For Flip
*Joanne Barton*

# Modern Management of Perinatal Psychiatric Disorders

## 2nd edition

Carol Henshaw

John Cox

Joanne Barton

RCPsych Publications

# CAMBRIDGE
## UNIVERSITY PRESS

University Printing House, Cambridge CB2 8BS, United Kingdom

One Liberty Plaza, 20th Floor, New York, NY 10006, USA

477 Williamstown Road, Port Melbourne, VIC 3207, Australia

314-321, 3rd Floor, Plot 3, Splendor Forum, Jasola District Centre, New Delhi - 110025, India

79 Anson Road, #06-04/06, Singapore 079906

Cambridge University Press is part of the University of Cambridge.

It furthers the University's mission by disseminating knowledge in the pursuit of education, learning and research at the highest international levels of excellence.

www.cambridge.org
Information on this title: www.cambridge.org/9781909726772

© The Royal College of Psychiatrists 2017

RCPsych Publications is an imprint of the Royal College of Psychiatrists,
21 Prescot Street, London E1 8BB
http://www.rcpsych.ac.uk

First published 2017
Reprinted 2018

*A catalogue record for this publication is available from the British Library*

ISBN 978-1-909-72677-2 Paperback

# Contents

Abbreviations | vi

The authors | viii

Preface | ix
Carol Henshaw, John Cox, Joanne Barton

Foreword | xi
Margaret Oates

1 Historical perspectives and classification issues | 1

2 Perinatal depression, anxiety, stress and adjustment | 10

3 Puerperal psychosis | 63

4 Childbearing in women with existing mental disorders | 84

5 Substance misuse | 108

6 Perinatal mental illness, children and the family | 139

7 Screening and prevention | 174

8 Physical treatments during pregnancy | 196

9 Physical treatments and breastfeeding | 245

10 Service provision | 267

11 Perinatal psychiatry in multi-ethnic societies | 278

Appendix I   Organisations offering support and information | 287

Appendix II   Edinburgh Postnatal Depression Scale | 289

Appendix III   Resources | 291

Index | 293

# Abbreviations

| | |
|---|---|
| ADHD | attention-deficit hyperactivity disorder |
| ART | assisted reproductive technology |
| BDI | Beck Depression Inventory |
| BDZ | benzodiazepine |
| CBT | cognitive–behavioural therapy |
| CEMD | Confidential Enquiry into Maternal Deaths |
| CNS | central nervous system |
| CSA | child sexual abuse |
| DSM | *Diagnostic and Statistical Manual of Mental Disorders* |
| ECT | electroconvulsive therapy |
| EDNOS | eating disorder not otherwise specified |
| EPDS | Edinburgh Postnatal Depression Scale |
| FASD | fetal alcohol spectrum disorder |
| GAD | generalised anxiety disorder |
| GP | general practitioner |
| HPA | hypothalamic–pituitary–adrenal |
| HRSD | Hamilton Rating Scale for Depression |
| ICD | International Classification of Diseases |
| IPT | interpersonal psychotherapy |
| LSD | lysergic acid diethylamide |
| MAOI | monoamine oxidase inhibitor |
| MDI | Mental Developmental Index |
| MDMA | methylenedioxymethamphetamine |
| NHS | National Health Service |
| NICE | National Institute for Health and Care Excellence |
| NICU | neonatal intensive care unit |

| | |
|---|---|
| NRT | nicotine replacement therapy |
| OCD | obsessive–compulsive disorder |
| O-DV | *O*-methyldesvenlafaxine |
| OR | odds ratio |
| PDSS | Postpartum Depression Screening Scale |
| PMDD | premenstrual dysphoric disorder |
| PNAS | poor neonatal adaptation syndrome |
| PTSD | post-traumatic stress disorder |
| RCT | randomised controlled trial |
| RR | relative risk |
| SNRI | serotonin–noradrenaline reuptake inhibitor |
| SSRI | selective serotonin reuptake inhibitor |
| STAI | Spielberger State–Trait Anxiety Inventory |
| TCA | tricyclic antidepressant |
| UKTIS | UK Teratology Information Service |
| VTE | venous thromboembolism |
| WHO | World Health Organization |
| Y-BOCS | Yale–Brown Obsessive Compulsive Scale |

# The authors

**Carol Henshaw** MB ChB MD FRCPsych FHEA was a Consultant in Perinatal Mental Health at Liverpool Women's NHS Foundation Trust, an Honorary Senior Lecturer at the University of Liverpool and a Visiting Fellow at Staffordshire University until her retirement in 2016. She was awarded a Winston Churchill Memorial Trust Fellowship in 2004 to study qualitative research methods at Victoria University of Technology in Melbourne, Australia, and was President of the Marcé Society from 2004 to 2006. She has sat on several Executive Committees of Faculties, Sections and Special Interest Groups of the Royal College of Psychiatrists and chaired the revision of College Report 164, 'Parents as Patients: addressing the needs, including the safety of children whose parents have mental illness'.

**John Cox** BM BChDM (Oxon) FRCPsych FRCP is Emeritus Professor of Psychiatry at Keele University, Staffordshire, a Past President of the Royal College of Psychiatrists and former Secretary General of the World Psychiatric Association. He is a founding member of the Marcé Society, and in 2014 was the first recipient of the John Cox Distinguished Service Marcé Medal. He developed the Edinburgh Postnatal Depression Scale (with Jennifer Holden and Ruth Sagovsky) when a Senior Lecturer in Edinburgh, following a 2-year lectureship at Makerere University in Uganda. In Stoke-on-Trent, he founded the first Parent and Baby Day Unit and, with Carol Henshaw, the Keele Perinatal Education Unit. He lives with his wife Karin in Cheltenham, where he continues to write and to enjoy singing as a trained soloist. He is a trustee of the Musical Brain and Patron of Listening Post.

**Joanne Barton** MB ChB PhD MRCPsych is a consultant Child and Adolescent psychiatrist who works for North Staffordshire Combined Healthcare NHS Trust, providing psychiatric input to a community-based child and adolescent mental health service. Her day-to-day work with children, young people and their families is a constant reminder of the importance of parental mental health to the well-being and development of children. Her interest in the impact of parental mental illness during the perinatal period developed during her PhD, which examined the role of maternal expressed emotion in the development and maintenance of child disruptive behavioural problems.

# Preface

The impetus to write this book over 5 years ago came from our concern, as clinicians, researchers and educators, that trainee psychiatrists required access to knowledge about the diagnosis and management of perinatal mental disorder which was not then readily available. We also had in mind general practitioners and obstetricians, and readers from other professional backgrounds such as psychology, nursing and management.

In this second edition we have rewritten and updated several chapters to reflect current practice and new knowledge in this now rapidly expanding field. We hope that readers from low and middle-income countries, where psychiatrists are few and far between, will find our approach, and the studies cited, helpful to their needs.

The development of active and informed advocacy groups in most regions of the world is a powerful synchrony of patient experience and professional expertise. We hope that this edition, although not including many clinical narratives, will nevertheless be of interest to parents and their carers.

Maternal mental disorder remains a risk factor for stunted growth and impairment of cognitive development in children throughout the world (Stein, 2014). Suicide remains a leading cause of maternal death in the UK (Knight *et al*, 2014). It is essential that clinicians in primary and secondary care are aware of these disabling conditions, and that women who suffer from them, or are at risk of doing so, are identified, assessed and treated.

It remains essential in our experience to approach the management of these women from a biopsychosocial perspective, and for health professionals to be fully aware of the sociocultural context and the 'meaning' of the illness for the mother and her family. The optimal management of parents with childbearing-related mental disorder, and of their developing relationship with their baby, requires clinical judgement of a high order. Psychiatry is an art and a science, and perinatal psychiatry is a person-centred, relationship-based specialty – and in this regard sets an example for the rest of medicine.

Our hope is that readers of this book will be encouraged to develop these broad clinical skills, and to hold together science and values – as well as the body, mind and spirit.

*Carol Henshaw*
*John Cox*
*Joanne Barton*

## Acknowledgements

We wish to thank Ilana Crome and Khaled Ismail for their help in writing Chapter 5 in the first edition, and Margaret Oates for her Foreword. Karin Cox has helped greatly over the years with research and writing. We are much indebted to our spouses and families for tolerating our labours – and especial thanks to all those parents and children who trusted us with their care and continue to inspire our work.

## References

Knight M, Kenyon S, Brocklehurst P, et al (eds) *Saving Lives, Improving Mothers' Care – Lessons Learned to Inform Future Maternity Care from the UK and Ireland Confidential Enquiries into Maternal Deaths and Morbidity 2009–12*. National Perinatal Epidemiology Unit, University of Oxford, 2014.

Stein A, Pearson RM, Goodman S, et al (2014) Effects of perinatal mental health disorders on the fetus and child. *Lancet*, **384**: 1800–1819.

# Foreword

This book is a testament to the increasing recognition that maternal mental health problems are the core business of both psychiatry and maternity care.

Perinatal psychiatry is now the internationally accepted term for conditions complicating pregnancy and the postpartum year. These include not only new-onset conditions following delivery, such as postnatal depression and puerperal psychosis, but also pre-existing conditions which may relapse, recur or continue during pregnancy and the postpartum period. It is concerned not only with the medical and psychosocial management of the mother, but also the impact of the disorder and its treatments on the developing infant before and after birth. Although in the UK, perinatal psychiatry is a subspecialty of adult psychiatry; it overlaps and shares common goals with child psychiatry and those concerned with infant development.

Why is perinatal psychiatry so important, and why has it achieved such recent prominence in national policy and practice guidelines? Postpartum psychiatric disorders have long been of great interest to researchers. Childbirth offers a unique research paradigm: a clearly defined cohort, and a mixture of neuroendocrine, psychosocial, anthropological, sociological and epidemiological factors which can be studied across time and across cultures, of interest to psychiatrists, obstetricians, psychologists and social scientists, and to adult and child workers. It poses and answers questions which are not only relevant to this life event but also can inform the aetiology and treatment of disorders, particularly affective disorders, at other times.

Although there has been prominent research interest in perinatal psychiatric disorders for over 40 years, with individual clinical centres of excellence, the provision of specialised services is patchy, inequitable and, at a national level, inadequate.

Over the past 10 years there has been an improvement in both quality and extent of the provision of specialised perinatal services. There are 18 mother and baby units in the UK, all meeting a single national service specification with common quality standards and criteria for access. There are at least 20 comprehensive community perinatal psychiatric teams, some linked with mother and baby units; this number is increasing, and they too operate to common service specifications and quality standards. Despite this, there is still a national shortfall of mother and baby unit beds, with many women being separated from their infants and admitted to general adult wards, and large areas of the UK where pregnant and postpartum women with mental health problems are cared for by general services rather than specialised services.

The need for specialised perinatal services, mother and baby units, community teams and maternity liaison services is underpinned by a number of factors. Pregnancy and childbirth are associated with considerable psychiatric morbidity. A small but significant number of women will develop a profound psychotic illness in the early weeks following childbirth, requiring specialist skills and resources for their and their infant's proper care. Although the number is small, it represents a substantial increase in the risk of developing a psychotic illness following childbirth compared to other times. A larger number of women will develop a severe non-psychotic affective disorder, and an even larger number will develop the mild-to-moderate affective disorder popularly known as postnatal depression. Overall, at least 10% of delivered women will suffer from a psychiatric disorder following childbirth. The more severe conditions will require the attention of specialised mental health services. The less severe conditions, while probably no more common than at other times, pose a major public health problem, with chronic maternal depression – particularly if associated with socioeconomic adversity – having adverse effects on infant and child development. The perinatal period is also very important because of the risk of recurrence in women with pre-existing serious mental illness, particularly bipolar disorder. Childbirth is unique in psychiatry as a major provoker of mental illness that comes with 9 months warning. The perinatal period poses particular problems for the management of psychiatric disorders. Many psychotropic medications, particularly mood stabilisers, are problematic in pregnancy. Acute psychotic episodes in pregnancy compromise maternal and infant health. The distinctive clinical presentation, rapid onset and deterioration can demand a different response from psychiatric services than at other times. Throughout the perinatal period, psychiatric professionals have to deal with two patients, both mother and infant.

Pregnancy and the early postpartum period is exceptional in the human lifespan for its level of surveillance by health professionals. This provides an opportunity not only for the early detection and prompt treatment of those who are ill, but also for the identification in early pregnancy of those at risk of developing an illness following delivery, and for secondary and perhaps primary prevention.

## The UK Confidential Enquiry into Maternal Deaths

Most of the UK national policies for perinatal mental health have been strongly influenced by the UK maternal mortality enquiries over the past

4 years. These reveal that suicide in particular, and psychiatric causes of maternal deaths in general, are a leading cause of maternal mortality. This is also likely to be true internationally. It is generally accepted that maternal mortality is the 'tip of the iceberg' and it is therefore reasonable to assume that psychiatric disorder is also a leading cause of maternal morbidity.

The UK Confidential Enquiry into Maternal Deaths (CEMD) combines both a maternal mortality surveillance and quantitative data analysis with an inquiry into individual cases' descriptions of the pathway of care and circumstances that were associated with an individual death. This combination of methods allows for the identification of themes and factors associated with poor outcomes, which in turn has led to the development of practice guidelines with demonstrable impact on the quality of maternity care. In addition, it allows for the emergence of new themes which reflect not only changes in reproductive epidemiology and technology (for example, increasing maternal age, rise in Caesarean sections, *in vitro* fertilisation) but also rapid societal changes such as the impact of asylum seekers and immigrants.

For the purposes of international comparison, it is important to understand how maternal mortality data are expressed. The maternal mortality rate refers to maternal deaths from 24 weeks of pregnancy to 42 days post-delivery. The causes are defined as direct (for example, haemorrhage, pre-eclampsia) and indirect (for example, pregnancy-exacerbated conditions, including suicide). The maternal mortality ratio is the number of maternal deaths compared to the number of births. ICD-10 pregnancy-related deaths are all deaths which occur during pregnancy and the postpartum year. The UK CEMD includes all deaths up to 1 year, but describe the data in such a way as to allow international comparison.

With each Enquiry, the case ascertainment increases and is generally regarded as being more complete than in other countries. This factor needs to be taken into account when comparing findings from the UK with other countries. Since 1997, case ascertainment has been enhanced by an Office of National Statistics linkage study, which identifies maternal deaths not reported directly to the Enquiry. These deaths have been, in the majority, late indirect and coincidental deaths, but have included a substantial number of suicides.

Over the past 20 years, suicide has remained a leading cause of maternal death. The numbers of maternal deaths due to suicide has not significantly changed, nor have their characteristics.

Over half of all maternal suicides were suffering from a serious mental illness (including postpartum psychosis). Half of these illnesses were occurring for the first time and half were a recurrence of a previous illness. These illnesses characteristically began in the early days and weeks following delivery and deteriorated very rapidly. All of the mothers suffering from serious mental illness were in contact with general adult psychiatric services at the time of their death. Half had a previous psychiatric history of serious mental illness and previous contact with psychiatric services. In the main, this was for serious affective disorder, including bipolar disorder and affective psychoses. In very few cases was this risk accurately identified at the booking clinic, and in even fewer was a management plan put in place. The apparent lack of awareness of the risk of recurrence of a serious affective disorder following childbirth was found not just in maternity and primary care services but also within mental health services.

The majority of maternal suicides were older, married or in stable cohabitation, employed and educated. This was particularly true of the women who were suffering from serious illness. The majority of women had been well in pregnancy, and many had been well for years previously, having fully recovered from a previous episode of serious illness. Because of their social characteristics and their prolonged period of well-being, these women would not have been recognised as 'vulnerable'. This serves as a reminder that serious illness can affect those in comfortable circumstances with no obvious personal or social problems.

Throughout the Enquiries it has been noted that midwives did not obtain or were not given information about a woman's previous history by the general practitioner or indeed by psychiatric services.

Over the past 20 years, very few mothers who died by suicide had been cared for by specialised perinatal psychiatric services, and even fewer had been admitted to a mother and baby unit – and those who had been admitted to a mother and baby unit died after their care had been taken over by general adult services. It is clear that in the majority of cases, the non-specialised services had not adapted to the maternity context and to the distinctive features of postpartum illness. They often responded too slowly, did not consider admission and underestimated the risk and severity of the condition. More recently it has been noted that the majority of maternal suicides suffered from discontinuity of care, receiving care from multiple psychiatric teams and mental health professionals.

The recommendations of the CEMD therefore remain that women should be asked at early pregnancy assessment for a previous psychiatric history and those with a history of serious mental illness should have a plan in place for the management of that risk. All women with serious mental illness in late pregnancy and the postpartum period should be managed by specialised perinatal psychiatric teams and, if admission is necessary, be admitted to a specialised mother and baby unit. In addition, the past two Enquiries recommend in their 'top 10 recommendations' that women with serious mental illness should be counselled prior to conception about the risk they face associated with pregnancy. Sadly, a constant finding of the CEMD since 1994 has been the violent method of suicide. In contrast to the method of female suicide at other times, 80% of maternal suicides used violent methods. The most common was hanging, followed by jumping from a height. Very few women died from an intentional overdose of prescribed or over-the-counter medication.

Suicide is not the only psychiatric cause of maternal death. Women also died from intentional or accidental overdoses of recreational drugs. A substantial number of women either died from medical conditions that were the consequence of their substance misuse exacerbated by pregnancy, or died because their psychiatric condition led to their medical conditions being missed or misattributed to psychiatric causes. These findings too have been constant over the past 20 years. A worrying theme to emerge from the Enquiries is the significant contribution to overall maternal mortality of substance misuse. Ten per cent of all maternal deaths occurred in substance misusers, and approximately half of all psychiatric deaths. Substance misuse was associated with avoiding antenatal care, high rates of removal of the infant into the care of local authorities and the subsequent absence of both psychiatric and maternity care for the mother. Very few of these women had had specialist care from drug addiction services during their pregnancies. This has led to the additional recommendations that specialised 'one-stop shop' services for pregnant substance misusers are provided, nested within the maternity services, with rapid access and active outreach as a principle of service provision.

The distinctive nature of perinatal psychiatric conditions and their consequences for the infant, as well as for mothers' future mental health, justify educating all those involved in the care of childbearing women and the provision of specialised services for those who are seriously mentally ill. If all psychiatrists discussed with their patients the implications of their conditions and treatments for pregnancy, if all women at risk of serious mental illness following childbirth had proactive management plans in place, and if those who became ill were treated by specialised services, then it is likely that there could be a reduction in maternal mortality and morbidity from psychiatric causes and an improvement in infant mental health. However, despite the increase in specialised service provision and the public profile of perinatal mental health problems, it sadly remains true that maternal suicide is not decreasing and many more suicides were avoidable.

*Margaret Oates OBE*

# Further reading

Cantwell R, Sisodia N, Oates M (2003) A comparison of mother & baby admission to a specialised inpatient service with postnatal admission to general services. *Archives of Women's Mental Health*, **6**: s83.

Cantwell R, Clutton-Brock T, Cooper G, *et al* (2011) Saving Mothers' Lives: reviewing maternal deaths to make motherhood safer: 2006–2008. *BJOG*, **118**: 1–203.

Cooper C, Jones L, Dunn E, *et al* (2007) Clinical presentation of postnatal and non-postnatal depressive episodes. *Psychological Medicine*, **37**: 1273–80.

Cox J, Murray D, Chapman G (1993) A controlled study of the onset, prevalence and duration of postnatal depression. *British Journal of Psychiatry*, **163**: 27–41.

Dean C, Kendell R (1981) The symptomatology of puerperal illness. *British Journal of Psychiatry*, **139**: 128–133.

Department of Health (2004) *National Service Framework: Children, Young People and Maternity Services*. DoH.

Department of Health (2009) *Improving Access to Psychological Therapies (IAPT): Perinatal Positive Practice Guide*. DoH.

Davies A, McIvor R, Kumar R (1995) Impact of childbirth on schizophrenic mothers. *Schizophrenic Research*, **16**: 25–31.

Elkin A, Gilburt H, Slade M, *et al* (2009) A national survey of psychiatric mother and baby units in England. *Psychiatric Services*, **5**: 629–633.

Heron J, McGuinness M, Blackmore E, *et al* (2008) Early postpartum symptoms in puerperal psychosis. *BJOG*, **115**: 348–353.

Howard L, Goss C, Leese M, *et al* (2003) Medical outcome of pregnancy in women with psychotic disorders and their infants in the first year after birth. *British Journal of Psychiatry*, **182**: 63–67.

Joint Commissioning Panel for Mental Health (2012) *Guidance for Commissioners of Perinatal Mental Health Services*. JCPMH.

Jones I, Craddock N (2005) Bipolar disorder and childbirth – the importance of recognising risk. *British Journal of Psychiatry*, **186**: 453–454.

Kendell R, Chalmers K, Platz C (1987) Epidemiology of puerperal psychoses. *British Journal of Psychiatry*, **150**: 662–673.

Knight M, Kenyon S, Brocklehurst P, *et al* (eds) *Saving Lives, Improving Mothers' Care*. MBRRACE-UK, 2014.

Leahy-Warren P (2007) Social support for first-time mothers: an Irish study. *American Journal of Maternal Child Nursing*, **32**: 368–374.

Morrell C, Slade P, Warner R, *et al* (2009) Clinical effectiveness of health visitor training in psychologically informed approaches for depression in postnatal women: pragmatic cluster randomised trial in primary care. *BMJ*, **338**: a3045.

Murray L, Hipwell A, Hooper R, *et al* (1996) The cognitive development of 5-year old children of postnatally depressed mothers. *Journal of Child Psychology and Psychiatry*, **37**: 927–935.

National Institute for Health and Care Excellence (2014) *Antenatal and Postnatal Mental Health* [CG45]. NICE.

National Institute for Health and Care Excellence (2011) *Caesarean Section* [CG132]. NICE.

NHS England (2013) *Specialised Perinatal Mental Health Services (Inpatient MBUs and Linked Outreach Teams)*. NHS England (http://www.england.nhs.uk/wp-content/uploads/2013/06/c06-spec-peri-mh.pdf).

O'Hara M, Swain A (1996) Rates and risk of postpartum depression – a meta-analysis. *International Review of Psychiatry*, **8**: 37–54.

Pawlby S, Fernyhough C, Meins E, *et al* (2010) Mind-mindedness and maternal responsiveness in infant–mother interactions in mothers with severe mental illness. *Psychological Medicine*, **40**: 1861–9.

Royal College of Obstetricians and Gynaecologists (2011) *Guidelines on the Management of Women with Mental Health Issues during Pregnancy and the Postnatal Period*. RCOG.

Royal College of Psychiatrists (2012) *Safe Patients and High Quality Services: A Guide to Job Descriptions and Job Plans for Consultant Psychiatrists* (CR174). RCPsych.

Royal College of Psychiatrists (2014) *Perinatal Mental Health Services* (CR88). RCPsych.

Scottish Intercollegiate Guidelines Network (2012) *Guideline 127: Management of Perinatal Mood Disorders*. SIGN.

# CHAPTER 1

# Historical perspectives and classification issues

## French pioneers and current opinion

Louis Victor Marcé, a brilliant pupil of Jean-Étienne Dominique Esquirol in Paris, in his seminal thesis in 1858, regarded the temporal association between postnatal illness and childbirth as its defining characteristic (Marcé, 1858). He also anticipated the development of endocrinology by delineating a 'morbid sympathie' between the postnatal mental state and bodily functions. A further observation by this scholarly 'ancien intern' was to identify certain symptoms of childbearing-related mental disorder that were rarely found together in non-puerperal mental disorders. Marcé recognised the specific forensic aspects of these case histories and, in particular, the risk to the infant and the mother of a severe puerperal psychosis. He may himself have suffered from bipolar disorder – and it is suggested by Luauté *et al* (2012) that he died by suicide. His pioneering work in his short life was honoured by the founders of the Marcé Society, which was named after him.

In this way, Marcé – and Esquirol, who in 1838 reported on a large study of postnatal illness in Paris – set the stage for further work in this field. It is regrettable that their work was largely lost to European psychiatry until the 1970s when the Marcé Society was founded.

Until the mid-20th century, puerperal psychosis continued to be regarded as a distinct condition. Numerous papers, comprehensively reviewed by Brockington (1996), were published; these described in detail the psychopathology of women with 'lactational psychosis', who experienced delusions about the baby and sexual infidelity, as well as religious themes. Confusion and perplexity were observed in many such women with non-infective psychoses, and such illnesses often resulted in the death of the mother and severe neglect of the baby. Menzies (1893) provided an account of many such women who were admitted to Rainhill asylum in Lancashire, and he made the customary distinction between lactational and other psychoses.

In the Middle Ages, madness after childbirth was more likely to be regarded as a religious than a medical problem. The mother was a 'witch' and her 'possession' was a punishment for misdemeanour. A postpartum mother was considered to be unclean, and a 'churching' cleansing ritual was therefore necessary to purify her. This ceremony was also attended by the midwife, and only after the churching had taken place could the mother again enter the church or attend Mass. In her autobiography, Margery Kempe (born 1373), who was a mediaeval mystic, described her recurrent postpartum mental disorders – which did not impair her ability to travel widely (Kempe, 1985).

In pre-Christian times, Greek physicians from the school of Hippocrates on the island of Kos were more holistic in their approach to mental disorder. Although they regarded mental disorders, including postnatal mental disorder, as having biological causes (milk diverted from the breast to the brain, or suppression of lochial discharge), prayers were also offered to gods such as Aesculapius or Apollo as part of the healing process.

It is apparent from this glimpse of medical history that postpartum mental disorders were thought to be different from those occurring at other times – and that the provision of healthcare varied according to the prevailing beliefs about causation. The choice of therapy was determined by the local culturally endorsed explanatory model. Deference to the now dominant scientific biomedical model for the causes of perinatal mental disorder might partially explain, for example, the still-popular beliefs that hormones are causal (e.g. Dalton, 1980) or, more recently, that receptor sensitivity (Wieck *et al*, 1991) or genetic vulnerability are the sole determinants.

## International classifications

International classifications of mental disorders – ICD-10 (World Health Organization, 1992) and DSM-V (American Psychiatric Association, 2013) – likewise reflect the dominant values of society, as well as the search for a common diagnostic language for clinicians and researchers across the world. Interestingly, the recently published DSM-V has re-emphasised the place of clinical judgement in psychiatric assessment, and the limitations of categorical operational approaches have been discussed (Maj, 2013). This more holistic integrative approach to diagnostic assessment is helpful and could facilitate increased understanding of the complex sociocultural context of perinatal mental disorder, and of the mother–baby relationship.

Despite the plethora of papers describing puerperal psychoses published in the late 19th and early 20th centuries, this diagnosis was nevertheless completely removed from ICD-9. Women with a postnatal onset of severe mental disorder were not thought to have any characteristics not found in mental disorders at other times – a consideration that remarkably overlooked the relevance of the development of the mother–infant relationship. This omission was partially corrected in ICD-10, when a 6-week postpartum onset specifier was introduced, and in DSM-IV (APA, 1994) by the addition of a 4-week specifier – but only for affective disorders. In ICD-10, the category of puerperal psychosis was to be used when the perinatal mental disorder could not be classified elsewhere, as might occur in a low-resource country. This limitation of ICD-10 for public health records, and for use by commissioners and providers of healthcare who wish to audit or cost a perinatal mental health service, was glaringly apparent. Currently, it is not possible to identify routinely from hospital records women at risk of a psychosis after childbirth, nor those who develop a mental disorder during pregnancy or the puerperium. A public enquiry following the deaths of the psychiatrist Daksha Emson and her baby, for example, recommended not only the establishment of specialist perinatal psychiatry services but also improved screening for women at high risk of puerperal psychosis (North East London Strategic Health Authority, 2003). These services will be greatly facilitated by a more inclusive ICD-11, which recognises the distinctive diagnoses of mental disorders that occur during pregnancy or following childbirth.

## Towards ICD-11 and DSM-V

The World Health Organization and the World Psychiatric Association have undertaken a radical critique of the existing international classifications, which is well summarised in a comprehensive and readable book edited by Salloum and Mezzich (2009). The authors recommend in their concluding chapter that psychiatric diagnosis should become more integrative. A comprehensive person-centred integrative diagnosis would include measures of positive health as well as illness, and consider quality of life and relationship problems which trigger mental disorder, as well as protective factors. Any new classification should make sense to patients as well as clinicians. International classifications should be a spur to creative thinking and should not restrict innovation (Cox, 2002). If a scientific evidence base for a classification is accepted uncritically, and values are ignored or the meaning of the illness for the patient is overlooked, then the classification can produce the 'mind-forg'd manacles' decried by William Blake rather than being a system of conceptual thought which provides a vehicle of communication for clinicians, researchers and patients. When J.C. worked in Uganda in the early 1970s, ICD-8 was being revised, and the exclusion of puerperal psychosis was in stark contrast to the experience of local psychiatrists – and contrary to the Kiganda classification of mental disorder, which included amakiro, a traditional puerperal illness (Orley, 1970).

It was recommended by the Royal College of Psychiatrists Perinatal Section Nosology Working Group that ICD-11 should include a new separate antenatal and postnatal onset specifier of 3 months for each ICD category of mood disorder, as well as for schizoaffective disorder and acute

---

**Box 1.1 ICD-10 F53 Mental and behavioural disorders associated with the puerperium**

This category is unusual and apparently paradoxical in carrying a recommendation that it should be used only when unavoidable. Its inclusion is a recognition of the very real practical problems in many developing countries that make the gathering of details about many cases of puerperal illness virtually impossible. However, even in the absence of sufficient information to allow a diagnosis of some variety of affective disorder (or, more rarely, schizophrenia), there will usually be enough known to allow diagnosis of a mild (F53.0) or severe (F53.1) disorder; this sub division is useful for estimations of workload, and when decisions are to be made about provision of services.

The inclusion of this category should not be taken to imply that, given adequate information, a significant proportion of cases of postpartum mental illness cannot be classified in other categories. Most experts in this field are of the opinion that a clinical picture of puerperal psychosis is so rarely (if ever) reliably distinguishable from affective disorder or schizophrenia that a special category is not justified. Any psychiatrist who is of the minority opinion that special postpartum psychoses do indeed exist may use this category, but should be aware of its real purpose.

Reproduced with permission from World Health Organization (1992): pp. 16–17.

---

and transient psychotic disorder. Austin (2010) has proposed that a code for mother–infant interaction difficulties should also be introduced into ICD-11 to encourage clinicians to consider the impact of maternal illness on the infant and to assist policy makers in this field. Brockington *et al* (2009) have similarly suggested that a category of disorder of mother–fetus and mother–infant relationship is considered for ICD-11, as difficulties in these relationships represent a high risk for child abuse and neglect. We suggest that ICD-11 should be inclusive of popular culturally conditioned categories such as puerperal psychosis and postnatal and antenatal depression, which – although lacking agreed diagnostic specificity – are nevertheless useful for patients and policy makers.

## Postmodern societies in transit

Any classification should be valid as well as reliable, and it should also be meaningful and understood by patients and their families. The World Psychiatric Association's International Guidelines for Diagnostic Assessment (Mezzich *et al*, 2002) innovatively included a narrative and descriptive approach to patient assessment and proposed that quality of life and the patient's belief system, including their religious beliefs, should be routinely considered.

The ICD-10 classification of mental and behavioural disorders concluded its preface with the apposite reflection that 'a classification is a way of seeing

---

**Box 1.2 ICD-10 F53 Mental and behavioural disorders associated with the puerperium, not elsewhere classified**

**F53.0**     Mild mental and behavioural disorders associated with the puerperium, not elsewhere classified

Includes: postnatal depression NOS

         postpartum depression NOS

**F53.1**     **Severe mental and behavioural disorders associated with the puerperium, not elsewhere classified**

Includes: puerperal psychosis NOS

**F53.8**     **Other mental and behavioural disorders associated with the puerperium, not elsewhere classified**

**F53.9**     **Puerperal mental disorder, unspecified**

This classification should be used only for mental disorders associated with the puerperium (commencing within 6 weeks of delivery) that do not meet the criteria for disorders classified elsewhere in this book, either because insufficient information is available, or because it is considered that special additional clinical features are present which make classification elsewhere inappropriate. It will usually be possible to classify mental disorders associated with the puerperium by using two other codes: the first is from elsewhere in Chapter V(F) and indicates the specific type of mental disorder (usually affective (F30–F39), and the second is 099.3 (mental diseases and diseases of the nervous system complicating the puerperium) of ICD-I0.

Reproduced with permission from World Health Organization (1992): pp. 195–196.

---

the world at a point in time'. In recent decades, this world has become globalised with increased migration, so that the classification of mental disorders in general, and perinatal mental disorders in particular, now need to be carefully reviewed (Box 1.1 and 1.2).

Although there was no specific category for puerperal psychosis in DSM-IV, some of the distinctive features of perinatal mental disorders were nevertheless usefully listed in the accompanying text (Box 1.3). The addition of the peripartum onset specifier in DSM-V is to be applied to the current or most recent depressive, manic or hypomanic episode in major depressive disorder, bipolar I or bipolar II disorder if the episode occurs during pregnancy or in the 4 weeks following delivery. This broadening of the scope of the specifier is welcome – but, as noted by Sharma & Mazmanian (2014), it is unfortunate that no distinction is made between prepartum and postpartum onset of mental disorder. Later editions of DSM-V should also reconsider the time period after childbirth when the specifier is applicable. We would suggest that it is extended to 6 months, a time interval that is consistent with the present evidence base.

---

**Box 1.3 DSM-V peripartum onset specifier**

**With peripartum onset:**

This specifier can be applied to the current or, if full criteria are not currently met for a major depressive episode, most recent episode of major depression if onset of mood symptoms occurs during pregnancy or in the 4 weeks following delivery.

**Note:** Mood episodes can have their onset either during pregnancy or postpartum.

Although the estimates differ according to the period of follow-up after delivery, between 3% and 6% of women will experience the onset of a major depressive episode during pregnancy or in the weeks or months following delivery. Fifty percent of 'postpartum' major depressive episodes actually begin prior to delivery. Thus, these episodes are referred to collectively as peripartum episodes. Women with peripartum major depressive episodes often have severe anxiety and even panic attacks. Prospective studies have demonstrated that mood and anxiety symptoms during pregnancy, as well as the 'baby blues,' increase the risk for a postpartum major depressive episode.

Peripartum-onset mood episodes can present either with or without psychotic features. Infanticide is most often associated with postpartum psychotic episodes that are characterized by command hallucinations to kill the infant or delusions that the infant is possessed, but psychotic symptoms can also occur in severe postpartum mood episodes without such specific delusions or hallucinations. Postpartum mood (major depressive or manic) episodes with psychotic features appear to occur in from 1 in 500 to 1 in 1,000 deliveries and may be more common in primiparous women. The risk of postpartum episodes with psychotic features is particularly increased for women with prior postpartum mood episodes but is also elevated for those with a prior history of a depressive or bipolar disorder (especially bipolar I disorder) and those with a family history of bipolar disorders.

Once a woman has had a postpartum episode with psychotic features, the risk of recurrence with each subsequent delivery is between 30% and 50%. Postpartum episodes must be differentiated from delirium occurring in the postpartum period, which is distinguished by a fluctuating level of awareness or attention. The postpartum period is unique with respect to the degree of neuroendocrine alterations and psychosocial adjustments, the potential impact of breast-feeding on treatment planning, and the long-term implications of a history of postpartum mood disorder on subsequent family planning.

Reproduced with permission from American Psychiatric Association (2013).

---

# What is special about perinatal mental disorders?

This question was considered at an international workshop in Sweden held in 1996, when the following characteristics of perinatal mental disorder were agreed:

- the birth context, which shapes experience and expression of the perinatal disorder

- the impact on the mother, which has the potential to damage self-image at a time of transition
- the impact on the child, partner and family, during a particularly sensitive period
- the high morbidity of untreated perinatal mental disorder, which has a cascading adverse effect on the family
- an increased readiness to provide assistance in the postnatal period
- better availability of systems to help, because community health services are organised to ensure frequent contact
- lower stigma in some countries because of high-profile public figures and successful advocacy groups
- high yield for intervention because of the preceding circumstances
- birth as a potential trigger
- distinctive biological components, relating to pregnancy and birth
- onset contrary to a cultural expectation of happiness.

Problems with the current classifications of perinatal mental disorder include:

- failure to include an obligatory antenatal and postnatal onset specifier
- failure to use a research-supported time period for onset after delivery; evidence from case-register studies indicates that the majority of excess presentations over expected rates occur within 3 months of delivery (Kendell et al, 1983; Munk-Olsen et al, 2006)

In addition, DSM-V does not allow easy coding for an acute mixed atypical psychosis, which is commonly seen by clinicians who treat severe postpartum disorders.

# Non-psychotic unipolar postnatal depression

Current diagnostic systems do not deal well with the milder (subsyndromal or subthreshold) depressions, which are increasingly recognised as being widely prevalent and of high associated morbidity. These are of particular importance in the postnatal period because of the risks they present to optimal child development and the frequency with which they develop into major depression. It is helpful to consider the perinatal mental disorders on a continuum from mild to severe; premonitory mild anxiety and depression can be a precursor of puerperal psychosis, bipolar disorder and a major depressive disorder. The popular term postnatal depression may be used as a category for a group of mood disorders that are exacerbated or triggered by childbirth. These are mostly unipolar disorders and can be subthreshold, or subsyndromal, because they are not usually characterised by delusions or obvious behavioural disturbances. Postnatal depression is a term commonly used by public health departments, by many advocacy groups and by the women themselves and should therefore be retained in ICD-11.

# Summary

This chapter has discussed the ways in which the classifications of perinatal mental disorder are partly derived from cultural assumptions and values, as well as from the findings of biomedical research. The debate about the optimal classification of perinatal mental disorder has illustrated that the birth event and its associated mental disorders can be fully understood only if there is a grasp of the individual within a cultural context, and that explanatory models which span the brain and the mind, and the mother and her infant, and which include existential dimensions, should be more actively considered.

It is our opinion, based on research and clinical work in this field, that it is in the best interest of these disturbed mothers with their need for skilled specialist help to include a mandatory prepartum and postpartum specifier in the revised classifications for all perinatal mental disorders. Furthermore, the diagnostic category of puerperal psychosis, because of its specific social context, its characteristic delusional content and its specific management, should be retained.

# References

American Psychiatric Association (1994) *Diagnostic and Statistical Manual of Mental Disorders* (4th edn) (DSM-IV): pp. 386–387. APA.

American Psychiatric Association (2013) *Diagnostic and Statistical Manual of Mental Disorders* (5th edn) (DSM-V). APA.

Austin M-P (2010) Classification of mental health disorders in the perinatal period: future directions for DSM-V and ICD-11. *Archives of Women's Mental Health*, **13**: 41–44.

Brockington I (1996) *Motherhood and Mental Health*. Oxford University Press.

Brockington I, Cox JL, Gloanec NG, *et al* (2009) Perinatal mental disorders. In *Psychiatric Diagnosis: Challenges and Prospects* (eds IM Saloum, JE Mezzich). Wiley Blackwell.

Cox JL (2002) Commentary: towards a more integrated international system of psychiatric classification. Psychopathology, **35**: 195–196.

Dalton K (1980) *Depression After Childbirth*. Oxford University Press.

Esquirol E (1838) *Des maladies mentales considérées sous les rapports médical, hygénique et médico-légal*. Baillière.

Kempe M (1985) *The Book of Margery Kempe*. Penguin Books.

Kendell RE, Rennie D, Clarke JA, *et al* (1983) The social and obstetric correlates of psychiatric admission in the puerperium. *Psychological Medicine*, **150**: 341–350.

Luauté JP, Lempérière T, Arnaud P (2012) Death of an alienist: Louis-Victor Marcé's final year. *History of Psychiatry*, **25**: 265–282.

Maj M (2013) "Clinical judgment" and the DSM-5 diagnosis of major depression. *World Psychiatry*, **12**: 89–91.

Marcé LV (1858) *Traité de la folie des femmes enceintes, des nouvelles accouchées et des nourrices*. Baillière.

Menzies WE (1893) Puerperal insanity. An analysis of 140 consecutive cases. *American Journal of Insanity*, **50**: 148–185.

Mezzich JE (2002) The WPA International Guidelines for Diagnostic Assessment. *World Psychiatry*, **1**: 36–39.

Munk-Olsen T, Laurenson T, Pederson C, *et al* (2006) New parents and mental disorders: a population-based register study. *JAMA*, **296**: 2582–2589.

North East London Strategic Health Authority (2003) *Report of an Independent Inquiry into the Care and Treatment of Daksha Emson M.B.B.S., MRCPsych, MSc. and her Daughter Freya.* North East London Strategic Health Authority.

Orley JH (1970) *Culture and Mental Illness: A Study from Uganda.* East African Publishing House.

Salloum IM, Mezzich JE (eds) (2009) *Psychiatric Diagnosis: Challenges and Prospects.* Wiley–Blackwell.

Sharma V, Mazmanian D (2014) The DSM-5 peripartum specifier: prospects and pitfalls. *Archives of Women's Mental Health,* **17**: 171–173.

Wieck A, Kumar R, Hirst AD, *et al* (1991) Increased sensitivity of dopamine receptors and recurrence of affective psychosis after childbirth. *BMJ,* **303**: 613–616.

World Health Organization (1992) *The ICD-10 Classification of Mental and Behavioural Disorders: Clinical Descriptions and Guidelines.* WHO.

# CHAPTER 2

# Perinatal depression, anxiety, stress and adjustment

Childbirth is a time of enormous upheaval and adjustment in biological, psychological and social terms. It is therefore not surprising that it is associated with considerable morbidity with respect to both depressive and anxiety disorders. This chapter looks at these disorders and their management.

## Postnatal depression

Gavin *et al* (2005) estimate the point prevalence of major depressive disorder to be 3.1–4.9% during pregnancy and 4.7% in the first 3 months postpartum, and the point prevalence including minor depression to be 11% during pregnancy and 13% in the first 3 months postpartum. The distress to the mother and her family is obvious, and some women who have experienced postnatal depression will change their plans for future pregnancies because of fears of recurrence, effects on the family or severity of the illness (Peindl *et al*, 1995). The consequences for partners and children are discussed in Chapter 6.

Postnatally depressed mothers and their infants consume more community care services than non-depressed mother–infant dyads (Petrou *et al*, 2002), and data from the USA indicate that just one emergency department visit for their infant distinguished depressed mothers from those who were not depressed (Mandl *et al*, 1999). Depressed mothers stop breastfeeding earlier (Henderson *et al*, 2003), and costs for community nursing, social care and paediatricians are higher (Roberts *et al*, 2001). Depressed mothers are more impaired on more dimensions of the Short Form Health Survey (SF-36) (Boyce *et al*, 2000) than age-appropriate normative data and non-depressed postpartum women. Role limitations due to physical problems are greater in primiparous than multiparous mothers (Boyce *et al*, 2000). A recent report estimated the cost of perinatal mental illness to UK society as £8.1 billion for each 1-year cohort of births (Bauer *et al*, 2014). Postnatal depression is clearly a major public health problem.

## Is postnatal depression a specific entity?

Whether or not postnatal depression is a specific concept still challenges researchers. In the late 1950s, researchers began to document non-psychotic illnesses which occurred after childbirth and observed that over a quarter of newly delivered women experienced emotional distress (e.g. Gordon & Gordon, 1959). Pitt's seminal paper in 1968 described many of the symptoms as atypical (Pitt, 1968). Subsequently, the general view became that if standardised rating scales and diagnostic interviews are employed, the symptomatic profile of postnatal depression does not differ from that of unipolar depression occurring at other times (although the content of negative or intrusive thoughts may focus on the maternal role and the infant). However, a case-record review of women with postnatal major depression and those with major depression unrelated to childbearing found that those depressed after delivery were more likely to present with anxiety features and took longer to recover (Hendrick et al, 2000).

There appears to be no difference in the prevalence of depression between puerperal and non-puerperal women, or between those who have adoptive and natural children and those who have only adoptive children (Cooper et al, 1988; Cox et al, 1993; Dean et al, 1995). However, onsets of postnatal episodes cluster in the first few weeks after delivery. Women whose first episode of depression is postnatal have an increased risk of further postnatal episodes – but not non-puerperal episodes – in the ensuing 5 years, whereas those whose first postnatal episode was recurrence of a disorder that had first occurred prior to becoming pregnant have an increased risk for non-puerperal but not puerperal recurrences. Postnatal episodes have a shorter duration (Cooper & Murray, 1995).

The rate of recurrence after a subsequent pregnancy, having been depressed after the first, is 27.3–48.9%, with the onset of recurrent

---

**Box 2.1 Risk factors for postnatal depression**

*Strong to moderate risk factors*

- Depression or anxiety during pregnancy
- Past history of mental disorder
- Life events
- Lack of or perceived lack of social support

*Moderate risk factors*

- Neuroticism
- A difficult marital relationship during pregnancy

*Small risk factors*

- Obstetric factors
- Socioeconomic status

---

episodes clustering close to delivery (Garfield *et al*, 2004; Wisner *et al*, 2004).

## Epidemiology

Although overall prevalence rates are generally similar for much of the world – including culturally quite diverse communities in Western Europe, the USA, Australia, rural India and Africa, Turkey and Hong Kong – variation is emerging as studies are carried out in settings that are more diverse. Malta (a very stable population where women have their extended families in close proximity) has a point prevalence of postnatal depression at 8 weeks postpartum of 8.7% (Felice *et al*, 2004), whereas in Khayelitsha township outside Cape Town in South Africa (where there is enormous social adversity) the rate is 34.7% (Cooper *et al*, 1999).

Immigrant women appear to be at a higher risk of postnatal depression in than women in their host country, with rates ranging from 24% to 42% (Collins *et al*, 2011). Halbreich & Karkun (2006), reviewing the available epidemiological studies, found rates ranging from almost zero to 60%. Prevalence figures are higher where self-report scales are used to define cases, as opposed to diagnostic interviews, but there are likely to be many other cross-cultural factors at work (see Chapter 11).

Most untreated episodes will last for a few weeks to a few months, but a third may last for up to a year and 10% continue into the second year of the infant's life (Feggetter *et al*, 1981; Watson *et al*, 1984). The social context is an important maintaining factor; persistent depression has been shown to be associated with poverty, and with having five or more children, an uneducated husband and no confidante (Rahman & Creed, 2007). Vliegen *et al* (2014) have reviewed 23 longitudinal studies published between 1985 and 2012. They reported that 30% of mothers with postnatal depression in community samples and 50% in clinical samples continue to suffer from depression in their child's first year and beyond.

Between one-third and half of all depressions occurring after birth will be continuations of episodes which had their onset during or before pregnancy (Watson *et al*, 1984; Gotlib *et al*, 1989; Wisner *et al*, 2013).

## Predictors of postnatal depression

Four meta-analyses of predictors have been conducted (Beck, 1996, 2001; O'Hara & Swain, 1996; Robertson *et al*, 2004). The last of these combined data from the previous three with other large-scale studies and calculated overall effect sizes. Strong to moderate and small risk factors are listed in Box 2.1. However, it should be noted that women in the included studies were mainly white, 25–35 years old and of mid-to-high socioeconomic status (Ross *et al*, 2006).

Factors that do not appear to have a relationship with postnatal depression in these meta-analyses are:

- parity or number of children
- level of education
- length of relationship with partner
- gender of the child (in Western societies).

A large prospective study in a more diverse population found low income to be the single largest significant predictor of postnatal depression (Segre *et al*, 2007).

Five systematic reviews have explored:

- the relationship between poverty and postnatal depression in low- and middle-income countries (Coast *et al*, 2012)
- prenatal and postnatal psychological well-being in Africa (Sawyer *et al*, 2010)
- postnatal depression in rural women in both high- and low-income countries (Villegas *et al*, 2011)
- poverty and common mental disorders in low- and middle-income countries (Lund *et al*, 2010)
- the prevalence and determinants of common perinatal mental disorders in women in low- and middle-income countries (Fisher *et al*, 2012). This study identified the following risk factors:
  - socioeconomic disadvantage
  - unintended pregnancy
  - being younger
  - being unmarried
  - lacking intimate partner support
  - having hostile in-laws
  - experiencing intimate partner violence.

In some settings, giving birth to a female child and having a history of mental health problems were risk factors, and having more education, having a job, being of the ethnic majority and having a kind and supportive partner were protective factors.

Several studies suggest that adolescent mothers are at increased risk of depression (e.g. Coletta, 1983; Hudson *et al*, 2000; Rubertsson *et al*, 2003; Nunes & Phipps, 2013). Barnett *et al* (1996) observed that stress and conflict with the infant's father were associated with depressive symptoms, whereas a supportive relationship with the infant's father was associated with fewer symptoms of depression. Additionally, support from a caseworker or support group can be protective (Thompson & Peebles-Wilkins, 1992). Social isolation, maternal competence and weight/shape concerns have also been identified as predictors of depressive symptoms in teenage mothers (Birkeland *et al*, 2005), as have prior depression and lack of social support (Nunes & Phipps, 2013).

Ross *et al* (2004) found that biological variables (progesterone and cortisol) did not have a direct effect on depressive symptoms during pregnancy but rather acted indirectly via psychosocial stressors and anxiety.

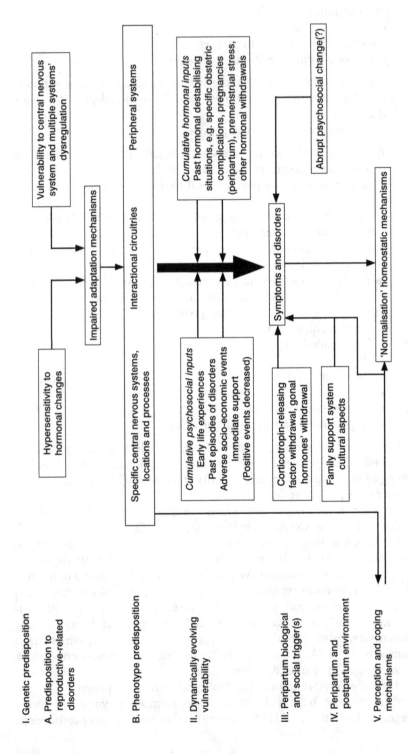

Fig. 2.1 A biopsychosociocultural model of the process leading to postpartum disorders. Reproduced with permission from Halbreich, 2005.

Halbreich (2005) proposed a biopsychosociocultural model of the processes that might lead to postpartum mental disorders (Figure 2.1).

## Past psychiatric history, mood during pregnancy and the early puerperium

A past history of depression is a clear risk factor for postnatal depression in both high- and low/middle-income countries (O'Hara & Swain, 1996, Sawyer et al 2010, Villegas et al, 2011, Fisher et al, 2012). Depressed or anxious mood during pregnancy (particularly in the last trimester) predicts depression postpartum and is also associated with increased reporting of somatic symptoms during pregnancy (Kelly et al, 2001; Sawyer et al, 2010; Villegas et al, 2011; Fisher et al, 2012). Anxiety disorder in the third trimester predicts high scores on the Edinburgh Postnatal Depression Scale (EPDS; see Appendix 2) postpartum, independently of the presence of major depressive disorder during pregnancy (Sutter-Dallay et al, 2004).

Boyce (2003) reported that those with a past history of psychopathology (particularly depression or anxiety) were at increased risk of developing depression after childbirth. A family history of mental illness (also O'Hara & Swain, 1996; Sawyer et al, 2010; Villegas et al, 2011; Fisher et al, 2012), a history of postnatal depression in the participant's mother and alcoholism in the participant's brother were also predictors. Bloch et al (2005) identified premenstrual dysphoric disorder (PMDD), mood symptoms on days 2–4 postpartum, a past history of depression and report of mood symptoms during past oral contraceptive use as being associated with major depression at 6–8 weeks postpartum. Others have also identified a history of premenstrual symptoms and PMDD as a risk factor for postnatal depression (Sylvén et al, 2012; Buttner et al, 2013; Craig, 2013).

Mood disturbance in the week after delivery is clearly related to the development of postnatal depression. Several retrospective and prospective studies have demonstrated links between postpartum blues and postnatal depression (for a review, see Henshaw, 2003). Subsequently, severe blues have been identified as an independent predictor of major and minor depression (Henshaw et al, 2004). Depression was almost three times more likely to occur in women with severe blues, the onset of depressive episodes was earlier in the puerperium, and these episodes lasted longer and were more likely to be major than minor depression. An association between blues and subsequent depression has also been demonstrated in Nigeria (Adewuya, 2006) and Japan (Watanabe et al, 2008). Reck and colleagues (2009) reported odds ratios (ORs) of 3.8 for depression and 3.9 for anxiety in the 3 months after delivery for women with blues. Women who are elated in the early puerperium are also more likely to become depressed later (Hannah et al, 1993; Glover et al, 1994). Heron et al (2005) have reviewed the literature on early postnatal euphoria and pose the question as to whether it is an indicator of bipolarity.

## Life events, adversity and social support

Stressful life events are known to trigger the onset of unipolar depression and, of course, pregnancy and childbirth are examples of such life events. Additional life events occurring during pregnancy were found to be strong predictors in the meta-analysis by O'Hara & Swain (1996), and women who suffer depression after delivery experience more life events and more negative life events in the preceding 12 months than those who do not become depressed (Oretti et al, 2003). Those with a prior history of major depression are more likely to relapse within 6 months of delivery if they experience a stressful life event in the 12 months before illness onset (Marks et al, 1992).

However, stressful life events have not been found to be predictors of postnatal depression in all countries and cultures; in some cases, there may be additional specific cultural factors which may be more important (see Chapter 11).

Several studies have reported a link between domestic violence and postnatal depression. A systematic review and meta-analysis of 67 studies reported an increased likelihood of depressive symptoms postpartum if partner violence is experienced during pregnancy (OR = 3.1) and increased odds of having experienced domestic violence in women who are experiencing depressive, anxiety or post-traumatic stress disorder (PTSD) symptoms during pregnancy (Howard et al, 2013). Another meta-analysis (Wu et al, 2012), which also included physical violence and sexual violence against women, reported a positive correlation between violence and postnatal depression (OR = 3.47). Hence, maternity and mental health services should ensure that they identify domestic violence experienced by women attending their services and respond to it.

Several systematic reviews have identified a consistent negative relationship between poor social support and postnatal depression (Beck, 1996, 2001; O'Hara & Swain, 1996; Robertson et al, 2004; Sawyer et al, 2010; Fisher et al, 2012).

There is some evidence that poor parenting is a risk factor (Boyce et al, 1991a). The prevalence of women with a history of child sexual abuse (CSA) ranges from 9% to 23%, and women with histories of CSA are overrepresented in psychiatric populations. Fifty per cent of women admitted to an Australian mother and baby unit (suffering from major depression or adjustment disorders) had histories of CSA (Buist, 1998), which was associated with higher scores on the Beck Depression Inventory (BDI), longer admissions and impaired mother–infant interactions. Follow up 2.5 to 3.5 years later found that those with histories of CSA had higher depression scores and more life stresses than controls (Buist & Janson, 2001). Battle et al (2006) reported 15% of perinatal psychiatric patients as having a history of physical abuse and 22% a history of CSA. A North American telephone survey of 200 postpartum women found that childhood emotional abuse (but not physical or sexual abuse) predicted postnatal depression (Cohen *et al*, 2002), a finding also reported by Ross & Dennis (2009) and Villegas *et al* (2011).

## Sociodemographic factors

Low family income, unemployment, lower social status and mother's occupation are associated with a significant increased risk of postnatal depression (Robertson *et al*, 2004; Segre *et al*, 2007; Lund *et al*, 2010; Sawyer *et al*, 2010, Villegas *et al*, 2011; Fisher *et al*, 2012).

## Obstetric factors

A prospective cohort study reported that unplanned pregnancy was associated with higher scores on the EPDS (Mercier *et al*, 2013). Obstetric factors, including pregnancy and delivery complications, have a small but significant effect on the development of depression after delivery (Blom *et al*, 2010; Vigod *et al*, 2010). However, some specific interventions may be important. It has been reported that women who conceive via assisted reproductive technologies (ART) are more likely to experience depressive symptoms postpartum. However, a systematic review of studies up to 2009 concluded that, although there were methodological problems with most of the studies, ART or multiple births did not appear to increase the risk of depression (Ross *et al*, 2011). In addition, a recent study which controlled for previous maternal psychiatric history, multiple birth and sociodemographic factors found no difference in the rates of depression in women who conceived naturally compared with those who conceived via ART (Listijono *et al*, 2014). Women delivered by Caesarean section have a more negative cognitive appraisal of delivery and higher level of post-traumatic stress symptoms (Ryding *et al*, 1997, 1998; Andersen *et al*, 2012; Furuta *et al*, 2012). However, despite earlier studies suggesting a relationship between Caesarean section and postnatal depression, a meta-analysis concluded that 'a link between Caesarean section and postpartum depression has not been established' (Carter *et al*, 2006), and a Canadian study reported that mode of delivery was not independently associated with depression postpartum (Sword *et al*, 2011). A prospective cohort study from China reported that women who had had epidural anaesthesia were less likely to suffer from depressive symptoms (Ding *et al*, 2014).

Physical health problems associated with depressive symptoms 7 to 9 months after delivery include tiredness, urinary incontinence, back pain, sexual problems, increased coughs and colds, and bowel problems (Brown & Lumley, 2000). There is an association between low haemoglobin levels on day 7 postpartum and depressive symptoms on day 28 (Corwin *et al*, 2003).

A large study examining outcomes in women who experienced severe obstetric morbidity (massive haemorrhage, pre-eclampsia, sepsis or uterine rupture) found that those with high EPDS scores took longer to resume sexual activity, and were more likely to cite fear of becoming pregnant again as a reason for this (Waterstone *et al*, 2003).

## Personality

Premorbid personality is an important vulnerability factor. In addition to neuroticism (O'Hara & Swain, 1996; Robertson *et al* 2004), hostility, anxiety, a perception of being out of control (rated during pregnancy) and a negative cognitive attributional style have been found to be associated with postnatal depressive symptoms (Hayworth *et al*, 1980; O'Hara *et al*, 1982; Cutrona, 1983; Martín-Santos *et al*, 2012), as has interpersonal sensitivity (Boyce *et al*, 1991*b*). Women scoring high on the Vulnerable Personality Scale are at increased risk of depression (Boyce, 2003), as are those with 'immature defence styles' and attachment styles that are characterised by anxiety over relationships (McMahon *et al*, 2005). Insecure avoidant attachment styles are associated with antenatal depression, whereas insecure enmeshed styles are associated with postnatal depression (Bifulco *et al*, 2004). Church *et al* (2005) have suggested that dysfunctional cognitions mediate the relationship between risk factors and postpartum depressive symptoms.

## Marital relationship

A poor marital relationship during pregnancy is a risk factor observed in many studies. Paykel *et al* (1980) found poor marital support to be a vulnerability factor leading to depression in the presence of life events. Women who report that their partners are not easy to talk to, do not give emotional support, provide low levels of care or are over-controlling, or who report global dissatisfaction with the relationship, are more likely to experience puerperal depression (Boyce *et al*, 1991*a*; Boyce, 2003).

## Social support

Poor social support during pregnancy is predictive of postnatal depression, with lack of support from the baby's father associated with high levels of symptoms. Lack of perceived support from a woman's primary support group and lack of support in relation to becoming pregnant are risk factors in first-time mothers (Brugha *et al*, 1998), but the size of a woman's primary social network does not seem to be important. Women reporting that they were unable to access satisfactory support in a crisis or were dissatisfied with the psychological support received after a crisis were at increased risk (Boyce, 2003). In India, where a woman often lives with her husband's family after marriage, a poor relationship with her mother-in-law has been identified as a risk factor for the development of postnatal depression (Chandran *et al*, 2002).

## Sleep deprivation and fatigue

Three studies have demonstrated that fatigue predicts depressed mood postpartum (Bozoky & Corwin 2002; Corwin *et al*, 2005; Dennis & Ross, 2005). A small study of 56 women reported that poor sleep quality after delivery predicted recurrence in women with previous histories of major depression (Okun *et al*, 2011), and another study found that poor sleep maintenance predicted higher scores on the EPDS in the last week of pregnancy and postpartum (Park *et al*, 2013). Ross *et al* (2005) reviewed the relationship between sleep and perinatal mood disorders, concluding that there was a significant relationship but that, at the time, the evidence base was limited. The links between sleep deprivation and puerperal psychosis are discussed in Chapter 3.

### Infant factors

It is clear that infant factors are independent risk factors for postnatal depression. Neonatal irritability and poor motor function have been shown to predict depression in first-time mothers (Murray *et al*, 1996). Infant sleep problems (Hiscock & Wake, 2001; Dennis & Ross, 2005) and inconsolable crying (Radesky *et al*, 2013) are associated with high EPDS scores. A systematic review has reported higher rates of postnatal depression in mothers of preterm, low-birth-weight infants (Vigod *et al*, 2010). There is evidence from randomised controlled trials (RCTs) of behavioural (Hiscock & Wake, 2002) and educational (Hiscock *et al*, 2014) interventions which improve both infant sleep and maternal depressive symptoms.

### Biological factors

The close temporal relationship between the rapid post-delivery decline in gonadal steroid hormones, cortisol and corticotrophin-releasing hormone (CRH), and the onset of early puerperal mood change, has led to the assumption that there must be a causal relationship with postnatal depression. Early studies of the role of biological risk factors that focused on hormone levels, correlating these with various measures of postnatal mood, were largely unfruitful (Bloch *et al*, 2003).

However, later studies have reported a higher cortisol response to a psychosocial stress test in women who scored >9 on the EPDS within 13 days of delivery (Nierop *et al*, 2006), dysregulation of the hypothalamic–pituitary–adrenal (HPA) axis in women with depressive symptoms (Jolley *et al*, 2007) and higher day 3 oestradiol levels in women with major depressive disorder (Klier *et al*, 2007). Others have demonstrated a higher mid-pregnancy CRH level in women depressed during pregnancy but not postpartum (Rich-Edwards *et al*, 2008), and a positive association between higher mid-pregnancy CRH levels and postpartum depressive symptoms (Yim *et al*, 2009). Glynn *et al* (2013) have reviewed the role of the HPA axis in postnatal depression, and Brummelte & Galea (2010) the contribution of the HPA axis and ovarian hormones to depression in pregnancy and the postpartum.

Challenge tests looking at functional neurotransmitter systems are more likely to yield positive findings. Replicating the rapid post-delivery fall in gonadal steroids by administering a gonadotrophin-releasing hormone agonist to women who did and did not have histories of postnatal depression and then administering supraphysiological doses of oestradiol and progesterone and withdrawing under double-blind conditions led to 62.5% of the women with a history developing mood symptoms during the withdrawal period (Bloch *et al*, 2000). This provides indirect evidence that women with previous postnatal depression are sensitive to the mood-destabilising effects of gonadal steroids. The same team later demonstrated that ovine CRH stimulation and supraphysiological oestradiol and progesterone, given as outlined above and then withdrawn, led to elevated basal cortisol levels and increased HPA axis sensitivity. The higher levels of cortisol were most marked in the women who had a history of postpartum depression (Bloch *et al*, 2005).

The growth hormone response to apomorphine is a measure of the functional state of dopamine ($D_2$) receptors. This was measured in 14 postpartum women who were currently well but had a history of major depression. The five who relapsed had enhanced growth hormone responses (suggesting increased sensitivity of $D_2$ receptors) that were particularly marked in those who had anxiety disorders (McIvor *et al*, 1996). Moses-Kolko *et al* (2012) used $D_{2/3}$ receptor neuroimaging in bipolar, unipolar and postpartum women. They reported lower [11]C raclopride binding in both unipolar depressed and postpartum women, primarily in the striatal dopaminergic system, which they postulate may contribute to the higher risk of mood disorders in the postpartum period. A small case–control study reported increased glutamate levels in the medial prefrontal cortex in women with postnatal depression (McEwan *et al*, 2012).

Newport *et al* (2004) identified alterations in serotonin transporter binding in women with postnatal depression (compared with healthy and depressed pregnant women and healthy postpartum women).

Lowering serum cholesterol is associated with violent death and suicide. Serum cholesterol rises during pregnancy and falls rapidly after delivery. This fall is associated with depressed mood in the first 4 days postpartum (Ploeckinger *et al*, 1996). Lower cholesterol levels are associated with fatigue and depressed mood (Nasta *et al*, 2002), anxiety, anger and irritability (Troisi *et al*, 2002). The latter group also found lower high-density lipoprotein concentrations to be associated with anxiety. However, van Dam and colleagues (1999), following 266 women from 32 weeks gestation until 34 weeks postpartum, found little to support the hypothesis that the rapidity of cholesterol decline is associated with postnatal depression.

Alterations in serum fatty acid composition have been observed in major depression. Several studies have reported lower levels in women who become depressed or have depressive symptoms postpartum (De Vriese *et al*, 2003; Otto *et al*, 2003; Markhus *et al*, 2013). Others have demonstrated higher levels of arachidonic acid and adrenic acid levels in pregnant women with suicidality and who had major depression (Vaz *et al*, 2014), and also the converse, no association between fatty acids and major depression in pregnancy (Bodnar *et al*, 2011).

There has been recent interest in whether low levels of maternal vitamin D in pregnancy are associated with an increased risk of depressive symptoms postpartum. An Australian study reported that women with serum vitamin D levels in the lowest quartile were more likely to report depressive symptoms at 3 days after delivery (Robinson *et al*, 2014). However, so soon after delivery, the symptoms are more likely to be attributable to postpartum blues, and the researchers used a non-validated 6-item version of the EPDS to measure depressive symptoms. A case–control study found no association between vitamin D levels in pregnancy and postpartum depressive symptoms (Nielsen *et al*, 2013).

A number of researchers have explored the relationship between mediators of inflammation and perinatal mood and anxiety symptoms. The theoretical background and the literature up to 2012 have been reviewed by Osborne & Monk (2013). Others have reported low oxytocin levels as a possible risk factor, and the data from animal and human research have been reviewed by Kim *et al* (2014).

Thyroid dysfunction is well-known to be associated with mood disturbance and follows around 10% of deliveries. Pop *et al* (1991) and Harris *et al* (1989) both found an association between thyroid dysfunction (measured by T3, T4 and thyroid-stimulating hormone) and depression after childbirth, but a later study (Lucas *et al*, 2001) failed to replicate this.

Around 10% of women of childbearing age are thyroid antibody positive. Those positive during pregnancy are more likely to develop clinical thyroid disease and depression after delivery (Harris *et al*, 1992; Kuijpens *et al*, 2001), but giving thyroxine daily to such women after delivery does not prevent the onset of depression (Harris *et al*, 2002). Pregnant women with total and free thyroxine concentrations in the lower euthyroid range may be more likely to develop depression postpartum (Pedersen *et al*, 2007).

## Genetics

It is estimated that genetic factors explain 38% of the variance in depressive symptoms postpartum and 25% of DSM-IV postpartum major depression (Treloar *et al*, 1999). Having a postpartum depressive episode predicts a sibling's depression after delivery (OR = 3.97; Murphy–Ebernez *et al*, 2006). Significant associations between tryptophan hydroxylase gene polymorphisms and depression, anxiety and comorbid depression and anxiety in postpartum women have been demonstrated (Sun *et al*, 2004), and familial factors appear to be important in vulnerability to triggering of narrowly defined postpartum episodes (onset within 6–8 weeks of delivery) in women with recurrent depressive disorder (Forty *et al*, 2006). Recent work includes a reported association between glucocorticoid and type 1 CRH receptor gene variants and depressive symptoms in pregnancy and postpartum (Engineer *et al*, 2013), and a small study suggests a role for the oestrogen receptor gene *ESR1*, which may interact with the serotonin transporter (Pinsonneault *et al*, 2013). There is also a systematic review of the role of the serotonergic transporter genotype and omega-3 fatty acid status, which are emerging as potential risk factors (Shapiro *et al*, 2012).

# Depression during pregnancy

The prevalence of depression during pregnancy is similar to the prevalence postpartum (Gavin *et al*, 2005). A systematic review and meta-analysis of prevalence studies (Bennett *et al*, 2004) confirmed rates of 7.4%, 12.8% and 12.0% in the first, second and third trimesters, respectively, whereas that of Gavin *et al* (2005) reported a period prevalence of 18.4% (major and minor depression) during pregnancy, with 12% of pregnant women suffering from major depression. A large Swedish study, which screened 1734 consecutive attenders at routine ultrasound screening, found 3.3% suffering from major depression, 6.9% minor depression and 6.6% anxiety disorders. Only 5.5% of those diagnosed had undergone any treatment (Andersson *et al*, 2003).

One systematic review of risk factors for depressive symptoms in pregnancy identified life stress, lack of social support and domestic violence as predictors, although most of the included studies had been undertaken in high-income countries (Lancaster *et al*, 2010). A later systematic review by Howard *et al* (2013) reporting a significant association between domestic violence and perinatal depression included studies from Asia, South America and the Middle East in addition to those from high-income countries.

Women reporting a history of CSA are more likely to experience depressive symptoms during pregnancy (Benedict *et al*, 1999), and those with a history of physical or sexual abuse or both are more likely to experience suicidal ideation (Farber *et al*, 1996).

In Kuwait, 16.9% of pregnant women had experienced assault or victimisation, with 9% suffering physical assault in the past month (Nayak *et al*, 1999). Assault history, marital conflict, family stress and stressful life events were all associated with depressive symptoms, and assault history remained a significant predictor even when the other variables were controlled for. A London study found that 23.5% of pregnant women had a lifetime history of domestic violence, with 3% reporting this during the current pregnancy. Those with a history of domestic violence were more likely to have depressive symptoms, to have smoked during and/or in the year prior to pregnancy, and to be single, separated or living alone (Mezey *et al*, 2005). Depressive, somatic and PTSD symptoms are higher in pregnant women who report intimate partner abuse or sexual coercion (Varma *et al*, 2007). These are often associated with alcohol misuse in the partner.

Depression in the year before delivery is an independent risk factor for sudden infant death syndrome, along with smoking and having a male infant (Howard *et al*, 2007). Depressive symptoms are associated with substance misuse, smoking and psychosocial difficulties (Pritchard, 1994; Pajulo *et al*, 2001). Women with depression find it harder to stop smoking when they become pregnant (Ludman *et al*, 2000). Depression and anxiety are associated with reduced adherence to vitamins during pregnancy, and increased use of hypnotics and nicotine, whereas depression only was associated with medication for physical symptoms (Newport *et al*, 2010). Substance misuse, depression and a history of physical or sexual abuse are closely related in pregnancy (Horrigan *et al*, 2000).

## Anxiety, stress and adjustment

Anxiety symptoms are probably more common than depression after delivery (Wynter *et al*, 2013) and possibly more prevalent during pregnancy (Ross & McLean, 2006). Anxiety during pregnancy has been identified as an independent predictor of childhood behavioural and emotional problems (O'Connor *et al*, 2002).

Rates of between 5 and 57% have been reported in postpartum populations (Stuart *et al*, 1998; Brockington *et al*, 2006), and between 4 and 16% of new mothers meet DSM-IV criteria for generalised anxiety disorder (GAD), panic or phobia (Wenzel *et al*, 2003). A study in the USA found postpartum prevalence rates of 8.2% for GAD (higher than in the general population of women), 1.4% for panic disorder and 4.1% for social phobia (Wenzel *et al*, 2005). Anxiety symptoms frequently coexist with depressive symptoms, and comorbid GAD and major depression is also common (Beeghly *et al*, 2002). An Australian study reported a 9.5% prevalence of GAD in pregnancy (Buist *et al*, 2011). Antenatal anxiety predicts postnatal depression at 8 weeks and 8 months, even after controlling for antenatal depression (OR=3.22, P<0.001; Heron *et al*, 2004).

Common themes of severe anxiety during pregnancy are fear of fetal loss (particularly if there is a history of reproductive loss or fertility problems) or abnormality, whereas after delivery the fear of cot death or of mothering skills being criticised are most common. A comprehensive review is found in Brockington *et al* (2006).

In depression not associated with childbirth, the presence of anxiety symptoms renders episodes more severe and long-lasting than episodes without anxiety symptoms. One small study suggests that this might also be the case for postnatal depression (Hendrick *et al*, 2000).

A large USA-based community study of postpartum women with depressive symptoms found 11% experiencing panic attacks, 8% obsessional thoughts and 9% compulsions (Wenzel *et al*, 2001); 2.3% had both subsyndromal panic and obsessive–compulsive disorder (OCD) symptoms, while 1.5% met DSM-IV (American Psychiatric Association, 1994) criteria for panic disorder and 3.9% for OCD. One per cent had comorbid major depressive disorder and panic disorder, and 2.4% had major depression comorbid with OCD. Ross & McLean (2006) have systematically reviewed the relationships between panic disorder, GAD, PTSD and OCD, and pregnancy and the postpartum period.

Around half of postnatally depressed mothers experience intrusive obsessional thoughts that are frequently aggressive in nature and directed towards their infant (Wisner *et al*, 1999a). Obsessions of infanticide have been reported in the literature since the late 1950s (Button & Reivich, 1972). Careful history-taking is essential in order to distinguish between obsessions of infanticide and thoughts of harming an infant, which a mother may be at risk of carrying out.

Hudak & Wisner (2012) report a case where the mother experienced obsessional thoughts of stuffing her baby into a microwave oven. The thoughts were ego-dystonic; there was no history of psychosis, no psychotic symptoms (e.g. hallucinations in any sensory modality or delusions) and no suicidal or homicidal ideation. She was treated with citalopram up to 40 mg daily, but remained symptomatic. She was then referred to a 12-week psycho-educational programme (2 sessions per week) including exposure and response prevention. Her citalopram was increased to 80 mg daily. She was helped by understanding that she was highly unlikely to harm her infant and responded well to treatment.

Obsessional symptoms are commonly centred on cleaning or hand-washing, and involve concerns that the infant might ingest something dirty or be contaminated with germs. Checking compulsions tend to focus on the infant's health, in particular whether he/she is still breathing during the night and has not died from sudden infant death syndrome (Weightman *et al*, 1998). The relationship between obsessive–compulsive symptoms, pregnancy and the puerperium has been reviewed by Abramowitz *et al* (2003).

Distress after delivery, measured by self-report scales, was found to occur in 37% of new mothers and 13% of new fathers, but only 9% of mothers and 2% of fathers reported severe intrusive stress (Skari *et al*, 2002). Rates had fallen to levels similar to those in the general population when measured at 6 weeks and 6 months after delivery. Being a single parent, multiparity and previous traumas in childbirth were predictors of severe distress.

PTSD in relation to childbirth has been described in the literature since the late 1970s. Three large studies have reported a prevalence of 1.3–2.4% 1–2 months postpartum, and 0.9–4.6% at 3–12 months after delivery (Söderquist *et al*, 2006, 2009; Alcorn *et al*, 2010). Adewuya *et al* (2006) reported a prevalence of 5.9% in postpartum Nigerian women. Andersen *et al* (2012) undertook a systematic review of predictors of PTSD and ranked them according to study quality. The top-ranked factors were:

- subjective distress in labour
- obstetric emergencies.

Intermediate factors were:

- infant complications
- anxiety or depression in pregnancy

- low level of support in childbirth
- previous psychological trauma, traumatic childbirth or sexual abuse.

Factors with a low impact on the development of PTSD were:

- psychosocial factors e.g. parity, unplanned pregnancy and low socioeconomic status
- obstetric factors including duration of labour, episiotomy and perineal lacerations.

Women who had previously delivered a stillborn infant had rates of PTSD of 21% in the third trimester of a subsequent pregnancy, which had dropped to 4% after one year postpartum. The likelihood of PTSD was increased with a shorter interval between the stillbirth and the current pregnancy (Turton *et al*, 2001). However, the sample followed by Söderquist *et al* (2006) had no reduction in symptoms over the course a year, and a study of parents bereaved by infant death reported 12.3% still symptomatic up to 18 years (mean 3.4 years) after the death of their infant (Christiansen *et al*, 2013).

Querulant (or complaining) disorder has also been described in relation to stressful deliveries, where women are so dissatisfied that they develop a morbid preoccupation and their mental health and functioning is substantially impaired. It is associated with PTSD (Brockington *et al*, 2006).

## Phobic anxiety

Sved-Williams (1992) reports that 13.6% of 66 mothers admitted to a mother and baby unit experienced phobic avoidance of their infant sufficiently severe to warrant management in its own right. A behavioural programme involving exposure is the recommended treatment.

Tokophobia is an intense dread of childbirth that can lead to women avoiding pregnancy, terminating an otherwise very much wanted pregnancy or demanding a Caesarean section in subsequent pregnancies (Hofberg & Brockington, 2000). It can be classified as:

- primary in a nulliparous woman
- secondary in a woman who has had previous traumatic deliveries

or

- secondary to a depressive illness or PTSD during pregnancy.

Heimstad *et al* (2006) and Sydsjö *et al* (2012) report the prevalence of serious fear as 3–5.5% and associated with elective Caesarean section delivery and instrumental delivery. The aetiology is multifactorial and may involve:

- transmission of fear of childbirth over generations
- a woman's appraisal of her last delivery and associated anxiety
- a history of sexual abuse or assault or traumatic gynaecological examination.

Women with a history of sexual abuse are less likely to have an uncomplicated vaginal delivery at term. The presence of anxiety or depression increases the risk of fear of childbirth, although around half the women studied by Storksen *et al* (2012) did not suffer from either disorder. Fear of childbirth is also a predictor of postnatal depression (Räisänen *et al*, 2013).

## Panic disorder

De Armond (1954) described a case series in which there was an onset of 'sudden panic-like fear without precipitating cause' shortly after leaving hospital. Panic disorder occurs for the first time in the postpartum period more often than is expected in the general population, with 10.9% of panic disorder sufferers reporting postpartum onset (age-corrected estimate = 0.92%; Sholomskas *et al*, 1993), but this was a retrospective study. A prospective study reported that 7.5% of pregnant women suffered from panic disorder, around half having comorbid depression or depressive symptoms (Marchesi *et al*, 2014). A prior history of anxiety predicted panic disorder without depressive comorbidity, whereas a history of depressive episodes and lack of family support predicted panic disorder with depressive comorbidity.

A qualitative study of mothers with postpartum-onset panic disorder described how it became a great struggle to manage their attacks, leading to negative changes in their lifestyles and lowered self-esteem (Beck, 1998). The impact of pregnancy and the postpartum period on pre-existing panic disorder is described in Chapter 4.

## Obsessive–compulsive disorder

OCD may occur for the first time during pregnancy or postpartum. Between 25 and 70% of parous women with OCD reported their first onset as occurring during pregnancy or after delivery, or that it was exacerbated by childbirth (Speisman *et al*, 2011). There is a report of a woman who experienced first-onset OCD after the birth of her first baby, going into remission after treatment. Three years later she had a recurrence after the birth of her second child (Hertzberg *et al*, 1997). There are two case reports of the onset of OCD in the fourth month of pregnancy that resolved spontaneously after delivery (Iancu *et al*, 1995; Kalra *et al*, 2005). Russell *et al* (2013) calculated in their meta-analysis that pregnant and postpartum women are at greater risk of experiencing OCD than the general population, with an aggregated risk ratio of 1.79.

A case series of 15 women with new-onset puerperal OCD found that all were experiencing intrusive thoughts of harming their infants and had developed some degree of avoidance of their babies (Sichel *et al*, 1993). None went on to harm their infants. Nine went on to develop a secondary depressive illness and ten were admitted during the acute phase of their illness. A year later, most were still taking medication (selective serotonin reuptake inhibitors (SSRIs) or clomipramine) and continued to have some intrusive thoughts. None had developed checking or other compulsions. A case–control study of women with postpartum-onset OCD found that the onset was within 4 weeks of delivery, and that these women reported significantly more aggressive obsessions (about harming the baby) than did controls who had not had a postpartum onset (Maina *et al*, 1999). Zambaldi *et al* (2009) reported that the most common obsessions were aggressive, contamination and miscellaneous, while the most frequent compulsions were for checking and washing/cleaning. Of the small sample, 38.9% had a comorbid depressive episode. Upadhyaya & Sharma (2012) reported the case of a tribal woman who developed pica (eating uncooked rice and wheat) resulting from obsessions in three pregnancies. It resolved spontaneously in the first two pregnancies but persisted in the third and responded to fluoxetine 40 mg daily for 3 months.

Postpartum-onset OCD can recur after later pregnancies, and therefore a woman with a previous history should be monitored closely and, if symptoms recur, rapid intervention offered. There is at present no evidence base to support the use of prophylactic medication, but this is recommended by Brandes *et al* (2004). Fathers have also been reported as experiencing a first onset of OCD coinciding with pregnancy or the birth of a child (Abramowitz *et al*, 2001). Speisman *et al* (2011) have reviewed the literature addressing postpartum OCD between 1950 and 2011. Pregnancy and the postpartum period in women with pre-existing OCD are described in Chapter 4.

## Adjustment and transition

Becoming a new mother or the mother of an additional child requires adjustment to a new set of personal and social circumstances. Cultural expectations that this is an inevitably easy and pleasurable experience may lead to idealised views of what motherhood should be like and render women vulnerable to depression when there is conflict between expectation and experience (Mauthner, 1998). Lack of comfort with the maternal role and low measures of maternal role attainment have been associated with postnatal depressive symptoms (Fowles, 1998).

The loss of ritual and traditional practices around birth and new motherhood has also been hypothesised as a causative factor (Seel, 1986; Cox, 1994). Psychologists writing from a feminist perspective argue that depression is a rational response to the loss and isolation resulting from childbirth and should not be medicalised. Nicolson (1998) argues that 'postnatal depression needs to be reconceptualised as part of the normal experience of motherhood'.

Cheryl Beck has undertaken a metasynthesis of 18 qualitative studies of postnatal depression from the 1960s to the 1990s (Beck, 2002). She identified common themes that brought together illustrate four different perspectives:

- incongruity between expectations and the reality of motherhood
- spiralling downward
- pervasive loss
- making gains.

## Pregnancy loss

Pregnancy loss is common, occurring after 15–20% of confirmed pregnancies and usually during the first trimester (Frost & Condon, 1996; Lee & Slade, 1996). Stillbirths after 24 weeks gestation account for 4.7 in every 1000 births in England and Wales (Office for National Statistics, 2013). Mental disorder, particularly affective illness and substance misuse, increase the risk of pregnancy loss (OR = 1.8; Gold *et al*, 2007).

Studies have shown that women who miscarry have higher levels of depressive and anxiety symptoms (Neugebauer *et al*, 1992*a*; Thapar & Thapar, 1992; Janssen *et al*, 1996; Brier, 2005), and have an increased risk of depression, anxiety and PTSD (Giannandrea *et al*, 2013). Those who are childless are at highest risk (Neugebauer *et al*, 1992*b*).

Women who miscarry are also at increased risk of minor (Klier *et al*, 2000) and major depression (Neugebauer *et al*, 1997) and a recurrent episode of OCD (Geller *et al*, 2001). In the study by Geller *et al* over half of the women with past histories of depression had a recurrence after miscarrying.

A study of mothers in the USA who had experienced stillbirth or neonatal death reported increased rates of depression, PTSD, GAD, social phobia and panic disorder (Gold & Johnson, 2014). Symptoms can persist for up to 30 months after the loss (Boyle *et al*, 1996). A comparison of attachment in infants born to mothers who had lost babies after 18 weeks gestation and controls found that those born subsequent to pregnancy loss had increased disorganised attachment to their mothers. This was predicted by maternal unresolved status with respect to loss (Hughes *et al*, 2001).

Women whose previous pregnancy ended in stillbirth experience higher levels of depressive and anxiety symptoms in the third trimester of the next pregnancy and a trend towards more depressive symptoms at 1 year post-partum if they became pregnant less than 12 months after the stillbirth (Hughes *et al*, 1999). Recent studies report an increase in low mood and anxiety in a pregnancy following pregnancy loss (Gong *et al*, 2013; Chojenta *et al*, 2014) but no increase in these symptoms after a subsequent birth. Fathers also report anxiety and depression after stillbirth or neonatal death, but at a lower level than mothers (Badenhorst *et al*, 2006; Cumming *et al*, 2007).

There is a non-significant trend towards having PTSD in the pregnancy after a stillbirth if the mother has been encouraged to see or to hold the dead infant (Turton *et al*, 2001). Therefore, this practice is not advised.

Community follow-up should be arranged for women who have experienced a stillbirth or neonatal death.

A large study of pregnant women reported that 121 out of 1370 miscarried, most before 20 weeks. One month later, the prevalence of DSM-IV PTSD was 25%. These women were more likely to report depression, and 4 months later 7% still met PTSD criteria. Length of gestation at the time of loss was associated with higher levels of PTSD symptoms (Engelhard *et al*, 2001). Seventy per cent of the women who miscarried reported peri-traumatic dissociation. This was predicted by prior low control of emotions, a tendency to dissociate and a lower educational level. It was not related to neuroticism or prior life events (Engelhard *et al*, 2003).

A UK study explored symptomatic women's experiences of miscarriage, the care they received and the views of primary healthcare professionals (Wong *et al*, 2003). The women felt a need for formal follow-up (there is currently no systematic follow-up for women who miscarry; they are expected to seek help if they need it). They felt unable to absorb information during their hospital stay and felt confused, wanted more specific information and answers to questions, and found the normalisation of miscarriage by healthcare professionals distressing. There was a tendency to feel guilty and have a sense of failure. The response to the care they received varied greatly, and the health professionals interviewed identified skills deficits as a factor contributing to this variation. The authors recommend that health visitors should be formally notified of a woman who has miscarried so that they can undertake a 6–8-week check of psychological and psychiatric morbidity, as they do with women who have delivered a live child.

How these risk factors might be incorporated into screening programmes and used during pregnancy to identify vulnerable women is discussed in Chapter 7.

The Miscarriage Association has information and support via its website for both women and health professionals (www.miscarriageassociation.org.uk), as does the Stillbirth and Neonatal Death Charity (www.uk-sands.org).

## Termination of pregnancy

One in five pregnancies in England and Wales are terminated on therapeutic grounds, the majority in early pregnancy. A large number of studies have addressed the issue of abortion and subsequent mental health (reviewed by Bellieni & Buonocore, 2013). Some seem to suggest that abortion increases the risk of depression, anxiety, suicidal behaviours and substance use disorders (e.g. Fergusson *et al*, 2006). However, the Fergusson study has limitations (as do many of the others), e.g. the comparison groups were women who had children and those who did not become pregnant. The authors are careful to say that their findings do not imply a causative link between abortion and mental health problems. Although the majority of women seeking termination may not be at risk, in the same way that

---

**Box 2.2 Risk factors for psychological disturbance after termination of pregnancy**

- Negative religious or cultural attitudes
- Lack of support from social network
- Unstable relationship with partner
- Past psychiatric history
- Older multiparous women with children
- Therapeutic abortion for fetal anomaly

From Zolese & Blacker (1992)

---

women vulnerable to depression after miscarriage might be identified and reviewed, those who are particularly vulnerable at the time of undergoing termination of pregnancy are also at risk. Those particularly at risk appear to be very young women, who are often multiply disadvantaged (Fergusson *et al*, 2006), those undergoing late termination for fetal anomaly (Davies *et al*, 2005; Korenromp *et al*, 2005; Kersting *et al*, 2007) and others (Box 2.2).

There are historical reports of psychosis following both termination and miscarriage (Brockington, 2005). One study found that admission rates for bipolar disorder were increased after abortion (Reardon *et al*, 2003), and there is a case report of a woman with bipolar II disorder experiencing a manic episode following a termination of pregnancy at 10 weeks gestation (Sharma *et al*, 2013). There appears to be no difference in depressive or anxiety symptoms between women who have a medical termination and those who have a surgical termination (Ashok *et al*, 2005).

## Impact of anxiety and depression during pregnancy on obstetric outcomes

A variety of poor outcomes have been reported as being associated with either depression or anxiety during pregnancy, including:

- pre-eclampsia
- increased nausea and vomiting, longer sick leave during pregnancy, an increased number of visits to the obstetrician
- elective Caesarean delivery and epidural analgesia during labour
- admission of the infant to neonatal care
- spontaneous preterm labour
- placental abruption
- preterm delivery
- low birth weight.

A meta-analysis of studies carried out between 1980 and 2009 concluded that depression in pregnancy is associated with an increased risk of preterm birth and low birth weight, but not intra-uterine growth retardation (Grote *et al*, 2010). Another meta-analysis, which included studies published up to June 2010, reported increased odds of preterm birth and decreased breastfeeding initiation (Grigoriadis *et al*, 2013). A Canadian study reported that depressed mothers were at higher risk of adverse obstetric outcomes if they attended fewer than seven antenatal appointments compared with depressed mothers who attended ten or more appointments (Chen & Lin, 2011). However, a meta-analysis of the association between pregnancy anxiety and gestational age at birth and birth weight failed to demonstrate a link (Littleton *et al*, 2007).

There is a growing literature describing the impact of depression during pregnancy on the fetus and neonate. Van den Bergh *et al* (2005) identified 14 independent studies showing a link between maternal anxiety and stress and cognitive, behavioural and emotional problems in the child. The links between maternal depression and anxiety during and after pregnancy and adverse child outcomes are further explored in Chapter 6.

## Assessment and management

This chapter addresses the community assessment and management of women with non-psychotic disorder. The assessment and treatment of those with psychosis or who require in-patient admission will be addressed in Chapter 3.

### Assessment

This is essentially the same as the standard psychiatric history and mental state examination, but it takes into consideration the context and the fact that there is a fetus or infant (and possibly other children) who must be accounted for in decisions relating to treatments and risk assessment. Hence, the social and psychological background to the pregnancy and the postpartum, the woman's physical health in relation to pregnancy and delivery and the relationship with the infant should all be systematically enquired about. In addition, screening for some symptoms requires adaptation when a woman is pregnant or has a baby. For example, when screening for obsessional intrusive thoughts, Brandes *et al* (2004) suggest that all postpartum women should be asked a simple screening question: 'It is not uncommon for new mothers to experience intrusive and unwanted thoughts that they might harm their baby. Have any thoughts like that happened to you?'

A positive answer should be followed up with probes for the frequency and intensity of thoughts, and for any thoughts or reports of actually harming the infant. A woman with active suicidal ideation should be considered as highly likely to involve her infant in any act of self-harm.

Questions relating to sleep, appetite, fatigue, activity levels and libido must take into consideration the norms for the stage of pregnancy or the postpartum.

As in any other situation, unusual symptoms should prompt consideration of alternative diagnoses. A 37-year-old postpartum woman presented with mood symptoms, then progressive hyperphagia, hypersexuality, disinhibition and impairment of judgement. She was treated for depression for months before a frontotemporal dementia was diagnosed (Dell & Halford, 2002). Women with serious physical illness have died owing to their symptoms being wrongly attributed to mental disorder, e.g. tachycardia of 140–160 bpm being attributed to panic attacks and anxiety, when in fact the patient had sepsis and cardiac arrhythmia (Lewis & Drife, 2004; Oates & Cantwell, 2011).

## Interventions for depression

There are several systematic reviews and meta-analyses (some from the Cochrane Collaboration) of a wide range of interventions for depression and anxiety during pregnancy and postpartum.

Bledsoe & Grote (2006) undertook one of the first meta-analyses. They found larger effect sizes (>0.95) when medication was combined with cognitive–behavioural therapy (CBT), interpersonal therapy (IPT), or group therapy with cognitive–behavioural, educational or transactional analysis components. Smaller effect sizes (<0.75) or no effect were observed when the interventions used counselling, educational or psychodynamic approaches. Postpartum implementations provided larger effect sizes than interventions delivered during pregnancy.

### Psychological and psychosocial therapies

Dennis & Hodnett (2007) carried out a Cochrane review of psychological and psychosocial interventions for the treatment of postpartum depression. The ten studies included consisted of trials of peer support (telephone-based), non-directive counselling and psychological therapies (CBT and ITP). All were individual interventions and, with the exception of peer support by telephone, were delivered face-to-face. All interventions were superior to usual care. A year later, Cuijpers and colleagues (2008) published a meta-analysis of psychological treatments for postpartum depression, including 17 studies of CBT, ITP, counselling and some social support interventions. They reported moderate effect sizes. A Cochrane review of psychological and psychosocial interventions for antenatal depression only included one small trial of ITP (Dennis & Hodnett, 2007).

Many UK health visitors offer Rogerian non-directive counselling as 'listening visits' (usually 4–8 sessions, each lasting around 1 h) to depressed postpartum women in their homes. However, training and supervision vary, as does the availability of specialist secondary services for women for whom this approach is unsuitable or who do not respond to the intervention.

Qualitative studies of women who had received interventions from their health visitor reveal that they felt positive about the intervention if they had a prior good relationship with their health visitor, but they were less positive and might decline the intervention if that relationship was poor, if they could not relate to the health visitor or if they did not know her (Shakespeare *et al*, 2006; Slade *et al*, 2010). Women perceived the intervention (listening visits) as supportive rather than therapeutic and attributed their recovery to other factors (Shakespeare *et al*, 2006). Morse *et al* (2004) evaluated the effectiveness of training Australian maternal and child health nurses (MCHNs) in the early detection and management of new mothers with mild distress. The MCHNs had access to a liaison psychiatric network that provided support and consultation. There was no difference in the rates or levels of distress or psychosocial functioning between the intervention group and those receiving routine care. However, satisfaction with the intervention was high. Nursing care (six weekly visits) was superior to problem solving when administered to women with high EPDS scores in the first week postpartum (Tezel & Gozum, 2006).

Health visitors can also be trained in cognitive–behavioural counselling (CBC) skills. The CBC intervention comprises childcare advice, reassurance, encouraging participation in enjoyable activities, accessing support from others and setting targets. Both CBC (Appleby *et al*, 1997) and cognitive therapy (Misri *et al*, 2004) have been shown to be as effective as antidepressant treatment for postnatal major depression, but CBC or cognitive therapy in addition to drug treatment did not confer any additional benefit. Training the health visitors in CBC not only improved their skills but also improved screening, treatment and increased referral rates to mental health services (Appleby *et al*, 2003). A large (over 4000 women) cluster-randomised trial of trained health visitors delivering sessions based either on cognitive–behavioural or person-centred approaches reported benefit over usual care at 6 and 12 months (Morrell *et al*, 2009). Neither approach was better than the other. Some of the above studies were included in a systematic review of six home-based interventions to treat postpartum depression (Leis *et al*, 2009). Four of the six studies reported statistically significant improvement.

IPT is a time-limited, manualised psychotherapy that focuses on four main problem areas: grief, interpersonal disputes, role transitions and interpersonal deficits. It consists of three phases. The initial phase covers assessment, psychoeducation, selection of a treatment focus and negotiation of a treatment agreement. The problems are then worked on in the intermediate phase, and a discussion of the progress made and how the patient feels about termination is carried out at the end.

IPT has been adapted to deal with issues facing women with postpartum depression, such as her relationship with the baby and her partner and returning to work. IPT has also been adapted for use in pregnant women suffering from depression with a focus on role transition in relation to pregnancy, interpersonal disputes related to pregnancy and motherhood, and complicated pregnancies (Spinelli & Endicott, 2003). A later RCT by Spinelli *et al* (2013) found IPT and a parenting education programme to be equally efficacious in a three-centre bilingual (English and Spanish) trial with equal numbers of white, African American and Hispanic women participating.

In a meta-analysis undertaken by Sockol and colleagues (2011) which included 27 studies treating perinatal depression, all interventions were superior to usual care and IPT was superior to interventions, including those with a CBT component. Miniati *et al* (2014) carried out a systematic review of 11 studies and concluded that the ideal time for IPT is during the acute depressive phase and that it leads to a better mid- and long-term outcome than intensive clinical management.

### Group interventions

Many interventions can be delivered in a group setting. Being part of a group can reduce the sense of isolation that many mothers with mental health problems feel and enable them to share experiences and coping strategies. It can also be a cost-effective way of delivering an intervention as several women can be treated at the same time. However, some mothers will have specific issues that may be better dealt with on a one-to-one basis, have difficulty talking openly in a group, may make negative social comparisons with others (Scope *et al*, 2012) and may require some individual work before they feel able to cope with a group.

The majority of group treatments consist of several components e.g. education, social support and CBT. They may involve partners in some or all sessions. Scope *et al* (2013) reviewed seven studies of group CBT compared to usual care or waiting-list groups for postnatal depression and report pooled effect sizes of $d = 0.57$ (95% CI 0.34–0.80; $P<0.001$) 10–13 weeks after randomisation, reducing to $d = 0.28$ (CI 0.03–0.53; $P = 0.025$) after 6 months. Stevenson *et al* (2010), in their systematic review, concluded that the evidence for the clinical effectiveness of group CBT for postnatal depression provides 'inconsistent and low quality information on which to base service provision' and found no studies on which to calculate cost-effectiveness.

Setting up, running and evaluating a group intervention has been described by Milgrom *et al* (1999). Their book includes material for all their group sessions. Reay and colleagues (2012) describe the development and content of IPT groups for postnatal depression.

Focused interventions can also be offered, e.g. a psycho-educational group has been shown to be superior to routine primary care in reducing depressive symptoms (Honey *et al*, 2002). An uncontrolled study examining counselling in the voluntary sector reported success in treating women both individually and in groups with therapy based on gestalt, person-centred and psychodynamic principles (Alder & Truman, 2002). Small studies suggest that group IPT is effective in treating postnatal depression (Clark *et al*, 2003; Reay *et al*, 2006). These and others were included in a systematic review of group treatment for postpartum depression undertaken by

Goodman & Santangelo (2011) and in a meta-analysis of IPT and relational therapies (both individual and group) in pregnant and postpartum women (Claridge, 2014). The latter study confirmed an overall effect size of 1.14 for one-group studies but lower effect sizes for treatment-control comparisons.

Two systematic reviews of interventions carried out in low- and middle-income countries have been published. Rahman et al (2013) undertook a systematic review and meta-analysis of interventions for common perinatal mental disorders in women in low- and middle-income countries. The pooled effect size was 0.38 (CI 0.56–0.21). The key features of effective interventions were culturally adapted approaches grounded in cognitive, problem-solving and educational techniques, and interventions applicable to individuals or groups and deliverable in women's homes (involving the extended family in crowded households. Supervised, non-specialist health and community workers delivered almost all the interventions with no training in mental healthcare. Clarke et al (2013) reported that interventions led to an overall reduction in symptoms compared to usual care, and that there were significantly larger effect sizes for psychological interventions than for health-promotion interventions. Both individual and group interventions were effective compared to usual care, although delivery method was not associated with effect size.

There is a pilot study of a mindfulness-based group intervention, which reduced symptoms of distress, depression and anxiety in pregnant women; however, numbers were small and there was a high attrition rate (Dunn et al, 2012). One meta-analysis of antenatal interventions to reduce subsyndromal maternal distress included four interventions (mindfulness, relaxation, acupuncture and a self-help workbook). They reported a standard mean difference of –0.29 (CI –0.54 to –0.04) for the treatments (Fontein-Kuipers et al, 2014).

Mothers can be trained in baby massage one-to-one or in a group setting, and this may improve mother–infant interaction (Onozawa et al, 2001). There is no evidence as yet that it has an impact on maternal mental disorder. Services may also offer groups (which are usually closed) targeted at mothers with specific problems, e.g. survivors of CSA, those who have been bereaved or adolescent mothers. Saisto et al (2006) describe a psycho-educational group approach for women with fear of childbirth, which led to withdrawn requests for Caesarean section.

Social support is often the main focus or an important component of group treatment. Many health visitors have set up such groups, with some becoming self-help groups beyond the lifetime of the original group. Groups may be open or closed; they may consist of just mothers, or fathers may attend some or all of the sessions. However, there are limited data relating to the efficacy of support groups, and it is not clear whether they are superior to other interventions.

There is evidence that exercise (group-based programmes or individual-ised home-based interventions) can reduce postpartum depressive symptoms (Heh *et al*, 2008; Da Costa *et al*, 2009; Ko *et al*, 2013). Physical exercise is beneficial for women during pregnancy and in the postpartum period, does not increases risks for the fetus or infant and can also lead to lifestyle changes which may confer long term health benefits (Nascimento *et al*, 2012).

## Information and education

Women with high EPDS scores 4 weeks after delivery were randomised to receive an information leaflet at 6 weeks postpartum or not. Those who received the leaflet had lower scores when re-assessed at 3 months (Heh & Fu, 2003). More than 90% of those who had received the booklet said that it was useful to them and their families. Many had not known about postnatal depression before reading it and, because of this information, those in the experimental group gained more practical help from their families.

## Telephone and internet interventions

Interventions can be delivered by telephone, and there is some trial evidence to support this. Interpersonal counselling (a shorter intervention aimed at distress rather than clinical depression) has been shown to reduce depressive symptoms in women with subsyndromal depression following a miscarriage when delivered by telephone (Neugebauer *et al*, 2007). A modified form of Gruen therapy, which encompasses relaxation techniques, problem-solving strategies and CBT, delivered by telephone over a 10-week period by nurse therapists is reported in a small pilot study (Ugarriza & Schmidt, 2006). It resulted in reduced BDI scores. Dennis & Kingston (2008) undertook a systematic review of telephone support for women during pregnancy and the early postpartum, concluding that such interventions can reduce depressive symptoms. This may be particularly suitable for housebound mothers or those in remote rural areas.

Pugh *et al* (2014) describe the successful assessment and treatment of a woman with postnatal depression with therapist-assisted internet-delivered CBT. O'Mahen and colleagues (2013) carried out a RCT of internet-based behavioural activation in 910 women scoring > 12 on the EPDS, recruited via a UK parenting website (Netmums). The intervention involved 11 weekly sessions lasting up to 40 min each, to be completed over a 15-week period. There were significant group differences between the intervention group and the treatment-as-usual group, with the intervention group having lower EPDS scores at follow-up. However, although there was a huge interest in participating, attrition was high and some women had difficulty accessing CBT, lacked privacy, had issues around speaking face-to-face and were concerned that their child would be taken away.

Wisner *et al* (2008) describe the development and implementation of a web-based educational resource for women and professionals, MedEdPPD (see further reading at the end of this chapter), which uses a variety of strategies to promote learning.

There are a number of organisations that provide information via literature or websites, or that run telephone support lines. Some also offer befriending or practical help in the home (see Appendix 1). However, caution must be exercised with respect to some websites, as several have been found not to contain much useful information, or to contain information that does not accurately reflect the evidence base and state of the science relating to postnatal depression (Summers & Logsdon, 2005).

## Antidepressants

Compared with the evidence base for major depressive disorder, the evidence base for depression during pregnancy and the postpartum is much smaller. It is growing with more trials and some systematic reviews. Efficacy is discussed here, and issues related to drug and other physical treatments in pregnant and breastfeeding women are described in Chapters 8 and 9.

There are several open-label studies. Eight postpartum women with DSM-IV major depressive disorder were treated for 8 weeks with bupropion SR, using a flexible dosing schedule of between 150 and 400 mg daily. This resulted in a significant reduction of scores on the Hamilton Rating Scale for Depression (HRSD), but only three women achieved remission. The women were permitted to use zolpidem for insomnia and lorazepam for anxiety, and some were receiving psychotherapy, so the improvement cannot be attributed to the antidepressant alone (Nonacs et al, 2005). Two of the women were breastfeeding.

An open-label study of nefazodone in doses up to 500 mg per day in 4 women (Suri et al, 2005) reported one dropping out due to lethargy and the others improving. Stowe et al (1995) treated 21 women with sertraline; 14 were reported to have achieved remission. Those with onsets less than 4 weeks postpartum appeared to respond more quickly and require less medication. Fifteen women received venlafaxine in a mean dose of 162.5 mg per day (Cohen et al, 2001), and 12 of these responded with an improvement in depressive and anxiety symptoms.

De Crescenzo and colleagues (2014) conducted a systematic review of six RCTs of SSRIs. They concluded that SSRIs are an effective treatment and may be more efficacious than psychological interventions at the conclusion of therapy, but that there was no difference in outcomes at the follow-up phase. There was no benefit of combining treatment modalities. Sharma & Sommerdyk (2013) reviewed the same studies and were much more cautious about claiming efficacy, given the small number of trials and their methodological flaws. Similar caution was advised by the authors of a Cochrane review (Molyneaux et al, 2014).

A chart review of women attending psychiatric out-patient services for treatment of postnatal depression noted that although they were as likely as non-postpartum women to respond to medication, their time to respond was longer and they were more likely to be receiving more than one antidepressant at a time (Hendrick et al, 2000).

A small naturalistic study compared response to SSRIs and tricyclic antidepressants in women with postnatal depression, and SSRIs appeared to be superior (Wisner *et al*, 1999*b*). Atypical antipsychotic augmentation of an SSRI when treating postpartum depression with intrusive obsessional thoughts resulted in resolution of resistant obsessional symptoms in a small case series (Corral *et al*, 2007*a*).

## Risks of discontinuing antidepressants during pregnancy

Some studies have reported that women who discontinue antidepressants on discovering they are pregnant, or who have taken them in the 2 years prior to conception and stopped, are more likely to report depressive symptoms during pregnancy (Marcus *et al*, 2005). They may even experience suicidal ideation or need admission (Einarson *et al*, 2001). Cohen *et al* (2004) followed up 32 women with histories of depression who were euthymic before discontinuing medication around the time of conception. Three-quarters relapsed during pregnancy – most in the first trimester – with 38% resuming taking their medication. However, the women participating in these three studies were in specialist psychiatric settings and more likely to have more severe depressive illnesses. Similar findings were reported from the same group when they followed 201 women from specialist centres: 26% of those who remained on medication relapsed, compared with 68% of those who did not (Cohen *et al*, 2006). A slightly larger study of women drawn from 137 community and hospital-based antenatal clinics in the USA found no difference in risk of becoming depressed in those who continued to take antidepressants and those who did not (Yonkers *et al*, 2011). Those who had four or more previous episodes of depression were more likely to become depressed.

Care must be taken when treating women with family histories of bipolar disorder with antidepressants, as there are reports of this triggering psychosis, a mixed affective episode or hypomania (Sharma, 2006). The issues in treating pregnant women with depression are clearly articulated by Yonkers *et al* (2012).

### Hormones

The assumption that postnatal depression must have a hormonal aetiology led to attempts to treat the disorder with oestrogens, progesterone and progestogens. Uncontrolled studies performed by Dalton (1985, 1989, 1995) claimed success with progesterone as a treatment and prevention; however, the studies have serious methodological problems and, as yet, there are no controlled data to support their conclusions. A Cochrane review concludes: 'Synthetic progestogens should be used with significant caution in the postpartum period. The role of natural progesterone in the prevention and treatment of postpartum depression has yet to be evaluated in a randomised, placebo-controlled trial' (Dennis *et al*, 2008).

Two small studies (one uncontrolled, one RCT) support the use of oestradiol in the treatment of severe postnatal depression (Gregoire *et al*, 1996; Ahokas *et al*, 2001). It should be noted that most of the women had previous or concurrent antidepressant or psychological therapy, so oestradiol has not been tested as a monotherapy. There are also concerns about using high doses of oestradiol in the postnatal period, owing to the increased risk of deep-vein thrombosis, difficulties with breastfeeding and endometrial hyperplasia. The optimum dose and route of administration has not been established. Until more data are available, the use of oestradiol is best limited to use as adjunct therapy for severe depressive disorders in women with no additional risk factors for thromboembolic disease or hormone-dependent tumours. For a review, see Gentile (2005). Dennis *et al* (2008) note that: 'Oestrogen therapy may be of modest value for the treatment of severe postpartum depression. Its role in the prevention of recurrent postpartum depression has not been rigorously evaluated. Further research is warranted'.

## Omega-3 fatty acids

There has been interest in exploring the role of omega-3 fatty acids in the treatment for perinatal depression, despite evidence that fish consumption and omega-3 status after childbirth are not associated with depression (Browne *et al*, 2006). Borja-Hart & Marino (2010) reviewed seven trials and observed that although scores on depression rating scales reduced, the difference was only significant in three studies. Four were RCTs and three were open-label studies. The most common adverse effects experienced were foul breath, an unpleasant taste and gastrointestinal complaints. There were no serious adverse events. They noted that many studies had small sample sizes and that the dosages and duration of treatment were variable. They describe the results as inconclusive. In their systematic review, Deligiannidis & Freeman (2014) recommend that perinatal women with depression take 1 g of eicosapentaenoic acid plus docosahexaenoic acid daily.

A Cochrane review (Dennis & Dowswell, 2013) concluded: 'The evidence is inconclusive to allow us to make any recommendations for depression-specific acupuncture, maternal massage, bright light therapy, and omega-3 fatty acids for the treatment of antenatal depression. The included trials were too small with non-generalisable samples, to make any recommendations'.

## Bright light therapy

There is an open trial of morning bright light therapy in pregnant women with major depression, reporting improvement in depression scores over 5 weeks and no adverse effects (Oren *et al*, 2002). A small RCT with 10 pregnant participants suffering from major depression reported an effect size similar to that of antidepressants during a 10-week period (Epperson *et al*, 2004). One woman experienced hypomania. Corral *et al* (2007*b*) randomised 15 women to 30 min each morning of bright light (10 000 lux) or dim light (600 lux) for 6 weeks. Both groups improved, with no difference between them. A slightly larger (n=27) RCT of bright light for depression in pregnancy randomised the women to 7000 lux fluorescent bright white or 70 lux dim red light (placebo) administered at home in the morning upon awakening for 1 h per day in a 5-week double-blind trial. Bright light produced a significantly greater reduction in depressive symptoms than dim red light (Wirz-Justice *et al*, 2011).

## Sleep deprivation

Sleep deprivation may help pregnant and postpartum women who are depressed. Parry *et al* (2000) exposed nine women with major depressive disorder who were either pregnant or postpartum to late (LSD) and early (ESD) sleep deprivation. More women responded to LSD and more responded after a night of recovery sleep. However, pregnant women responded to ESD and not to LSD. Clearly, further research with controlled conditions is needed.

## Complementary therapies

Deligiannidis & Freeman (2014) carried out a review of complementary and alternative therapies. In addition to omega-3 fatty acids, bright light therapy and exercise (see above), they reviewed the evidence for folate, S-adenosylmethionine, St John's wort, massage and acupuncture. There is no evidence to support the use of folate as a treatment for perinatal depression and only one non-randomised placebo-controlled study of S-adenosylmethionine (Cerutti *et al*, 1993), which reported it to be superior to placebo in reducing symptoms of anxiety and depression. St John's wort has not been evaluated for safety and efficacy in a perinatal population. There is some evidence that massage is effective when combined with group psychotherapy, but the authors concluded that 'it is premature to recommend acupuncture as a first line treatment for perinatal major depressive disorder'.

Over one-third of women use herbal medicine during pregnancy (Forster *et al*, 2006). Thirty per cent reported currently using complementary therapies. The most commonly used were massage, herbal medicine and acupuncture. One-third were using more than one treatment. Schnyer *et al* (2003) have described a conceptual framework for the use of acupuncture to treat depression in pregnancy and two case studies, and there is a case report of a woman successfully treated with hypnosis (Yexley, 2007).

Some of the psychological interventions described above, particularly CBT, can be adapted for anxiety symptoms. In addition, some specific interventions have been developed for perinatal anxiety disorders; the literature remains limited but is growing. Arch *et al* (2012) asked whether exposure-based CBT was safe in pregnancy. They concluded that it probably was and provided guidelines for adapting the most common exposures to feared bodily sensations for pregnancy, e.g. monitoring maternal heart rate.

There are interventions for fear of delivery. One study gave those in the intervention group support from a psychosomatic gynaecologist (mean 3.4 sessions) and some received brief psychotherapy (mean 7.4 sessions) during pregnancy. Before the intervention, 68% had requested Caesarean section. Afterwards, this dropped to 38%. Obstetric outcomes in those who had vaginal deliveries were similar to controls, but they were more likely to have had induction of labour, epidural anaesthesia or a pudendal nerve block (Sjögren & Thomasson, 1997).

An RCT of an intervention comprising information, education and cognitive therapy delivered to pregnant women with fear of vaginal delivery produced a reduction in unnecessary Caesarean sections, a reduction in pregnancy and birth-related concerns and shorter labours when compared with a control group who received information only (Saisto *et al*, 2001).

Forty women randomised to video and verbal feedback during ultrasound examinations or usual care had reduced scores on the Spielberger State–Trait Anxiety Inventory (STAI), reduced fetal activity and fewer delivery complications (Field *et al*, 1985). Another study compared seven sessions of applied relaxation therapy to usual antenatal care in pregnant women with high scores on the STAI. The intervention group had significant reductions in anxiety symptoms and perceived stress (Bastani *et al*, 2005).

In Sweden, 'fear of childbirth teams' have been established to meet the needs of women with fears of delivery and/or who had previous traumatic labours. Midwives trained in counselling talked to the women and invited them to express their fears, and individual birth plans were devised. Although women were very satisfied with their care, those in the intervention group had more frightening experiences of delivery and higher rates of post-traumatic stress symptoms than those in the control group (Ryding *et al*, 2003).

Others have devised an intervention for women diagnosed with fetal malformation, which ran from pregnancy to delivery and reduced anxiety and depression symptoms (Gorayeb *et al*, 2013), although the numbers in each group were small. The authors note that this type of psychological intervention and support may be very important in countries where termination of pregnancy for fetal malformation is only permitted in very extreme situations.

Kersting *et al* (2013) conducted an RCT of an internet-based intervention using exposure techniques and cognitive restructuring designed to target PTSD symptoms and prolonged grief following pregnancy loss. Participants (228 in total) were randomised to the intervention (a 5-week, CBT-based treatment) or waiting-list control. Significant improvement was observed in both PTSD symptoms and prolonged grief post-treatment and at 12-month follow-up. There is also a planned RCT of eye-movement desensitisation and reprocessing treatment for women who suffered PTSD after childbirth planned in France (George *et al* 2013).

Marc et al (2011) undertook a systematic review of mind–body interventions which might benefit women's anxiety during pregnancy. They reviewed 8 trials with 556 participants (1 trial of hypnotherapy, 5 of imagery, 1 of autogenic training and 1 of yoga) and concluded that 'there is some but no strong evidence for the effectiveness of mind-body interventions for the management of anxiety during pregnancy', particularly imagery and autogenic training. The main limitations of the studies were the lack of blinding and insufficient details on the methods used for randomisation. The studies were often small and with a high risk of bias.

## Interventions for OCD

There is no RCT evidence to guide the clinician in treating postpartum-onset OCD. However, as at any other time, the management is likely to include CBT with exposure and response-prevention and/or thought-stopping. This might also be the treatment of choice in pregnant women to avoid fetal exposure to drugs. Support for the patient, and for her partner and family, is essential. Women with OCD may be afraid of being left alone with the infant in case they harm the baby. This can lead to pressures on the extended family, and there are reports of fathers giving up work to be with their partner (Jennings et al, 1999). Challacombe & Salkovskis (2011) describe the use of intensive CBT in a small case series of women with postpartum OCD.

SSRIs, venlafaxine and clomipramine all have a substantial evidence base behind their use in OCD, and there are small open-label trials in postpartum-onset OCD. Sichel et al (1993) treated the women in their study with fluoxetine, clomipramine, desipramine or a combination of these and reported significant improvement in symptoms. Buttolph & Holland (1990) describe four women successfully treated with fluoxetine, and Arnold (1999) reported a case series of seven women, of whom three entered into an open-label trial of fluvoxamine 50–300 mg daily. Two of the three had more than 30% improvement in their score on the Yale–Brown Obsessive Compulsive Scale (Y-BOCS). A small, uncontrolled study of women with OCD (most of whom had new onsets postpartum) who had not responded to 8 weeks of antidepressant therapy (SSRIs and serotonin-noradrenaline reuptake inhibitors (SNRIs)) found that adding quetiapine produced a full response (assessed using the Y-BOCS and the Clinical Global Impressions Scale) in 11 out of 17 patients (Misri & Milis, 2004).

## What do women think about treatments?

There is a growing literature exploring women's views on treatments for perinatal depression. Concerns about treatment may stem from a reluctance to be labelled as suffering from depression. More than 90% of mothers interviewed by Whitton et al (1996) recognised there was something wrong, but only one-third believed they were suffering from postnatal depression. Primiparous women and those from social classes I (professional), II (semi-professional, e.g. teachers) and III (skilled manual) were less likely to recognise themselves as depressed. Over 80% had not reported their symptoms to any health professional, and 81% said they would not consider antidepressants. A more recent study from Wales found that mothers had little knowledge of postnatal depression before pregnancy, felt that it happened to 'other people' and tended to hide their emotions from their family (Hanley & Long, 2006).

In a German study, only 18% of those offered a variety of interventions took up the offer. Thirty-nine per cent refused for what were described as 'factual reasons', e.g. not thinking that psychiatric or psychotherapeutic treatments would help (von Ballestrem et al, 2005). There may also be stigma attached to accessing mental healthcare. One study found that 50% of women with depressive symptoms who were offered a psychiatric assessment by the clinic staff refused it. The staff reported spending up to an hour with women after they had been told there was a strong suggestion that they were depressed. They suggested that important factors in the women's decisions were stigma, differing expectations of well-being and the inconvenience of attending appointments. Women also preferred not to see a psychologist (Robinson & Young, 1982).

However, a US study reports that although only 5% of pregnant women with anxiety or depressive symptoms had discussed this with their obstetrician, 82.4% said they would be willing to and would accept a referral to a mental health professional (Birndorf et al, 2001). The study did not follow the women through to see if this actually happened. Women with PTSD may also not want treatment. A variety of factors inform their decision, including avoidance of reminders of the trauma, expensive and difficult to access services, childcare difficulties and the stigma of mental health treatments (Loveland Cook et al, 2004).

Women suffering from postnatal depression have worries about antidepressants. Of 35 who had been prescribed antidepressants, 4 chose not to take them because they were breastfeeding, 20 found them helpful but 11 did not. As well as the four women who reported that they did not take them, others missed doses or did not increase the dose when advised to do so, suggesting some degree of self-regulation. Most did not take them beyond remission (Boath et al, 2004a). Being provided with more information about treatments does not appear to increase the acceptability of antidepressants (Chabrol et al 2001, 2004), but experience of taking them and discussing this with a clinician may lead to women viewing them as beneficial (Turner et al, 2008). Office-based therapies were more acceptable than those delivered at home, but very few women found antidepressants acceptable. Being provided with more information about the interventions made little difference to the acceptability rating of psychotherapy and reduced that of antidepressants further.

However, Pearlstein *et al* (2006) found that most women chose IPT, with or without sertraline, and observed a trend towards those with a history of depression being more likely to opt for the antidepressant.

A study comparing the satisfaction of women suffering from postnatal depression with treatment in primary care and that in a specialist multidisciplinary parent and baby day unit (PBDU) offering individualised programmes of care found overall levels of satisfaction greater in women who had attended the PBDU. They particularly valued the peer support received (Boath *et al*, 2004*b*). More of these mothers reported that they would like the same treatment again, would recommend it to a friend and felt better informed about postnatal depression. There were a few negative comments about the PBDU, but there were many more made by the women who had been treated in primary care. These most often related to the short length of time they had in consultations with their GP. One-third were dissatisfied with the treatment they received from their GP, and one-fifth with the treatment they received from their health visitor. These women were less likely to recommend the care they had received to a friend. An Australian study found that women scoring high on the EPDS were more likely to visit a GP and other professionals than those with low scores, but that they were less satisfied with the care they received from their GP. This mostly related to lack of information and not feeling listened to (Webster *et al*, 2001). These findings raise concern, as specialist services are limited and not uniformly accessible across the UK. Most women with perinatal depression will be treated by primary care professionals, and it appears that a significant minority of those women will not be satisfied with that care.

Women with postnatal depression may also have practical reasons for not taking up treatment offers. They may have multiple roles: 26% of those offered self-help, out-patient treatment, out-patient psychotherapy or in-patient therapy did not take up any, saying they did not have time (von Ballestrem *et al*, 2005). There may be difficulty accessing services by public transport or attending appointments that take place outside school hours, or in accessing services that do not provide childcare.

# References

Abramowitz J, Moore K, Carmin C, *et al* (2001) Acute onset of obsessive–compulsive disorder in males following childbirth. *Psychosomatics*, **42**: 429–431.

Abramowitz JS, Schwartz SA, Moore KM, *et al* (2003) Obsessive–compulsive symptoms in pregnancy and the puerperium: a review of the literature. *Anxiety Disorders*, **17**: 461–478.

Adewuya AO (2006) Early postpartum mood as a risk factor for postnatal depression in Nigerian women. *American Journal of Psychiatry*, **163**: 1435–1437.

Adewuya AO, Ologun YA, Ibigami OS (2006) Post-traumatic stress disorder after childbirth in Nigerian women: prevalence and risk factors. *BJOG*, **113**: 284–288.

Ahokas A, Kaukoranta J, Wahlbeck K, *et al* (2001) Estrogen deficiency in severe postpartum depression: successful treatment with sublingual physiologic 17-beta-estradiol: a preliminary study. *Journal of Clinical Psychiatry*, **62**: 332–336.

Alcorn KL, O'Donovan A, Patrick C, *et al* (2010) A prospective study of the prevalence of post-traumatic stress disorder resulting from childbirth events. *Psychological Medicine,* **40**: 1849–1859.

Alder E, Truman J (2002) Counselling for postnatal depression in the voluntary sector. *Psychology and Psychotherapy,* **75**: 207–220.

American Psychiatric Association (1994) *Diagnostic and Statistical Manual of Mental Disorders* (4th edn) (DSM-IV). APA.

Andersen LB, Melvaer LB, Videbech P, *et al* (2012) Risk factors for developing post-traumatic stress disorder following childbirth: a systematic review. *Acta Obstetricia et Gynecologica Scandinavica,* **91**: 1261–1272.

Andersson L, Sundström-Poromaa I, Bixo M, *et al* (2003) Point prevalence of psychiatric disorders during the second trimester of pregnancy: a population-based study. *American Journal of Obstetrics & Gynecology,* **189**: 148–154.

Appleby L, Warner R, Whitton A, *et al* (1997) A controlled study of fluoxetine and cognitive–behavioural counselling in the treatment of postnatal depression. *BMJ,* **314**: 932–936.

Appleby L, Hirst E, Marshall S, *et al* (2003) The treatment of postnatal depression by health visitors: impact of brief training on skills and clinical practice. *Journal of Affective Disorders,* **77**: 261–266.

Arch JA, Dimidjian S, Chessick C (2012) Are exposure-based cognitive behavioral therapies safe during pregnancy? *Archives of Women's Mental Health,* **15**: 445–457.

de Armond M (1954) A type of postpartum anxiety reaction. *Diseases of the Nervous System,* **15**: 26–29.

Arnold LM (1999) A case-series of women with postpartum onset obsessive–compulsive disorder. *Primary Care Companion to the Journal of Clinical Psychiatry,* **1**: 103–108.

Ashok PW, Hamoda H, Flett GM, *et al* (2005) Psychological sequelae of medical and surgical abortion at 10–13 weeks gestation. *Acta Obstetricia Gynecologica Scandinavica,* **84**: 761–766.

Badenhorst W, Riches S, Turton P, *et al* (2006) The psychological effects of stillbirth and neonatal death on fathers: systematic review. *Journal of Psychosomatic Obstetrics & Gynecology,* **27**: 245–256.

von Ballestrem CL, Strauss M, Kaechele H (2005) Contribution to the epidemiology of postnatal depression in Germany – implications for the utilization of treatment. *Archives of Women's Mental Health,* **8**: 29–35.

Barnet B, Joffe A, Duggan AK, *et al* (1996) Depressive symptoms, stress, and social support in pregnant and postpartum adolescents. *Archives of Pediatrics and Adolescent Medicine,* **150**: 64–69.

Bastani F, Hidarnia A, Kazemnejad A, *et al* (2005) A randomized controlled trial of the effects of applied relaxation training on reducing anxiety and perceived stress in pregnant women. *Journal of Midwifery and Women's Health,* **50**: 36–40.

Battle CL, Zlotnick C, Miller IW, *et al* (2006) Clinical characteristics of perinatal patients: a chart review study. *Journal of Nervous and Mental Disease,* **194**: 369–377.

Bauer A, Parsonage M, Knapp M, *et al* (2014) *Costs of Perinatal Mental Health Problems.* Centre for Mental Health & London School of Economics.

Beck CT (1996) A meta-analysis of predictors of postpartum depression. *Nursing Research,* **45**: 297–303.

Beck CT (1998) Postpartum onset of panic disorder. *Journal of Nursing Scholarship,* **30**: 131–135.

Beck CT (2001) Predictors of postpartum depression. *Nursing Research,* **50**: 275–285.

Beck CT (2002) Postpartum depression: a meta-synthesis. *Qualitative Health Research,* **12**: 453–472.

Beeghly M, Weinberg MK, Olson KL, *et al* (2002) Stability and change in level of maternal depressive symptomatology during the first postpartum year. *Journal of Affective Disorders,* **71**: 169–180.

Bellieni CV, Buonocore G (2013) Abortion and subsequent mental health: review of the literature. *Psychiatry and Clinical Neuroscience*, **67**: 301–310.

Benedict MI, Paine LL, Paine LA, *et al* (1999) The association of childhood sexual abuse with depressive symptoms during pregnancy, and selected pregnancy outcomes. *Child Abuse and Neglect*, **23**: 659–670.

Bennett HA, Einarson A, Taddio A, *et al* (2004) Prevalence of depression during pregnancy: systematic review. *Obstetrics & Gynecology*, **103**: 698–709.

Bifulco A, Figueiredo B, Guedeney N, *et al* (2004) Maternal attachment style and depression associated with childbirth: preliminary results from a European and US cross-cultural study. *British Journal of Psychiatry*, **184**: s31–s37.

Birkeland R, Thompson JK, Phares V (2005) Adolescent motherhood and postpartum depression. *Journal of Clinical Child and Adolescent Psychology*, **34**: 292–300.

Birndorf CA, Madden A, Portera L, *et al* (2001) Psychiatric symptoms, functional impairment and receptivity towards mental health treatment among obstetrical patients. *International Journal of Psychiatry in Medicine*, **31**: 355–365.

Bledsoe SE, Grote NK (2006) Treating depression during pregnancy and the postpartum: a preliminary meta-analysis. *Research in Social Work Practice*, **16**: 109–120.

Bloch M, Schmidt PJ, Danaceau M, *et al* (2000) Effects of gonadal steroids in women with a history of postpartum depression. *American Journal of Psychiatry*, **157**: 924–930.

Bloch M, Daly RC, Rubinow DR (2003) Endocrine factors in the etiology of postpartum depression. *Comprehensive Psychiatry*, **44**: 234–236.

Bloch M, Rotenberg N, Koren D, *et al* (2005) Risk factors associated with the development of postpartum mood disorders. *Journal of Affective Disorders*, **88**: 9–18.

Bloch M, Rubinow DR, Schmidt PJ, *et al* (2005) Cortisol response to ovine corticotrophin-releasing hormone in a model of pregnancy and parturition in euthymic women with and without a history of postpartum depression. *Journal of Clinical Endocrinology and Metabolism*, **90**: 695–699.

Blom EA, Jansen PW, Verhulst FC, *et al* (2010) Perinatal complications increase the risk of postpartum depression. *The Generation R Study. BJOG*, **117**: 1390–1398.

Boath E, Bradley E, Henshaw C (2004a) Women's views of antidepressants in the treatment of postnatal depression. *Journal of Psychosomatic Obstetrics & Gynecology*, **25**: 221–236.

Boath E, Bradley E, Anthony P (2004b) Users' views of two alternative approaches to the treatment of postnatal depression. *Journal of Reproductive and Infant Psychology*, **22**: 13–24.

Bodnar LM, Wisner KL, Luther JF, *et al* (2011) An exploratory factor analysis of nutritional biomarkers associated with major depression in pregnancy. *Public Health Nutrition*, **15**: 1078–1086.

Borja-Hart D, Marino J (2010) Role of omega-3 fatty acids for prevention or treatment of perinatal depression. *Pharmacotherapy*, **30**: 210–216.

Boyce P (2003) Risk factors for postnatal depression: a review and risk factors in Australian populations. *Archives of Women's Mental Health*, **6**: S43–S50.

Boyce P, Hickie I, Parker G (1991a) Parents, partners or personality? Risk factors for post-natal depression. *Journal of Affective Disorders*, **21**: 245–255.

Boyce PG, Parker G, Barnett B, *et al* (1991b) Personality as a vulnerability factor to depression. *British Journal of Psychiatry*, **159**: 106–114.

Boyce P, Johnstone SA, Hickey AR, *et al* (2000) Functioning and well-being at 24 weeks postpartum of women with postnatal depression. *Archives of Women's Mental Health*, **3**: 91–97.

Boyle FM, Vance JC, Najman JM, *et al* (1996) The mental health impact of stillbirth, neonatal death or SIDS: prevalence and patterns of distress among mothers. *Social Science and Medicine*, **43**: 1273–1282.

Bozoky IE, Corwin J (2002) Fatigue as a predictor of postpartum depression. *Journal of Obstetric, Gynecologic, and Neonatal Nursing*, **31**: 436–443.

Brandes M, Soares CN, Cohen LS (2004) Postpartum onset obsessive-compulsive disorder: diagnosis and management. *Archives of Women's Mental Health*, **7**: 99–110.

Brier N (2005) Anxiety after miscarriage: a review of the empirical literature and implications for clinical practice. *Birth*, **31**: 138–142.

Brockington IF (2005) Post-abortion psychosis. *Archives of Women's Mental Health*, **8**: 53–54.

Brockington IF, Macdonald E, Wainscott G (2006) Anxiety, obsessions and morbid preoccupations in pregnancy and the puerperium. *Archives of Women's Mental Health*, **9**: 253–263.

Brown S, Lumley J (2000) Physical health problems after childbirth and maternal depression at six to seven months postpartum. *BJOG*, **107**: 1194–1201.

Browne JC, Scott KM, Silvers M (2006) Fish consumption in pregnancy and omega-3 status after birth are not associated with postnatal depression. *Journal of Affective Disorders*, **90**: 131–139.

Brugha TS, Sharp HM, Cooper SA, *et al* (1998) The Leicester 500 project: social support and the development of postnatal depressive symptoms, a prospective cohort study. *Psychological Medicine*, **28**: 63–79.

Brummelte S, Galea LAM (2010) Depression during pregnancy and postpartum: contribution of stress and ovarian hormones. *Progress in Neuro-Psychopharmacology and Biological Psychiatry*, **34**: 766–776.

Buist A (1998) Childhood abuse, parenting and postpartum depression. *Australian and New Zealand Journal of Psychiatry*, **32**: 479–487.

Buist A, Janson H (2001) Childhood sexual abuse, parenting and postpartum depression – a 3-year follow-up study. *Child Abuse & Neglect*, **25**: 909–921.

Buist A, Gotman N, Yonkers KA (2011) Generalized anxiety disorder: course and risk factors in pregnancy. *Journal of Affective Disorders*, **131**: 277–283.

Buttner M, Mott SL, Pearlstein T, *et al* (2103) Examination of premenstrual symptoms as a risk factor for depression in postpartum women. *Archives of Women's Mental Health*, **16**: 219–225.

Buttolph LM, Holland AD (1990) Obsessive compulsive disorders in pregnancy and childbirth. In *Obsessive Compulsive Disorders: Theory and Management* (eds M Jenike, L Baer, W Minichiello): pp. 89–97. Year Book Medical.

Button JH, Reivich RS (1972) Obsessions of infanticide. *Archives of General Psychiatry*, **27**: 235–240.

Carter FA, Frampton CMA, Mulder RT (2006) Caesarean section and postpartum depression: a review of the evidence examining the link. *Psychosomatic Medicine*, **68**: 321–330.

Cerutti R, Sichel MP, Brintz CE, *et al* (1993) Psychological distress during the puerperium: a novel approach using S-adenosyl methionine. *Current Therapeutic Research*, **53**: 701–716.

Chabrol H, Teissedre F, Santrisse K, *et al* (2001) Acceptabilité des antidépresseurs et des psychotherapies dans les depressions du post-partum: enquête chez 198 accouchées. *Encéphale*, **27**: 380–382.

Chabrol H, Teissedre F, Armitage J, *et al* (2004) Acceptability of psychotherapy and antidepressants for postnatal depression among newly delivered mothers. *Journal of Reproductive and Infant Psychology*, **22**: 5–12.

Challacombe FL, Salkovskis PM (2011) Intensive cognitive–behavioural treatment for women with postnatal obsessive–compulsive disorder: a consecutive case series. *Behaviour Research and Therapy*, **49**: 422–426.

Chandran M, Tharyan P, Muliyil J, *et al* (2002) Post-partum depression in a cohort of women from a rural area of Tamil Nadu, India. *British Journal of Psychiatry*, **181**: 499–504.

Chen C-H, Lin H-C (2011) Prenatal care and adverse pregnancy outcomes among women with depression: a nationwide population-based study. *Canadian Journal of Psychiatry*, **56**: 273–280.

Chojenta C, Harris S, Reilly N, *et al* (2014) History of pregnancy loss increases the risk of mental health problems in subsequent pregnancies but not in the postpartum. *PLoS ONE*, **9**: e95038.

Christiansen DM, Elkit A, Olff M (2013) Parents bereaved by infant death: PTSD symptoms up to 18 years after the loss. *General Hospital Psychiatry*, **35**: 605–611.

Church NF, Brechman-Toussaint ML, Hine DW (2005) Do dysfunctional cognitions mediate the relationship between risk factors and postnatal depression symptomatology? *Journal of Affective Disorders*, **87**: 65–72.

Claridge AM (2014) Efficacy of systemically oriented psychotherapies in the treatment of perinatal depression: a meta-analysis. *Archives of Women's Mental Health*, **17**: 3–15.

Clark R, Tluczek A, Wenzel A (2003) Psychotherapy for postpartum depression: a preliminary report. *American Journal of Orthopsychiatry*, **73**: 441–454.

Clarke K, King M, Prost A (2013) Psychosocial interventions for perinatal common mental disorders delivered by providers who are not mental health specialists in low- and middle-income countries: a systematic review and meta-analysis. *PLoS Medicine*, **10**: e1001541.

Coast E, Leone T, Hirose A, *et al* (2012) Poverty and postnatal depression: a systematic mapping of the evidence from low and lower middle-income countries. *Health & Place*, **18**: 1188–1197.

Cohen LS, Viguera VC, Bouffard SM, *et al* (2001) Venlafaxine in the treatment of postpartum depression. *Journal of Clinical Psychiatry*, **62**: 592–596.3

Cohen LS, Nonacs RM, Bailey JW, *et al* (2004) Relapse of depression during pregnancy following antidepressant discontinuation: a preliminary prospective study. *Archives of Women's Mental Health*, **7**: 217–221.

Cohen LS, Altschuler LL, Harlow BL, *et al* (2006) Relapse of major depression during pregnancy in women who maintain or discontinue antidepressant treatment. *Journal of the American Medical Association*, **295**: 499–507.

Cohen MM, Schei B, Ansara D, *et al* (2002) A history of personal violence and postpartum depression: is there a link? *Archives of Women's Mental Health*, **4**: 83–92.

Coletta ND (1983) At risk for depression: a study of young mothers. *Journal of Genetic Psychology*, **142**: 301–310.

Collins CH, Zimmerman C, Howard LM (2011) Refugee, asylum seeker, immigrant women and postnatal depression: rates and risk factors. *Archives of Women's Mental Health*, **14**: 3–11.

Cooper PJ, Campbell EA, Day A, *et al* (1988) Non-psychotic psychiatric disorder after childbirth: a prospective study of prevalence, incidence, course and nature. *British Journal of Psychiatry*, **152**: 799–806.

Cooper PJ, Murray L (1995) Course and recurrence of postnatal depression. Evidence for the specificity of the concept. *British Journal of Psychiatry*, **166**: 191–195.

Cooper PJ, Tomlinson M, Swartz L, *et al* (1999) Post-partum depression and the mother–infant relationship in a South African peri-urban settlement. *British Journal of Psychiatry*, **175**: 554–558.

Corwin EJ, Murray-Kolb LE, Beard JL (2003) Low hemoglobin level is a risk factor for postpartum depression. *Journal of Nutrition*, **133**: 4139–4142.

Corwin EJ, Brownstead J, Barton N, *et al* (2005) The impact of fatigue on the development of postpartum depression. *Journal of Obstetric, Gynecologic, and Neonatal Nursing*, **34**: 577–586.

Corral M, Misri S, Wardrop A. (2007) Atypical augmentation of postpartum depression complicated with obsessions. *Archives of Women's Mental Health*, **9**: 161–171.

Corral M, Wardrop A, Zhang A, *et al*. (2007) Morning light therapy for postpartum depression. *Archives of Women's Mental Health*, **10**: 221–224.

Da Costa D, Lowenstyn I, Abramowicz M, *et al* (2009) A randomized clinical trial of exercise to alleviate postpartum depressed mood. *Journal of Psychosomatic Obstetrics & Gynecology*, **30**: 191–200.

Cox J, Murray D, Chapman G (1993) A controlled study of the onset, duration and prevalence of postnatal depression. *British Journal of Psychiatry*, **163**: 27–31.

Cox JL (1994) Prevention of postnatal mental illness: sociocultural facets. *Topics in Preventive Psychiatry*, **165**: 40–48.

Craig MC (2013) Should psychiatrists be prescribing oestrogen therapy to their female patients? *British Journal of Psychiatry*, **202**: 9–13.

De Crescenzo F, Perelli F, Armando M, *et al* (2014) Selective serotonin reuptake inhibitors (SSRIs) for post-partum depression (PPD): a systematic review of randomized clinical trials. *Journal of Affective Disorders*, **152–154**: 39–44.

Cuijpers P, Brännmark JG, van Straten A (2008) Psychological treatment of postpartum depression: a meta-analysis. *Journal of Clinical Psychology*, **64**: 103–118.

Cumming G, Klein S, Bolsover D, *et al* (2007) The emotional burden of miscarriage for women and their partners: trajectories of anxiety and depression over 13 months. *BJOG*, **114**: 1138–1145.

Cutrona CE (1983) Causal attributions and perinatal depression. *Journal of Abnormal Psychology*, **92**: 161–172.

Dalton K (1985) Progesterone prophylaxis used successfully in postnatal depression. *Practitioner*, **229**: 507–508.

Dalton K (1989) Successful progesterone prophylaxis for idiopathic postnatal depression. *International Journal of Prenatal Perinatal Studies*, **1**: 322–327.

Dalton K (1995) Progesterone prophylaxis for postnatal depression. *International Journal of Prenatal Perinatal Psychology Medicine*, **7**: 447–450.

van Dam RM, Schuit AJ, Schouten G, *et al* (1999) Serum cholesterol decline and depression in the postpartum period. *Journal of Psychosomatic Research*, **46**: 385–390.

Davies V, Gledhill J, McFadyen A, *et al* (2005) Psychological outcome in women undergoing termination of pregnancy for ultrasound-detected fetal anomaly in the first and second trimesters: a pilot study. *Ultrasound in Obstetrics & Gynecology*, **25**: 389–392.

Dean C, Dean NR, White A, *et al* (1995) An adoption study comparing the prevalence of psychiatric illness in women who have adoptive and natural children and women who have adoptive children only. *Journal of Affective Disorders*, **34**: 55–60.

Deligiannidis KM, Freeman MP (2014) Complementary and alternative medicine therapies for perinatal depression. *Best Practice & Research Clinical Obstetrics & Gynecology*, **28**: 85–95.

Dell DL, Halford JJ (2002) Dementia presenting as postpartum depression. *Obstetrics & Gynecology*, **99**: 925–928.

Dennis CL, Dowswell T (2013) Interventions (other than pharmacological, psychosocial or psychological) for treating antenatal depression. *Cochrane Database of Systematic Reviews*, **7**: CD006795.

Dennis CL, Hodnett ED (2007) Psychosocial and psychological interventions for treating postpartum depression. *Cochrane Database of Systematic Reviews*, **4**: CD006116.

Dennis C-L, Kingston D (2008) A systematic review of telephone support for women during pregnancy and the early postpartum period. *Journal of Obstetric, Gynecologic, and Neonatal Nursing*, **37**: 301–314.

Dennis C-L, Ross L (2005) Relationships among infant sleep patterns, maternal fatigue, and development of depressive symptomatology. *Birth*, **32**: 187–193.

Dennis CL, Ross LE, Herxheimer A (2008) Oestrogens and progestins for preventing and treating postpartum depression. *Cochrane Database of Systematic Reviews*, **4**: CD001690.

Ding T, Wang D-X, Qu Y, *et al* (2014) Epidural labour analgesia is associated with a decreased risk of postpartum depression: a prospective cohort study. *Anesthesia and Analgesia*, **119**: 383–392.

Dunn C, Hanich E, Roberts R (2012) Mindful pregnancy and childbirth: effects of a mindfulness-based intervention on women's psychological distress and well-being in the perinatal period. *Archives of Women's Mental Health*, **15**: 139–143.

Einarson A, Selby P, Koren G (2001) Abrupt discontinuation of psychotropic drugs during pregnancy: fear of teratogenic risk and impact of counselling. *Journal of Psychiatry and Neuroscience*, **26**: 44–48.

Engelhard IM, van den Hout MA, Amtz A (2001) Posttraumatic stress disorder after pregnancy loss. *General Hospital Psychiatry*, **23**: 62–66.

Engelhard IM, van den Hout MA, Kindt M, *et al* (2003) Peritraumatic dissociation and posttraumatic stress after pregnancy loss: a prospective study. *Behaviour Research and Therapy*, **41**: 67–78.

Engineer N, Darwin L, Nishigandh D, *et al* (2013) Association of glucocortoid and type 1 corticotrophin-releasing hormone receptors gene variants and risk for depression during pregnancy and post-partum. *Journal of Psychiatric Research*, **47**: 1166–1173.

Epperson CN, Terman M, Terman JS, *et al* (2004) Randomized trial of bright light therapy for antepartum depression: preliminary findings. *Journal of Clinical Psychiatry*, **65**: 421–425.

Farber EW, Herbert SE, Reviere SL (1996) Childhood sexual abuse and suicidality in obstetrics patients in a hospital-based urban prenatal clinic. *General Hospital Psychiatry*, **18**: 56–60.

Feggetter G, Cooper P, Gath D (1981) Non-psychotic psychiatric disorders in women one year after childbirth. *Journal of Psychosomatic Research*, **25**: 369–372.

Felice E, Saliba J, Grech V, *et al* (2004) Prevalence rates and psychosocial characteristics associated with depression in pregnancy and postpartum in Maltese women. *Journal of Affective Disorders*, **82**: 297–301.

Fergusson DM, Horwood, LJ, Ridder EM (2006) Abortion in young women and subsequent mental health. *Journal of Child Psychology and Psychiatry*, **47**: 16–24.

Field T, Sandberg D, Quetel TA, *et al* (1985) Effects of ultrasound feedback on pregnancy anxiety, fetal activity and neonatal outcome. *Obstetrics & Gynaecology*, **66**: 525–528.

Fisher J, Cabral de Mello M, Patel V, *et al* (2012) Prevalence and determinants of common perinatal mental disorders in women in low- and lower-middle-income countries: a systematic review. *Bulletin of the World Health Organization*, **90**: 139–149.

Fontein-Kuipers YJ, Nieuwenhuijze MJ, Ausems M, *et al* (2014) Antenatal interventions to reduce maternal distress: a systematic review and meta-analysis of randomised trials. *BJOG*, **121**: 389–397.

Forster DA, Denning A, Wills G, *et al* (2006) Herbal medicine use during pregnancy in a group of Australian women. *BMC Pregnancy & Childbirth*, **6**: 21.

Forty L, Jones L, Macgregor S, *et al* (2006) Familiality of postpartum depression in unipolar disorder: results from a family study. *American Journal of Psychiatry*, **163**: 1549–1553.

Fowles, ER (1998) The relationship between maternal role attainment and postpartum depression. *Health Care for Women International*, **19**: 83–94.

Frost M, Condon JT (1996) The psychological sequelae of miscarriage: a critical review of the literature. *Australian and New Zealand Journal of Psychiatry*, **30**: 54–62.

Furuta M, Sandall J, Bick, D (2012) A systematic review of the relationship between severe maternal morbidity and post-traumatic stress disorder. *BMC Pregnancy & Childbirth*, **12**: 125.

Garfield P, Kent A, Paykel ES, *et al* (2004) Outcome of postpartum disorders: a 10 year follow-up of hospital admissions. *Acta Psychiatrica Scandinavica*, **109**: 434–439.

Gavin NI, Gaynes BN, Lohr KN, *et al* (2005) Perinatal depression: a systematic review of prevalence and incidence. *Obstetrics & Gynecology*, **106**: 1071–1083.

Geller PA, Klier CM, Neugebauer R (2001) Anxiety disorders following miscarriage. *Journal of Clinical Psychiatry*, **62**: 432–438.

Gentile S (2005) The role of estrogen therapy in postpartum psychiatric disorders. *CNS Spectrums*, **10**: 944–952.

George A, Thilly N, Rydberg J, *et al* (2013) Effectiveness of eye movement desensitization and reprocessing treatment in post-traumatic stress disorder after childbirth: a randomized controlled trial protocol. *Acta Obstetricia et Gynecologica*, **92**: 866–868.

Giannandrea SAM, Cerulli C, Anson E, *et al* (2013) Increased risk for postpartum psychiatric disorders among women with past pregnancy loss. *Journal of Women's Health*, **22**: 750–768.

Glover V, Liddle P, Taylor A, *et al* (1994) Mild hypomania (the highs) can be a feature of the first postpartum week. Association with later depression. *British Journal of Psychiatry*, **164**: 517–521.

Glynn LM, Davis EP, Sandman CA (2013) New insights into the role of perinatal HPA-axis dysregulation in postpartum depression. *Neuropeptides*, **47**: 363–370.

Gold KJ, Dalton VK, Schwenk TL, *et al* (2007) What causes pregnancy loss? Preexisting mental illness as an independent risk factor. *General Hospital Psychiatry*, **29**: 207–213.

Gold KJ, Johnson TR (2014) Mothers at risk: maternal and mental health outcomes after perinatal death. *Obstetrics & Gynecology*, **123** (Suppl 1): 6S.

Gong X, Hao J, Tao F, *et al* (2013) Pregnancy loss and anxiety and depression in subsequent pregnancies: data from the C-ABC study. *European Journal of Obstetrics & Gynecology and Reproductive Biology*, **166**: 30–36.

Goodman JH, Santangelo G (2011) Group treatment for postpartum depression: a systematic review. *Archives of Women's Mental Health*, **14**: 277–293.

Gorayeb R, Gorayeb R, Berzowski AT, *et al* (2013) Effectiveness of psychological intervention for treating symptoms of anxiety and depression among women diagnosed with fetal malformation. *International Journal of Gynecology & Obstetrics*, **121**: 123–126.

Gordon REG, Gordon KK (1959) Social factors in the prediction and treatment of emotional disorders of pregnancy. *American Journal of Obstetrics & Gynecology*, **77**: 1074–1083.

Gotlib IH, Whiffen VE, Mount JH, *et al* (1989) Prevalence rates and demographic characteristics associated with depression in pregnancy and the postpartum. *Journal of Consulting and Clinical Psychology*, **57**: 269–274.

Gregoire AJP, Kumar R, Everitt B, *et al* (1996) Transdermal oestrogen for treatment of severe postnatal depression. *Lancet*, **347**: 930–933.

Grigoriadis S, VonderPorten EH, Mamisashvili L, *et al* (2013) The impact of maternal depression during pregnancy on perinatal outcomes: a systematic review and meta-analysis. *Journal of Clinical Psychiatry*, **74**: e321–e341.

Grote NK, Bridge JA, Gavin AR, *et al* (2010) A meta-analysis of depression during pregnancy and the risk of preterm birth, low birth weight, and intrauterine growth restriction. *Archives of General Psychiatry*, **67**: 1012–1024.

Halbreich U (2005) Postpartum disorders: multiple interacting underlying mechanisms and risk factors. *Journal of Affective Disorders*, **88**: 1–7.

Halbreich U, Karkun, S (2006) Cross-cultural and social diversity of prevalence of postpartum depression and depressive symptoms. *Journal of Affective Disorders*, **91**: 97–111.

Hanley J, Long B (2006) A study of Welsh mothers' experience of postnatal depression. *Midwifery*, **22**: 147–157.

Hannah P, Cody D, Glover V, *et al* (1993) The tyramine test is not a marker for postnatal depression: early postpartum euphoria may be. *Journal of Psychosomatic Obstetrics & Gynecology*, **14**: 295–304.

Harris B, Fung H, Johns S, *et al* (1989) Transient postpartum thyroid dysfunction and postnatal depression. *Journal of Affective Disorders*, **17**: 243–249.

Harris B, Othman S, Davies JA, *et al* (1992) Association between postpartum thyroid dysfunction and thyroid antibodies and depression. *BMJ*, **305**: 152–156.

Harris B, Oretti R, Lazarus J, *et al* (2002) Randomised trial of thyroxine to prevent postnatal depression in thyroid-antibody-positive women. *British Journal of Psychiatry*, **180**: 327–330.

Hayworth J, Little BC, Bonham-Carter S, *et al* (1980) A predictive study of post-partum depression: some predisposing characteristics. *British Journal of Medical Psychology*, **53**: 161–167.

Heh S-S, Fu Y-Y (2003) Effectiveness of informational support in reducing the severity of postnatal depression in Taiwan. *Journal of Advanced Nursing*, **42**: 30–36.

Heh S-S, Huang L-H, Ho S-M, *et al* (2008) Effectiveness of an exercise support program in reducing the severity of postnatal depression in Taiwanese women. *Birth: Issues in Perinatal Care*, **35**: 60–65.

Heimstad R, Dahloe R, Laache I, *et al* (2006) Fear of childbirth and history of abuse: implications for pregnancy and delivery. *Acta Obstetricia et Gynecologica Scandinavica*, **85**: 435–440.

Henderson JJ, Evans SF, Straton JA, *et al* (2003) Impact of postnatal depression on breastfeeding duration. *Birth*, **30**: 175–180.

Hendrick V, Altshuler L, Strouse T, *et al* (2000) Postpartum and nonpostpartum depression: differences in presentation and response to pharmacologic treatment. *Depression and Anxiety*, **11**: 66–72.

Henshaw C (2003) Mood disturbance in the early puerperium: a review. *Archives of Women's Mental Health*, **6**: S33–S42.

Henshaw C, Foreman D, Cox J (2004) Postnatal blues: a risk factor for postnatal depression. *Journal of Psychosomatic Obstetrics & Gynecology*, **25**: 267–272.

Heron J, O'Connor TG, Evans J, *et al* (2004) The course of anxiety and depression through pregnancy and the postpartum in a community sample. *Journal of Affective Disorders*, **80**: 65–73.

Heron J, Craddock N, Jones I (2005) Postnatal euphoria – are 'the highs' an indicator of bipolarity? *Bipolar Disorders*, **7**: 103–110.

Hertzberg T, Leo RJ, Kim KY (1997) Recurrent obsessive–compulsive disorder associated with pregnancy and childbirth. *Psychosomatics*, **38**: 386–388.

Hiscock H, Wake M (2001) Infant sleep problems and postnatal depression: a community-based study. *Pediatrics*, **107**: 6.

Hiscock H, Wake M (2002) Randomised controlled trial of behavioural infant sleep intervention to improve infant sleep and maternal mood. *BMJ*, **324**: 1062–1065.

Hiscock H, Cook F, Bayer J, *et al* (2014) Preventing early infant sleep and crying problems and postnatal depression: a randomized trial. *Pediatrics*, **133**: e346.

Hofberg K, Brockington I (2000) Tokophobia: an unreasoning dread of childbirth. *British Journal of Psychiatry*, **176**: 83–85.

Honey KL, Bennett P, Morgan M (2002) A brief psycho-educational group intervention for postnatal depression. *British Journal of Clinical Psychology*, **41**: 405–409.

Horrigan TJ, Schroeder AV, Schaffer RM (2000) The triad of substance abuse, violence, and depression are interrelated in pregnancy. *Journal of Substance Abuse Treatment*, **18**: 55–58.

Howard LM, Kirkwood G, Latinovic, R (2007) Sudden infant death syndrome and maternal depression. *Journal of Clinical Psychiatry*, **68**: 1279–1283.

Howard LM, Oram S, Galley H, *et al* (2013) Domestic violence and perinatal mental health disorders: a systematic review and meta-analysis. *PLoS Medicine*, **10**: e1001452.

Hudak R, Wisner KL (2012) Diagnosis and treatment of postpartum obsessions and compulsions that involve infant harm. *American Journal of Psychiatry*, **169**: 360–363.

Hudson DB, Elek SM, Campbell-Grossman C (2000) Depression, self-esteem, loneliness, and social support among adolescent mothers participating in the new parents project. *Adolescence*, **35**: 445–453.

Hughes PM, Turton P, Evans CD (1999) Stillbirth as risk factor for depression and anxiety in the subsequent pregnancy: cohort study. *BMJ*, **318**: 1721–1724.

Hughes P, Turton P, Hopper E, *et al* (2001) Disorganised attachment behaviour among infants born subsequent to stillbirth. *Journal of Child Psychology and Psychiatry & Allied Disciplines*, **42**: 791–801.

Iancu I, Lepkifker E, Dannon P, *et al* (1995) Obsessive–compulsive disorder limited to pregnancy. *Psychotherapy and Psychosomatics*, **64**: 109–112.

Janssen HJ, Cusinier MC, Hoogduin KA (1996) Controlled prospective study on the mental health of women following pregnancy loss. *American Journal of Psychiatry*, **153**: 226–230.

Jennings KD, Ross S, Popper S, *et al* (1999) Thoughts of harming infants in depressed and nondepressed mothers. *Journal of Affective Disorders*, **54**: 21–28.

Jolley SN, Elmore S, Barnard KE, *et al* (2007) Dysregulation of the hypothalamic–pituitary–adrenal axis in postpartum depression. *Biological Research for Nursing*, **8**: 210–222.

Kalra H, Tandon R, Trivedi JK, *et al* (2005) Pregnancy-induced obsessive compulsive disorder: a case-report. *Annals of General Psychiatry*, **4**: 12.

Kelly RH, Russo J, Katon, W (2001) Somatic complaints among pregnant women cared for in obstetrics: normal pregnancy or depressive and anxiety symptom amplification revisited? *General Hospital Psychiatry*, **23**: 107–113.

Kersting A, Kroker K, Steinhard J, *et al* (2007) Complicated grief after traumatic loss: a 14 month follow up study. *European Archives of Psychiatry and Clinical Neuroscience*, **257**: 437–443.

Kersting A, Dolemeyer R, Steining J, *et al* (2013) Brief internet-based intervention reduces posttraumatic stress and prolonged grief in parents after the loss of a child during pregnancy: a randomized controlled trial. *Psychotherapy and Psychosomatics*, **82**: 372–381.

Kim S, Soeken TA, Cromer SJ, *et al* (2014) Oxytocin and postpartum depression: delivering on what's known and what's not. *Brain Research*, **1580**: 219–232.

Klier CM, Geller PA, Neugebauer R (2000) Minor depressive disorder in the context of miscarriage. *Journal of Affective Disorders*, **59**: 13–21.

Klier CM, Muzik M, Dervic K, *et al* (2007) The role of estrogen and progesterone in depression after birth. *Journal of Psychiatric Research*, **41**: 273–279.

Ko YL, Yang CL, Fang CL, *et al* (2013) Community-based postpartum exercise programme. *Journal of Clinical Nursing*, **22**: 2122–2131.

Korenromp MJ, Christiaens GCML, van den Bout J, *et al* (2005) Long-term psychological consequences of pregnancy termination for fetal abnormality: a cross-sectional study. *Prenatal Diagnosis*, **25**: 253–260.

Kuijpens JL, Vader HL, Drexhage HA, *et al* (2001) Thyroid peroxidase antibodies during gestation are a marker for subsequent depression postpartum. *European Journal of Endocrinology*, **145**: 579–584.

Lancaster CA, Gold KJ, Flynn HA, *et al* (2010) Risk factors for depressive symptoms during pregnancy: a systematic review. *American Journal of Obstetrics & Gynecology*, **202**: 5–14.

Lee C, Slade, P (1996) Miscarriage as a traumatic event: a review of the literature and new implications for intervention. *Journal of Psychosomatic Research*, **40**: 235–244.

Leis JA, Mendelson T, Tandon DS, *et al* (2009) A systematic review of home-based interventions to prevent and treat postpartum depression. *Archives of Women's Mental Health*, **12**: 3–13.

Lewis G, Drife J (2004) *Why Mothers Die 2002-2004. The Sixth Report of the Confidential Enquiries into Maternal Death in the United Kingdom.* RCOG Press.

Listijono DR, Mooney S, Chapman M (2014) A comparative analysis of postpartum maternal mental health in women following spontaneous or ART conception. *Journal of Psychosomatic Obstetrics & Gynecology*, **35**: 51–54.

Littleton HL, Breitkopf CR, Berenson AB (2007) Correlates of anxiety symptoms during pregnancy and association with perinatal outcomes: a meta-analysis. *American Journal of Obstetrics & Gynecology*, **196**: 424–432.

Loveland Cook CA, Flick LH, Homan SM, *et al* (2004) Posttraumatic stress disorder in pregnancy: prevalence, risk factors, and treatment. *Obstetrics & Gynecology*, **103**: 710–717.

Lucas A, Pizarro E, Granada ML, *et al* (2001) Postpartum thyroid dysfunction and postpartum depression: are they two linked disorders? *Clinical Endocrinology*, **55**: 809–814.

Ludman EJ, McBride CM, Nelson JC *et al* (2000) Stress, depressive symptoms, and smoking cessation among pregnant women. *Health Psychology*, **19**: 21–27.

Lund C, Breen A, Flisher AJ, *et al* (2010) Poverty and common mental disorders in low and middle income countries: a systematic review. *Social Science and Medicine*, **71**: 517–528.

McEwan AM, Burgess DT, Hanstock CC, *et al* (2012) Increased glutamate levels in the medial prefrontal cortex in patients with postpartum depression. *Neuropsychopharmacology*, **37**: 2428–2435.

McIvor R, Davies R, Wieck A, *et al* (1996) The growth hormone response to apomorphine at 4 days postpartum in women with a history of major depression. *Journal of Affective Disorders*, **40**: 131–136.

McMahon C, Barnett B, Kowalenko N, *et al* (2005) Psychological factors associated with persistent postnatal depression: past and current relationships, defence styles and the mediating role of insecure attachment style. *Journal of Affective Disorders*, **84**: 15–24.

Maina G, Albert U, Bogetto F, *et al* (1999) Recent life events and obsessive–compulsive disorder (OCD): the role of pregnancy/delivery. *Psychiatry Research*, **89**: 49–58.

Mandl KD, Tronick EZ, Brennan TA, *et al* (1999) Infant health care use and maternal depression. *Archives of Pediatrics and Adolescent Medicine*, **153**: 808–813.

Marc I, Toureche N, Ernst E, *et al* (2011) Mind–body interventions during pregnancy for preventing or treating women's anxiety. *Cochrane Database of Systematic Reviews*, **7**: CD007559.

Marchesi C, Ampollini P, Paraggio C, *et al* (2014) Risk factors for panic disorder in pregnancy: a cohort study. *Journal of Affective Disorder*, **156**: 134–138.

Marcus SM, Flynn HA, Blow F, *et al* (2005) A screening study of antidepressant treatment rates and mood symptoms in pregnancy. *Archives of Women's Mental Health*, **8**: 25–27.

Markhus MW, Skotheim S, Graff IE, *et al* (2013) Low omega-3 index in pregnancy is a possible biological risk factor for postpartum depression. *PLoS ONE*, **8**: e6717.

Marks M, Wieck A, Checkley SA, *et al* (1992) Contribution of psychological and social factors to psychotic and non-psychotic relapse after childbirth in women with previous histories of affective disorder. *Journal of Affective Disorder*, **29**: 253–264.

Martín-Santos R, Gelabert E, Subirá S, *et al* (2012) Is neuroticism a risk factor for postpartum depression? *Psychological Medicine*, **42**: 1559–1565.

Mauthner NS (1998) 'It's a woman's cry for help': a relational perspective on postnatal depression. *Feminism and Psychology*, **8**: 325–355.

Mercier JR, Garrett J, Thorp J, *et al* (2013) Pregnancy intention and postpartum depression: secondary data analysis from a prospective cohort. *BJOG*, **120**: 1116–1122.

Mezey G, Bacchus L, Bewley S, *et al* (2005) Domestic violence, lifetime trauma and psychological health of childbearing women. *BJOG*, **112**: 197–204.

Milgrom J, Martin PR, Negri LM (1999) *Treating Postnatal Depression: A Psychological Approach for Health Care Practitioners*. Wiley.

Miniati M, Callari A, Calugi S, *et al* (2014) Interpersonal psychotherapy for postpartum depression: a systematic review. *Archives of Women's Mental Health*, **17**: 257–268.

Misri S, Milis L (2004) Obsessive–compulsive disorder in the postpartum: open-label trial of quetiapine augmentation. *Journal of Clinical Psychopharmacology*, **24**: 624–627.

Misri S, Reebye P, Corral M, *et al* (2004) The use of paroxetine and cognitive–behavioral therapy in postpartum depression and anxiety: a randomized controlled trial. *Journal of Clinical Psychiatry*, **65**: 1236–1241.

Molyneaux E, Howard LM, McGeown HR, *et al* (2014) Antidepressant treatment for postnatal depression. *Cochrane Database of Systematic Reviews*, **9**: CD002018.

Morrell J, Slade P, Warner R, *et al* (2009) Clinical effectiveness of health visitor training in psychologically informed approaches for depression in postnatal women: pragmatic cluster randomised trial in primary care. *BMJ*, **338**: a3045.

Morse C, Durkin S, Buist A, *et al* (2004) Improving the postnatal outcomes of new mothers. *Journal of Advanced Nursing*, **45**: 465–474.

Moses-Kolko E, Price JC, Wisner KL, *et al* (2012) Postpartum and depression status are associated with lower [11C] raclopride BPND in reproductive age women. *Neuropsychopharmacology*, **37**: 1422–1432.

Murphy-Ebernez K, Zandi PP, March D, *et al* (2006) Is perinatal depression familial? *Journal of Affective Disorders*, **90**: 49–55.

Murray L, Stanley C, Hooper R, *et al* (1996) The role of infant factors in postnatal depression and mother–infant interactions. *Developmental Medicine and Child Neurology*, **38**: 109–119.

Nascimento SL, Surita FG, Cecatti JG (2012) Physical exercise during pregnancy: a systematic review. *Current Opinion in Obstetrics and Gynecology*, **24**: 387–394.

Nasta MT, Grussu P, Quatraro RM, *et al* (2002) Cholesterol and mood states at 3 days after delivery. *Journal of Psychosomatic Research*, **52**: 61–63.

Nayak MB, Al-Yattama M (1999) Assault victim history as a factor in depression during pregnancy. *Obstetrics & Gynecology*, **94**: 204–208.

Neugebauer R, Kline J, O'Connor P, *et al* (1992*a*) Depressive symptoms in women in the six months after miscarriage. *American Journal of Obstetrics & Gynecology*, **166**: 104–109.

Neugebauer R, Kline J, O'Connor P, *et al* (1992*b*) Determinants of depressive symptoms in the early weeks after miscarriage. *American Journal of Public Health*, **82**: 1332–1339.

Neugebauer R, Kline J, Shrout P, *et al* (1997) Major depressive disorder in the 6 months after miscarriage. *JAMA*, **277**: 383–388.

Neugebauer R, Kline J, Bleiberg K, *et al* (2007) Preliminary open trial of interpersonal counseling for subsyndromal depression following miscarriage. *Depression and Anxiety*, **24**: 219–222.

Newport DJ, Owens MJ, Knight DL, *et al* (2004) Alterations in platelet serotonin transporter binding in women with postpartum onset major depression. *Journal of Psychosomatic Research*, **38**: 467–473.

Newport DJ, Ji S, Long Q, *et al* (2010) Maternal depression and anxiety differentially impact fetal exposures during pregnancy. *Journal of Clinical Psychiatry*, **73**: 247–251.

Nicolson P (1998) *Post-Natal Depression: Psychology, Science and the Transition to Motherhood*. Routledge.

Nielsen NO, Strøm M, Boyd HA, *et al* (2013) Vitamin D status in pregnancy and the risk of subsequent postpartum depression: a case-control study. *PLoS ONE*, **8**: e80686.

Nierop A, Bratiskas A, Zimmerman R, *et al* (2006) Are stress induced cortisol changes during pregnancy associated with postpartum depressive symptoms? *Psychosomatic Medicine*, **68**: 931–937.

Nonacs RM, Soares CN, Viguera AC, *et al* (2005) Bupropion SR for the treatment of postpartum depression: a pilot study. *International Journal of Psychopharmacology*, **8**: 445–449.

Nunes AP, Phipps MG (2013) Postpartum depression in adolescent and adult mothers: comparing prenatal risk factors and predictive models. *Maternal and Child Health*, **17**: 1071–1079.

Oates M, Cantwell R (on behalf of the Centre for Maternal and Child Enquiries) (2011) Saving Mothers' Lives: reviewing maternal deaths to make motherhood safer: 2006–2008. *BJOG*, **118** (Suppl 1): 134–144.

O'Connor TG, Heron J, Glover V, *et al* (2002) Antenatal anxiety predicts child behavioral/emotional problems independently of postnatal depression. *Journal of the American Academy of Child & Adolescent Psychiatry*, **41**: 1470–1477.

Office for National Statistics (2013) *Births in England and Wales: 2013*. ONS (http://www.ons.gov.uk/ons/rel/vsob1/birth-summary-tables--england-and-wales/2013/index.html).

O'Hara M, Rehm LP, Campbell S (1982) Predicting depressive symptomatology cognitive–behavioral models and postpartum depression. *Journal of Abnormal Psychology*, **91**: 457–461.

O'Hara MW, Swain AM (1996) Rates and risks of postpartum depression: a meta analysis. *International Review of Psychiatry*, **8**: 37–54.

Okun ML, Prather AA, Perel JM, *et al* (2011) Changes in sleep quality, but not hormones predict time to postpartum depression recurrence. *Journal of Affective Disorders*, **130**: 378–384.

O'Mahen HA, Woodford J, McGinley J, *et al* (2013) Internet-based behavioral activation – treatment for postnatal depression (Netmums): a randomized controlled trial. *Journal of Affective Disorders*, **150**: 814–822.

Onozawa K, Glover V, Adams D, *et al* (2001) Infant massage improves mother–infant interaction for mothers with postnatal depression. *Journal of Affective Disorders*, **63**: 201–207.

Oren DA, Wisner KL, Spinelli M, *et al* (2002) An open trial of morning light therapy for treatment of antepartum depression. *American Journal of Psychiatry*, **159**: 666–669.

Oretti RG, Harris B, Lazarus IH, *et al* (2003) Is there an association between life events, postnatal depression and thyroid dysfunction in thyroid antibody positive women? *International Journal of Social Psychiatry*, **49**: 70–76.

Osborne, LM, Monk C (2013) Perinatal depression: the fourth inflammatory morbidity of pregnancy? Theory and literature review. *Psychoneuroendocrinology*, **38**: 1929–1952.

Otto SJ, de Groot RH, Hornstra G (2003) Increased risk of postpartum depressive symptoms is associated with slower normalization after pregnancy of the functional docosahexaenoic acid status. *Prostaglandins, Leukotrienes, and Essential Fatty Acids*, **69**: 237–243.

Pajulo M, Savonlahti E, Sourander A, *et al* (2001) Antenatal depression, substance dependency and social support. *Journal of Affective Disorders*, **65**: 9–17.

Park EM, Meltzer-Brody S, Stickgold R (2013) Poor sleep maintenance and subjective sleep quality are associated with postpartum maternal depression symptom severity. *Archives of Women's Mental Health*, **16**: 539–547.

Parry BL, Curran ML, Stuenkel CA, *et al* (2000) Can critically timed sleep deprivation be useful in pregnancy and postpartum depressions? *Journal of Affective Disorders*, **60**: 201–212.

Paykel E, Emms E, Fletcher J, *et al* (1980) Life events and social support in puerperal depression. *British Journal of Psychiatry*, **136**: 339–346.

Pearlstein TB, Zlotnick C, Battle CL, *et al* (2006) Patient choice of treatment for postpartum depression. *Archives of Women's Mental Health*, **9**: 303–308.

Pedersen CA, Johnson JL, Silva S, *et al* (2007) Antenatal thyroid correlates of postpartum depression. *Psychoneuroendocrinology*, **32**: 235–245.

Peindl KS, Wisner KL, Zolnik EJ, *et al* (1995) Effects of postpartum psychiatric illness on family planning. *International Journal of Psychiatry in Medicine*, **25**: 291–300.

Petrou S, Cooper P, Murray L, *et al* (2002) Economic costs of post-natal depression in a high-risk British cohort. *British Journal of Psychiatry*, **181**: 505–512.

Pinsonneault JK, Sullivan D, Sadee W, *et al* (2013) Association study of the estrogen receptor gene ESR1 with postpartum depression. *Archives of Women's Mental Health*, **16**: 499–509.

Pitt B (1968) 'Atypical' depression following childbirth. *British Journal of Psychiatry*, **114**: 1325–1335.

Ploeckinger B, Dantendorfer K, Ulm M, *et al* (1996) Rapid decrease of serum cholesterol concentration and postpartum depression. *BMJ*, **313**: 664.

Pop VJ, de Rooy HA, Vader HL (1991) Postpartum thyroid dysfunction and depression in an unselected population. *New England Journal of Medicine*, **324**: 1815–1816.

Pritchard CW (1994) Depression and smoking in pregnancy in Scotland. *Journal of Epidemiology and Community Health*,**48**: 377–382.

Pugh NE, Hadjiustavropoulos HD, Fuchs CM (2014) Internet therapy for postpartum depression: a case illustration of e-mailed therapeutic assistance. *Archives of Women's Mental Health*, **17**: 327–337.

Radesky JS, Zuckerman B, Silverstein M, *et al*, (2013) Inconsolable infant crying and maternal postnatal depressive symptoms. *Pediatrics*, **131**: e1857–e1864.

Rahman A, Creed F (2007) Outcome of prenatal depression and risk factors associated with persistence in the first postnatal year: prospective study from Rawalpindi, Pakistan. *Journal of Affective Disorders*, **100**: 115–121.

Rahman A, Fisher J, Bower P, *et al* (2013) Interventions for common mental disorders in women in low-and middle-income countries: a systematic review and meta-analysis. *Bulletin of the World Health Organization*, **91**: 593–601.

Räisänen S, Lehto SM, Nielsen HS, *et al* (2013) Fear of childbirth predicts postpartum depression: a population-based analysis of 511 422 singleton births in Finland. *BMJ Open*, **3**: e004047.

Reardon DC, Cougle JR, Rue VM, *et al* (2003) Psychiatric admission of low-income women following abortion and childbirth. *Canadian Medical Association Journal*, **168**: 1253–1256.

Reay R, Fisher Y, Robertson M, *et al* (2006) Group interpersonal psychotherapy for postnatal depression: a pilot study. *Archives of Women's Mental Health*, **9**: 31–39.

Reay RE, Mulcahy R, Wilkinson RB, *et al* (2012) The development and content of an interpersonal psychotherapy group for postnatal depression. *International Journal of Group Psychotherapy*, **62**: 221–251.

Reck C, Stehle E, Reinig K, *et al* (2009) Maternity blues as a predictor of DSM-IV depression and anxiety disorders in the first three months postpartum. *Journal of Affective Disorders*, **113**; **77–87**.

Rich-Edwards JW, Mohllajee AP, Kleinman K, *et al* (2008) Elevated midpregnancy corticotropin-releasing hormone is associated with prenatal but not postpartum depression. *Journal of Clinical Endocrinology and Metabolism*, **93**: 1496–1951.

Roberts J, Sword W, Watt S, *et al* (2001) Costs of postpartum care: examining associations from the Ontario mother and infant survey. *Canadian Journal of Nursing Research*, **33**: 19–34.

Robertson E, Grace S, Wallington T, *et al* (2004) Antenatal risk factors for postpartum depression: a synthesis of recent literature. *General Hospital Psychiatry*, **26**: 289–295.

Robinson M, Whitehouse JO, Newnham JP, *et al* (2014) Low maternal serum vitamin D during pregnancy and the risk for postpartum depression symptoms. *Archives of Women's Mental Health*, **17**: 213–219.

Robinson R, Young J (1982) Screening for depression and anxiety in the postnatal period: acceptance or rejection of a subsequent treatment offer. *Australian and New Zealand Journal of Psychiatry*, **16**: 47–51.

Ross LE, Dennis C-L (2009) The prevalence of postpartum depression among women with substance use, an abuse history, or chronic illness: a systematic review. *Journal of Women's Health*, **18**: 475–486.

Ross LE, McLean LM (2006) Anxiety disorders during pregnancy and the postpartum period: a systematic review. *Journal of Clinical Psychiatry*, **67**: 1285–1298.

Ross LE, Sellers EM, Gilbert Evans SE, *et al* (2004) Mood changes during pregnancy and the postpartum period: development of a biopsychosocial model. *Acta Psychiatrica Scandinavica*, **109**: 457–466.

Ross LE, Murray BJ, Steiner M (2005) Sleep and perinatal mood disorders: a critical review. *Journal of Psychiatry and Neuroscience*, **30**: 247–256.

Ross LE, Campbell VL, Dennis C-L, *et al* (2006) Demographic characteristics of participants in studies of risk factors, prevention and treatment of postpartum depression. *Canadian Journal of Psychiatry*, **51**: 704–710.

Ross LE, McQueen K, Vigod S, *et al* (2011) Risk for postpartum depression associated with assisted reproductive technologies and multiple births: a systematic review. *Human Reproduction Update*, **17**: 96–106.

Rubertsson C, Waldenström U, Wickberg, B (2003) Depressive mood in early pregnancy: prevalence and women at risk in a national Swedish sample. *Journal of Reproductive and Infant Psychology*, **21**: 113–123.

Russell EJ, Fawcett JM, Mazmanian D (2013) Risk of obsessive–compulsive disorder in pregnant and postpartum women: a meta-analysis. *Journal of Clinical Psychiatry*, **74**: 377–385.

Ryding EL, Wijma B, Wijma K (1997) Posttraumatic stress reactions after emergency cesarean section. *Acta Obstetricia et Gynecologica Scandinavica*, **76**: 856–861.

Ryding EL, Wijma K, Wijma B (1998) Psychological impact of emergency Cesarean section, instrumental and normal vaginal delivery. *Journal of Psychosomatic Obstetrics & Gynecology*, **19**: 135–144.

Ryding EL, Persson A, Onell C, *et al* (2003) An evaluation of midwives' counseling of pregnant women in fear of childbirth. *Acta Obstetricia et Gynecologica Scandinavica*, **82**: 10–17.

Saisto T, Salmela Aro K, Nurmi J-E, *et al* (2001) A randomized controlled trial of intervention in fear of childbirth. *Obstetrics & Gynecology*, **98**: 820–826.

Saisto T, Toivanen R, Samela-Arp K, *et al* (2006) Therapeutic group psychoeducation and relaxation in treating fear of childbirth. *Acta Obstetricia et Gynecologica Scandinavica*, **85**: 1315–1319.

Sawyer A, Ayers S, Smith H (2010) Pre- and postnatal psychological wellbeing in Africa: a systematic review. *Journal of Affective Disorders*, **123**: 17–29.

Schnyer RN, Manber R, Fitzcharles AJ (2003) Acupuncture treatment for depression during pregnancy: conceptual framework and two case reports. *Complementary Health Practice Review*, **8**: 40–53.

Scope A, Booth A, Sutcliffe P (2012) Women's perceptions and experiences of group cognitive behaviour therapy and other group interventions for postnatal depression: a qualitative synthesis. *Journal of Advanced Nursing*, **68**: 1909–1919.

Scope A, Leaviss J, Kalthenthaler E, *et al* (2013) Is group cognitive behaviour therapy for postnatal depression evidence-based practice? A systematic review. *BMC Psychiatry*, **13**: 321.

Seel RM (1986) Birth Rite. *Health Visitor*, **59**: 182–184.

Segre LS, O'Hara MW, Arndt S., *et al* (2007) The prevalence of postpartum depression: the relative significance of three social indices. *Social Psychiatry and Psychiatric Epidemiology*, **42**: 316–321.

Shakespeare J, Blake F, Garcia J (2006) How do women with postnatal depression experience listening visits in primary care? A qualitative interview study. *Journal of Reproductive and Infant Psychology*, **24**: 149–162.

Shapiro GD, Fraser WD, Séguin JR (2012) Emerging risk factors for postpartum depression: serotonin transporter genotype and omega-3 fatty acid status. *Canadian Journal of Psychiatry*, **57**: 704–712.

Sharma V (2006) A cautionary note on the use of antidepressants in postpartum depression. *Bipolar Disorders*, **8**: 411–414.

Sharma V, Sommerdyk C (2013) Are antidepressants effective in the treatment of postpartum depression? A systematic review. *Primary Care Companion for CNS Disorders*, **15**: e1–e7.

Sharma V, Sommerdyk C, Sharma S (2013) Post-abortion mania. *Archives of Women's Mental Health*, **16**: 167–169.

Sholomskas DE, Wickamaratne PJ, Dogolo L, *et al* (1993) Postpartum onset of panic disorder: a coincidental event? *Journal of Clinical Psychiatry*, **54**: 476–480.

Sichel DA, Cohen LS, Dimmock JA, *et al* (1993) Postpartum obsessive compulsive disorder: a case series. *Journal of Clinical Psychiatry*, **54**: 156–159.

Sjögren B, Thomasson P (1997) Obstetric outcome in 100 women with severe anxiety over childbirth. *Acta Obstetricia et Gynecologica Scandinavica*, **76**: 948–952.

Skari H, Skreden M, Malt UF, *et al* (2002) Comparative levels of psychological distress, stress symptoms, depression and anxiety after childbirth – a prospective population-based study of mothers and fathers. *BJOG*, **109**: 1154–1163.

Slade P, Morrell CJ, Rigby A, *et al* (2010) Postnatal women's experiences of management of depressive symptoms: a qualitative study. *British Journal of General Practice*, **60**: e440–e448.

Sockol LE, Epperson CN, Barber J (2011) A meta-analysis of treatments for perinatal depression. *Clinical Psychology Review*, **31**: 839–849.

Söderquist J, Wijma B, Wijma K (2006) The longitudinal course of post-traumatic stress after childbirth. *Journal of Psychosomatic Obstetrics & Gynecology*, **27**: 113–119.

Söderquist J, Wijma B, Thorbert G (2009) Risk factors in pregnancy for post-traumatic stress and depression after childbirth. *BJOG*, **116**: 672–680.

Speisman BB, Storch EA, Abramowitz JS (2011) Postpartum obsessive–compulsive disorder. *Journal of Obstetric, Gynecological and Neonatal Nursing*, **40**: 680–690.

Spinelli MG, Endicott J (2003) Controlled clinical trial of interpersonal psychotherapy versus parenting education program for depressed pregnant women. *American Journal of Psychiatry*, **160**: 555–562.

Spinelli MG, Endicott J, Leon AC, *et al* (2013) A controlled clinical treatment trial of interpersonal psychotherapy for depressed pregnant women at 3 New York City sites. *Journal of Clinical Psychiatry*, **74**: 393–399.

Stevenson MA, Scope A, Slade P, *et al* (2010) Group cognitive behavioural therapy for postnatal depression: a systematic review of clinical effectiveness, cost-effectiveness and value of information analyses. *Health Technology Assessment*, **14**: 1–107.

Storksen HT, Eberhard-Gran M, Garthus-Niegel S, *et al* (2012) Fear of childbirth: the relation to anxiety and depression. *Acta Obstetricia et Gynecologica Scandinavica*, **91**: 237–242.

Stowe ZN, Casarella J, Landry J, *et al* (1995) Sertraline in the treatment of women with postpartum major depression. *Depression*, **3**: 49–55.

Stuart S, Couser G, Schilder K, *et al* (1998) Postpartum anxiety and depression: onset and comorbidity in a community sample. *Journal of Nervous and Mental Disease*, **186**: 420–424.

Summers AL, Logsdon MC (2005) Web sites for postpartum depression: convenient, frustrating, incomplete, and misleading. *American Journal of Maternal Child Nursing*, **30**: 88–94.

Sun HS, Tsai H-W, Ko H-C, *et al* (2004) Association of tryptophan hydroxylase polymorphisms with depression, anxiety and comorbid depression and anxiety in a population-based sample of postpartum Taiwanese women. *Genes, Brain and Behavior*, **3**: 328–336.

Suri R, Burt VK, Altshuler LL (2005) Nefazodone for the treatment of postpartum depression. *Archives of Women's Mental Health*, **8**: 55–56.

Sutter-Dallay AL, Giaconne-Marchese V, Glatigny-Dallay E, *et al* (2004) Women with anxiety disorders during pregnancy are at increased risk of intense postnatal depressive symptoms: a prospective survey of the MATQUID cohort. *European Psychiatry*, **19**: 459–463.

Sved-Williams AE (1992) Phobic reactions of mothers to their own babies. *Australian and New Zealand Journal of Psychiatry*, **26**: 631–638.

Sword W, Kurtz Landy C, Thabane L, *et al* (2011) Is mode of delivery associated with postpartum depression at 6 weeks: a prospective cohort. *BJOG*, **118**: 966–977.

Sydsjö G, Sydsjö A, Gunnervik C, *et al* (2012) Obstetric outcome for women who received individualised treatment for fear of childbirth during pregnancy. *Acta Obstetricia et Gynecologica Scandinavica*, **91**: 44–49.

Sylvén SM, Ekselius L, Sundström-Poromaa I, *et al* (2012) Premenstrual syndrome and dysphoric disorder as risk factors for postpartum depression. *Acta Obstetricia et Gynecologica Scandinavica*, **92**: 178–184.

Tezel A, Gozum S (2006) Comparison of effects of nursing care to problem solving training on levels of depressive symptoms in post partum women. *Patient Education and Counseling*, **63**: 64–73.

Thapar AK, Thapar A (1992) Psychological sequelae of miscarriage: a controlled study using the general health questionnaire and the hospital anxiety and depression scale. *British Journal of General Practice*, **42**: 94–96.

Thompson MS, Peebles-Wilkins W (1992) The impact of formal, informal and societal support networks on the psychological well-being of black adolescent mothers. *Social Work*, **37**: 322–328.

Treloar SA, Martin NG, Bucholz KK, *et al* (1999) Genetic influences on post-natal depressive symptoms: findings from an Australian twin sample. *Psychological Medicine*, **29**: 645–654.

Troisi A, Moles A, Panepuccia L, *et al* (2002) Serum cholesterol levels and mood symptoms in the postpartum period. *Psychiatry Research*, **109**: 213–219.

Turner KM, Sharp D, Folkes L, *et al* (2008) Women's views and experiences of antidepressants as a treatment for postnatal depression: a qualitative study. *Family Practice*, **25**: 450–455.

Turton P, Hughes P, Evans CD, *et al* (2001) Incidence, correlates and predictors of post-traumatic stress disorder in the pregnancy after stillbirth. *British Journal of Psychiatry*, **178**: 556–560.

Ugarriza DN, Schmidt L (2006) Telecare for women with postpartum depression. *Journal of Psychosocial Nursing and Mental Health Services*, **44**: 37–45.

Upadhyaya SK, Sharma A (2012) Onset of obsessive compulsive disorder in pregnancy with pica as the sole manifestation. *Indian Journal of Psychological Medicine*, **34**: 276–278.

Van den Bergh BRH, Mulder EJH, Mennes M, *et al* (2005) Antenatal maternal anxiety and stress and the neurobehavioural development of the fetus and child: links and possible mechanisms. A review. *Neuroscience and Biobehavioral Reviews*, **29**: 237–258.

Varma D, Chandra PS, Thomas T, *et al* (2007) Intimate partner violence and sexual coercion among pregnant women in India: Relationship with depression and post-traumatic stress disorder. *Journal of Affective Disorders*, **102**: 227–235.

Vaz JS, Kac G, Nardi AE, *et al* (2014) Omega-6 fatty acids and greater likelihood of suicide risk and major depression in early pregnancy. *Journal of Affective Disorders*, **152–154**: 76–82.

Vigod SN, Villegas L, Dennis C-L, *et al* (2010) Prevalence and risk factors for postpartum depression among women with preterm and low-birth-weight infants: a systematic review. *BJOG*, **117**: 540–550.

Villegas L, McKay K, Dennis C-L, *et al* (2011) Postpartum depression among rural women from developed and developing countries: a systematic review. *Journal of Rural Health*, **27**: 278–288.

Vliegen N, Casalin S, Lutyen P (2014) The course of postpartum depression: a review of longitudinal studies. *Harvard Review of Psychiatry*, **22**: 1–22.

De Vriese SR, Christophe AB, Maes M, *et al* (2003) Lowered serum n-3 polyunsaturated fatty acid (PUFA) levels predict the occurrence of postpartum depression: Further evidence that lowered n-PUFA are related to major depression. *Life Sciences*, **73**: 3181–3187.

Watanabe M, Wada K, Sakata Y, *et al.* (2008) Maternity blues as predictor of postpartum depression: a prospective cohort study among Japanese women. *Journal of Psychosomatic Obstetrics & Gynecology*, **29**: 206–212.

Waterstone M, Wolfe C, Hooper R, *et al* (2003) Postnatal morbidity after childbirth and severe obstetric morbidity. *BJOG*, **110**: 128–133.

Watson J, Elliott S, Rugg A, *et al* (1984) Psychiatric disorder in pregnancy and the first postnatal year. *British Journal of Psychiatry*, **144**: 453–462.

Webster J, Pritchard MA, Linnane JWJ, *et al* (2001) Postnatal depression: Use of health services and satisfaction with health-care providers. *Journal of Quality in Clinical Practice*, **21**: 144–148.

Weightman H, Dalal BM, Brockington IF (1998) Pathological fear of cot death. *Psychopathology*, **31**: 246–249.

Wenzel A, Gorman L, O'Hara M, *et al* (2001) The occurrence of panic and obsessive compulsive symptoms in women with postpartum dysphoria: a prospective study. *Archives of Women's Mental Health*, **4**: 5–12.

Wenzel A, Haugen E, Jackson LC, *et al* (2003) Prevalence of generalised anxiety at eight weeks postpartum. *Archives of Women's Mental Health*, **6**: 43–49.

Wenzel A, Haugen E, Jackson LC, *et al* (2005) Anxiety symptoms and disorders at eight weeks postpartum. *Anxiety Disorders*, **19**: 295–311.

Whitton A, Warner R, Appleby L (1996) The pathway to care in post-natal depression: women's attitudes to post-natal depression and its treatment. *British Journal of General Practice*, **46**: 427–428.

Wirz-Justice A, Bader A, Frisch U, *et al* (2011) A randomized, double-blind, placebo-controlled study of light therapy for antepartum depression. *Journal of Clinical Psychiatry*, **72**: 986–993.

Wisner KL, Peindl KS, Gigliotti TV, *et al* (1999a) Obsessions and compulsions in women with postpartum depression. *Journal of Clinical Psychiatry*, **60**: 176–180.

Wisner KL, Peindl KS, Gigliotti TV, *et al* (1999b) Tricyclics vs SSRIs for postpartum depression. *Archives of Women's Mental Health*, **1**: 189–191.

Wisner KL, Perel JM, Peindl KS, *et al* (2004) Timing of depression recurrence in the first year after birth. *Journal of Affective Disorders*, **78**: 249–252.

Wisner KL, Logsdon CL, Shanahan BR (2008) Web-based education for postpartum depression; conceptual development and impact. *Archives of Women's Mental Health*, **11**: 377–385.

Wisner KL, Sit DKY, McShea MC, *et al* (2013) Onset timing, thoughts of self-harm, and diagnoses in postpartum women with screen-positive depression findings. *JAMA Psychiatry*, **70**: 490–498.

Wong MKY, Crawford T, Gask L, *et al* (2003) A qualitative investigation into women's experiences after a miscarriage: implications for the primary healthcare team. *British Journal of General Practice*, **53**: 697–702.

Wu Q, Chen H-L, Xu X-J (2012) Violence as a risk factor for postpartum depression in mothers: a meta-analysis. *Archives of Women's Mental Health*, **15**: 107–114.

Wynter K, Rowe H, Fisher J (2013) Common mental disorders in women and men in the first six months after the birth of their first infant: A community study in Victoria, Australia. *Journal of Affective Disorders*, **151**: 980–985.

Yexley M (2007) Treating postpartum depression with hypnosis: addressing specific symptoms presented by the client. *American Journal of Clinical Hypnosis*, **49**: 219.

Yim IS, Glynn LM, Schetter CD, *et al* (2009) Risk of postpartum depressive symptoms with elevated corticotropin-releasing hormone in human pregnancy. *Archives of General Psychiatry*, **66**: 162–169.

Yonkers KA, Ramin SM, Rush AJ, *et al* (2011) Does antidepressant use attenuate the risk of a major depressive episode in pregnancy? *Epidemiology*, **22**: 848–854.

Yonkers KA, Gotman N, Smith MV, *et al* (2012) The management of depression during pregnancy: a report from the American Psychiatric Association and the American College of Obstetricians and Gynecologists. *Focus: the Journal of Lifelong Learning in Psychiatry*, **10**: 78–89.

Zambaldi CF, Cantalino A, Montenegro AC, *et al* (2009) Postpartum obsessive-compulsive disorder: prevalence and clinical characteristics. *Comprehensive Psychiatry*, **50**: 503–509.

Zolese G, Blacker CV (1992) The psychological complications of therapeutic abortion. *British Journal of Psychiatry*, **160**: 742–749.

# Further reading

Raphael-Leff J, Malberg N, Shai D, *et al* (2012) *Working with Teenage Parents: Handbook of Theory and Practice for Practitioners Working with Pregnant Teenagers and Their Children*. Anna Freud Centre.

Raphael-Leff J (1991) *Psychological Processes of Childbearing*. Chapman and Hall.

Stowe ZN, McCreary P, Hostetter A, *et al* (2001) Management of treatment-resistant depression during pregnancy and the postpartum period. In *Treatment-Resistant Mood Disorders* (eds JD Amsterdam, M Hornig, AA Nierenberg): pp. 321–349. Cambridge University Press.

Williams C, Cantwell R, Robertson K (2008) *Overcoming Postnatal Depression: A Five Areas Approach*. Hodder Arnold.

## *www.mededppd.org*

A website supported by the US National Institute of Mental Health providing information to help screen, diagnose and treat women with postnatal depression. There are sections for professionals (which include continuing professional development material), and for women with postnatal depression and their families.

# CHAPTER 3

# Puerperal psychosis

Early studies suggested that the few weeks after delivery are the time in a woman's life when she is at highest risk of a psychotic illness. Kendell *et al* (1987) demonstrated that in the 3 months following childbirth, a woman is more than 20 times more likely to be admitted with this diagnosis. However, Terp & Mortensen (1998), using women from the general population as controls, found that the relative risk (RR) of all admissions was only increased slightly (RR = 1.09) but that for a first admission with functional psychosis between days 2 and 28 after delivery the RR was 3.21. Harlow *et al* (2007) found a similar incidence of hospital admission in first-time mothers (0.01%), noting that this was largely confined to women who had previously had a psychotic or bipolar illness and that most of the postpartum episodes occurred within 4 weeks of delivery. Munk-Olsen *et al* (2006), using women who had delivered in the previous 11 to 12 months as controls, found the risk to be raised in the first 3 months; the highest risk for first-time mothers was 10–19 days postpartum (RR = 7.31). Similarly the risk of psychiatric out-patient contact for first-time mothers was increased in the first 3 months and highest 10–19 days after delivery (RR = 2.67). The prevalence for the first 3 months was 1.03 per 1000 births. Women with schizophrenia-like disorders were more likely to be admitted within the first month after delivery, and those with bipolar disorder in the first 2 months. Kendell *et al* (1976) identified a later peak of admissions from the 10th to the 24th month after delivery.

Puerperal psychoses are severe illnesses, which have their onset within 2–4 weeks of delivery and usually require admission. Affective illnesses predominate, most often fulfilling diagnostic criteria for major depression with psychotic features, mania or schizoaffective psychosis (Dean & Kendell, 1981; Meltzer & Kumar, 1985; Pfuhlmann *et al*, 1998). A proportion can only be classified as 'unspecified functional psychosis', and around half meet Leonhard's criteria for cycloid psychosis (Pfuhlmann *et al*, 1998).

Organic psychoses occurring in relation to childbirth have been recognised and documented since the time of Hippocrates and include idiopathic confusional states, stupor, post-eclamptic psychosis, infective delirium, and delirium associated with anaemia and alcohol withdrawal (Brockington, 1996).

There are reports of subdural haematoma (Campbell & Varma, 1993), meningioma (Khong *et al*, 2007; Schwartz *et al*, 2013), acute encephalitis (Shaaban *et al*, 2012) and atypical posterior reversible encephalopathy syndrome (Kitabayashi *et al*, 2007) presenting with psychotic symptoms postpartum. Dhasmana *et al* (2010) describe a postpartum woman who presented with a mixed presentation of euphoria and aggressive behaviour, declaring that her baby possessed special powers and that she wished to harm her baby and herself. She later became mute and withdrawn, lacking insight. Platelets, fibrinogen and C-reactive protein were raised. A magnetic resonance imaging (MRI) brain scan revealed a transverse sinus thrombosis. A woman with memory problems, sensations of *déja vu* and mild headaches who became increasingly anxious with delusions that her baby was dying was admitted to a psychiatric unit with a diagnosis of puerperal psychosis. She was treated with olanzapine and electroconvulsive therapy (ECT) but after 3 days developed tonic–clonic seizures and was later diagnosed as having paraneoplastic encephalitis (Yu & Moore, 2011). Another woman with more marked confusion and who was less delusional than is usually seen in puerperal psychosis was subsequently found to have a late-onset urea cycle disorder (Fassier *et al*, 2011).

Organic psychoses, particularly infective psychoses, may be a common cause of puerperal psychosis in some low-income countries, or they may be a comorbidity (Ndosi & Mtawali, 2002). Forty-four per cent of mothers in a Tanzanian sample of mothers with puerperal psychosis had an infection, such as malaria, HIV, tuberculosis or infectious diarrhoea. Clinicians should therefore bear in mind that there might be an alternative diagnosis when assessing a woman with psychotic symptoms postpartum.

## Phenomena

The early signs of illness are often non-specific, e.g. insomnia, agitation, perplexity and odd behaviour. Such symptoms can easily be overlooked or attributed to postpartum blues and their significance not recognised. However, the patient may be floridly psychotic within a few hours, as the onset is frequently very rapid and often occurs only a few days after delivery. Such symptoms occurring in a woman with a history of puerperal psychosis or bipolar disorder should be taken seriously as possibly indicating the onset of a recurrence.

When the symptoms of 58 patients with puerperal psychosis and 52 women with non-puerperal psychotic illnesses (including schizophrenia) were compared, the puerperal group were found to be less likely to have persecutory or systematised delusions, auditory hallucinations, odd affect and social withdrawal than the non-puerperal controls. However, they were more likely to have manic features such as elation, lability of mood, rambling speech and distractibility, as well as having more confusion and an increased need to be supervised during tasks (Brockington et al, 1981). Conversely, in a South African study comparing 20 puerperal women with psychosis and 20 age-matched controls with mania (Oosthuizen et al, 1995), the puerperal group had more delusions of control, auditory hallucinations, blunted affect and emotional turmoil. However, these findings were limited by the following considerations: many women with puerperal psychosis have a depressive illness, but these individuals were excluded from the study; the patients were not randomly selected; and one-third of the puerperal group had a history of treatment for schizophrenia. Others have reported more anxiety and depressive symptoms, and increased lability of mood and disorientation in puerperal mania compared with non-puerperal mania (Ganjekar et al, 2013). Four cases meeting the criteria for delusional misidentification, as in the Fregoli syndrome, have been described (O'Sullivan & Dean, 1991).

Apparent cognitive deficits are not unusual. An American study compared 21 women who had childbearing-related affective psychoses with 96 women whose psychosis was not related to delivery. They found that the recently delivered group had 'more prominent symptoms relating to cognitive impairment and bizarre behaviour' and more homicidal ideas than the control group (Wisner et al, 1994).

Mood-incongruent delusions are not infrequent, e.g. delusions of reference or persecution – for example, the woman may believe that the nurses are trying to hurt her (Viguera et al, 2008). There may also be visual, tactile or olfactory hallucinations which again suggest an organic syndrome. Catatonic symptoms such as waxy flexibility, stupor, mutism, immobility and negativism have been reported in the literature (Hanson & Brown, 1973; Lai & Huang, 2004) and observed in clinical practice, but their true prevalence in the postpartum population is not known. One reported case of a postpartum woman with catatonic stupor was found to have an encephalopathy (Kitabayashi et al, 2007).

# Epidemiology

The past few decades have seen a fall in mortality and morbidity from childbirth; however, this has not been paralleled by a fall in the incidence of puerperal psychosis, which has remained remarkably stable at 1–2 per 1000 deliveries (Meltzer & Kumar, 1985; Terp & Mortensen, 1998; Munk-Olsen et al, 2006; Harlow et al, 2007). However, if a woman has had a past episode, the risk rises to 1 in 7 (Kendell et al, 1987).

Risk factors for admission in the puerperium include being primiparous, being single, and having had a Caesarean section (Kendell et al, 1976, 1981, 1987; Meltzer & Kumar, 1985). This last study found an association with a history of perinatal death not found in the others. Paffenbarger (1964) also identified being older, having longer intervals between pregnancies, and having had fertility problems as being risk factors. A large study of first-time mothers in Sweden ($n = 502\,767$), identified older age and being single as risk factors (Nager *et al*, 2005). Analyses on the same data-set found that those living in the poorest neighbourhoods had a significantly higher risk of admission (Nager *et al*, 2006). In a within-subject comparative study of 129 women with bipolar affective puerperal psychosis, Blackmore *et al* (2006) identified primiparity (odds ratio (OR) = 3.76) and delivery complications (OR = 2.68) as independent risk factors. More recent work has confirmed the association between primiparity and admissions for psychosis/mania (Bergink *et al*, 2011; Di Florio *et al*, 2014) and onset of recurrent major depression within 6 weeks of delivery (Di Florio *et al*, 2014).

There are differences in the sleep patterns of women in late pregnancy and the postpartum period that are more marked in first-time mothers. Women with puerperal psychosis may have had a longer labour and be more likely to have delivered at night than controls (Sharma *et al*, 2004), and sleep loss has been suggested as a final common pathway for various causal factors in the development of psychosis in vulnerable women (Sharma & Mazmanian, 2003).

In low- and middle-income countries (LMIC), there is high comorbidity with physical health problems, including anaemia, infection and edema proteinuria hypertension gestosis (Agrawal *et al*, 1990; Ndosi & Mtawali, 2002). However, some authors have noted the close match between the incidence, pattern of illness and associated findings in a Black African population and those described in the literature in populations in the Western world (Allwood *et al*, 2000). A recent study in the USA reported that women admitted to hospital with puerperal psychosis had 2.3 times higher odds of having complications such as infection, anaemia and venous or lactation problems, and that their infants had a 4.1 times higher odds of death within the first year of life (Hellerstedt *et al*, 2013).

## Onset, course and prognosis

Paffenbarger (1964) reported that there was usually a 'lucid interval' after delivery, before the development of symptoms. One-third of his sample developed symptoms within the first week, 68% within the first month and 80% within 6 weeks. In a study of women admitted to hospital in Japan, half had an onset of illness in the first week postpartum and 56% in the second week; 80% became ill within the first month (Okano *et al*, 1998). However, a more recent study refutes the notion of a latent period, with 50% of bipolar women with a puerperal psychotic illness first experiencing symptoms on days 1–3, with 22% of onsets on day 1 (Heron *et al*, 2007). Early symptoms include feeling excited, elated or high, not sleeping, feeling energetic or active, and talking more (Heron *et al*, 2008). Others have reported a median onset at 8 days postpartum but with prodromal symptoms present earlier (Bergink *et al*, 2011).

There is often a time lag between onset of illness and admission. Several studies indicate that women with manic episodes are admitted more quickly than those with depressive psychoses (Dean & Kendell, 1981; Meltzer & Kumar, 1985; Okano *et al*, 1998), and that psychotic depressions onset earlier than non-psychotic illnesses (Meltzer & Kumar, 1985).

The course of illness can fluctuate and may involve very severe disturbance, but the prognosis for the acute episode is good, with most women making a good recovery (92.2% reported by Bergink *et al*, 2011) and returning to premorbid functioning. In the longer term, however, there is a risk of further episodes, both after subsequent pregnancies and at other times.

Brockington *et al* (1982) summed the findings of six studies published between 1956 and 1972 and estimated the combined risk of recurrence to be about one in five for each subsequent pregnancy. Others estimate it at 25–50%. For example, Pfuhlmann *et al* (2000) followed up women 6–26 years after a first-episode puerperal psychosis and observed a 47% recurrence rate after later deliveries. Puerperal recurrence after subsequent pregnancies in a 10-year follow-up was 75–80% for women whose index illness was a psychosis and 27.3% for those in whom it was depression (Garfield *et al*, 2004). The risk of non-puerperal episodes appears to be higher.

Da Silva & Johnstone (1981) found 50% of a sample of women admitted to hospital remaining well after 1–6 years' follow-up. Of the remainder, 2 had died by suicide, 3 were long-term in-patients, 14 were in out-patient care, 1 was on lithium but well, and 3 were unwell but not in treatment. They noted a poorer outcome in women with an index schizophrenic illness. Dean *et al* (1989) observed a 36% recurrence rate if the index episode was puerperal but 50% if it was not. Similar findings were reported by Schöpf & Rust (1994); others found a higher recurrence rate in those with index puerperal episodes (40% *v.* 31%), although this was a smaller sample (Hunt & Silverstone 1995). Videbech & Gouliaev (1995) followed up 50 women 7–14 years after their first psychotic episode, which was puerperal. Forty per cent of the women were not working to full capacity owing to mental disorder, and 60% had had recurrences, and schizophreniform symptoms in the index episode predicted incapacity to work. Only 4% of women had exclusively puerperal episodes.

Garfield *et al* (2004) followed up 66 women 10 years after hospital admission with a puerperal illness. The recurrence rate was 87.2% and the readmission rate 63.3%. The strongest predictor of recurrence was a past psychiatric history. Women with no previous psychiatric history or who had only experienced previous puerperal episodes did better at follow up (only 38.9% relapsed) than those who had a prior history of non-puerperal illness (70.9% relapsed). Most of the women in this study had a diagnosis of major depression. Of 61 women reviewed after 25 years since a puerperal psychotic episode (various diagnoses), 63.9% had had further episodes, with the average number of episodes being 4.8 (Rohde & Marneros, 1993). A 9-year follow-up of women with clearly defined bipolar affective puerperal psychosis found 57% experiencing additional puerperal illnesses and 62% non-puerperal episodes (Robertson *et al*, 2005). A recent study of women a mean of 12 years after discharge reported diagnostic stability, with those who initially presented with an a unipolar or bipolar disorder having affective recurrences, and those whose postpartum diagnosis was a brief or cycloid psychosis shifting to a clear bipolar disorder with further recurrences (Kapfhammer *et al*, 2014).

In a retrospective study of 116 women (Blackmore *et al*, 2013), only 58% of those who experienced puerperal psychosis had a second pregnancy. Eighteen per cent of marriages ended after the puerperal psychosis episode. One-third of the women in this study had a past history of bipolar disorder (34%) or unipolar depression (55%). The recurrence rate of puerperal psychosis was 54%. A long duration of the first episode and a longer interval between the first and subsequent pregnancies were predictors. The rate of non-puerperal episodes (all bipolar) was 69%. Nager *et al* (2013) confirmed the high rate of non-puerperal readmission in a large study ($n = 3140$) but noted that this declined over time: 76% by the second year, 50% in years 6–10 and 29% after more than 20 years. Women with admissions prior to puerperal psychosis, lower levels of education and a diagnosis of schizophrenia were at highest risk of recurrence.

## Psychosis in pregnancy

There are case reports of psychosis occurring (Brockington *et al*, 1990) and recurring during pregnancy (Glaze *et al*, 1991). Howe & Srinavasan (1999) report a case of Cotard's syndrome occurring around the 33rd week of pregnancy. The woman jumped out of the upstairs window of the obstetric unit, sustaining multiple fractures. Her baby was delivered by Caesarean section and she was treated with ECT. Friedman & Rosenthal (2003) reported a case of delusional disorder and borderline personality disorder in the third trimester. The patient was treated successfully with olanzapine and psychotherapy. Another report describes a woman presenting at 28 weeks gestation with symptoms initially appearing like eclampsia but becoming floridly psychotic within 48 h of Caesarean delivery of her infant. It was then assumed that her initial presentation had in fact been catatonic stupor (Ranzini *et al*, 1996). Menick (2005) reports 12.5% of women presenting to a hospital in Cameroon with childbirth-related psychotic disorders having become acutely ill while pregnant.

As with postpartum presentations, some acute neurological disorders may present with psychotic symptoms in pregnancy. McCarthy *et al* (2012) describe a case of anti-NMDA (*N*-methyl-D-aspartate) receptor encephalitis in a woman who was 8 weeks pregnant, presenting with visual and auditory hallucinations and paranoid delusions. She later developed catatonia, tachycardia, fever and labile blood pressure.

There are also case reports of psychosis occurring after termination of pregnancy or miscarriage (Da Silva & Johnstone 1981; Brockington, 2005), hydatidiform mole (Hopker & Brockington, 1991) and male-to-female gender reassignment (Mallett *et al*, 1989). Many of these women have gone on to suffer from puerperal psychoses after subsequent pregnancies that went to term, suggesting a link between late pregnancy, post-abortion and postpartum triggers.

# Relationship to bipolar disorder

Chaudron & Pies (2003) reviewed the evidence base from 1966 to 2002, which includes the follow-up studies cited above, and concluded that it 'supported a link between postpartum psychosis and bipolar disorder', with many but not all puerperal psychotic episodes falling within the bipolar spectrum. The evidence base to support this is growing. Chapter 4 includes a discussion of the high risk of recurrence of bipolar disorder after delivery, and its management.

# Aetiology

## Genetics

In the early 19th century, Esquirol noted that puerperal psychosis tended to run in families (Esquirol, 1838). Dean *et al* (1989) observed a significantly and substantially higher incidence of affective morbidity in first-degree relatives of women who had experienced puerperal psychosis compared with the relatives of women with bipolar disorder who had not had a puerperal episode. Puerperal psychosis has a close relationship with bipolar disorder and there is compelling evidence from family, twin and adoption studies that genes influence susceptibility to bipolar disorder, although the mode of inheritance appears to be complex and it is likely that interaction of several susceptibility genes is required. There are case reports of monozygotic twin pairs concordant for puerperal psychosis (e.g. Kane, 1968) and a familial clustering where there was consanguinity (Craddock *et al*, 1994). Jones & Craddock (2001) have demonstrated that women with bipolar disorder who have a first-degree relative who has had an episode of puerperal psychosis are more likely to experience a puerperal episode following subsequent pregnancies, compared with those who have no first-degree relatives with a history of puerperal psychosis. In addition, bipolar women who have had a puerperal episode are more likely to have a first-degree relative with an affective disorder than those without a history of puerperal episodes (Jones & Craddock, 2001).

Variation at the serotonin transporter gene is influenced by oestradiol. The presence of one allele (Stin2.12) was associated with almost four times the risk of puerperal psychosis (OR = 3.9), an effect that increased when the phenotype was restricted to women who had experienced multiple episodes (Coyle *et al*, 2000). Subsequent work has shown linkage with chromosomes 16p13 and 8q24 (Jones *et al*, 2007).

## Dopamine

Oestrogen modulates monoamine neurotransmitter systems, including the dopaminergic system. The rapid fall of circulating gonadal steroid hormones after delivery, which occurs in parallel with the often acute onset of symptoms, led to the hypothesis that women who become psychotic may have supersensitive dopamine receptors, particularly $D_2$ receptors. Two cases in which the patients' puerperal psychosis was accompanied by abnormal extrapyramidal movements support this idea (Vinogradov & Csernansky, 1990), and there are case reports of puerperal psychosis following treatment with bromocriptine (e.g. Canterbury *et al*, 1987; Reeves & Pinkofsky, 1997; Pinardo Zabala *et al*, 2003). Wieck and colleagues (1991) tested this by giving the dopamine agonist apomorphine to postpartum women with a history of psychosis and to a control group 4 days after delivery. The women who had recurrences of psychosis had greater growth hormone responses than the controls and those who remained well. However, a later study was unable to replicate these findings and found no difference between those at high risk of recurrence and controls (Meakin *et al*, 1995).

Wieck *et al* (2003) demonstrated that women predisposed to bipolar relapses in the puerperium had greater growth hormone responses than controls in the midluteal phase of the menstrual cycle but not in the follicular phase.

## Thyroid function

The relationship between nonpsychotic puerperal depression and thyroid function has been described in Chapter 2. The literature relating to psychotic puerperal illnesses and thyroid abnormalities is limited to a case report of a woman who developed a psychotic depression at 3 months postpartum and who also had thyroiditis. Her symptoms resolved when she became biochemically euthyroid (Bokhari *et al*, 1998).

## Immune system dysregulation

Abnormal activation of the immune system (which has been suggested as contributing to the pathogenesis of mood disorders) is evidenced by elevated serum cytokines and chemokines, activation of circulating monocytes demonstrated via profiling of inflammatory gene expression, and activation of the T cell system. Bergink *et al* (2013) analysed immune system activation in a sample of women with first-onset puerperal psychosis, healthy postpartum women and non-postpartum women. They observed elevated T cell levels in healthy postpartum women compared to controls and a lack of this normal postpartum elevation in women with puerperal psychosis. In women with puerperal psychosis, monocyte gene expression was upregulated compared to both control groups and monocyte levels were elevated. They propose that this immune dysregulation via increased macrophage activity and reduced T cell numbers might be the trigger for the onset of puerperal psychosis in women who have an underlying genetic susceptibility to bipolar disorder or psychosis.

## Obstetric factors

Di Florio *et al* (2014) demonstrated that puerperal psychosis or mania were more likely to occur in primiparous women with bipolar I disorder. Blackmore and colleagues (2006) studied 129 women who had suffered bipolar puerperal psychosis and found that primiparity and delivery complications were independently associated with recurrence.

# Women's experiences

There is a growing qualitative literature exploring the experience of puerperal psychosis for women and their partners. Women who have suffered from the disorder feel very strongly that it is different from other mental illnesses, as it is precipitated by childbirth and has a biological aetiology. As such, they feel that it requires specialised treatment. Those who had been treated in general psychiatric services felt frustrated and angry that their specific needs were not met and that they had been treated like everyone else. Other important themes were loss – of aspects of motherhood, of control and of future pregnancies – and disruption of social roles and relationships (Robertson & Lyons, 2003). Others stress that the experience cannot be fully shared with others who have not experienced it themselves (Engqvist & Nilsson, 2013). Hanzak (2005) has written a vivid account of her illness, admission to hospital and recovery, and Martini (2008) has described her experience of familial puerperal psychosis. More recent studies have focused on the recovery process, the need for professionals to provide reassurance and appropriate information and to understand that it will take time. The need for specialist support following discharge to continue long enough to allow women and their families to rebuild their lives has been highlighted. Informal support groups can lack knowledge of the illness, and fathers may struggle to identify their support needs (Doucet *et al*, 2012; Heron *et al*, 2012; McGrath *et al*, 2013).

# Suicide, self-harm and infanticide

## Suicide

*Why Mothers Die 2000–2002* (Lewis & Drife, 2004), like the two triennial UK Confidential Enquiry into Maternal Deaths (CEMD) reports before it, highlighted suicide as a major cause of maternal death. Like the 1997–1999 report, it found suicide to be the leading cause of indirect or late indirect deaths in the year following delivery. The majority of these deaths appeared to be of women suffering from psychosis or a very severe depressive illness. Oates (2003) has estimated the suicide rate for puerperal psychosis to be 2 per 1000 sufferers. Lindahl *et al* (2005) estimate that suicide accounts for 20% of maternal deaths, even though the rate for all delivered women in the year after birth is lower than that of the general population. *Saving Mothers' Lives* (Lewis, 2007) found a decrease in the numbers of maternal suicide, which was mostly accounted for by a fall in the number of suicides between 6 months and 1 year after delivery. In the 2005–2008 triennium (Oates & Cantwell, 2011), there was a non-significant rise in the number of suicides before 6 months postpartum. From 2011 to 2013, 1 in 7 maternal deaths was a suicide and 23% of the women who died between 6 weeks and 1 year postpartum died from psychiatric causes (Knight *et al*, 2015).

The most common profile of a woman who is at risk of suicide in late pregnancy or after delivery is a white, well-educated older woman in her second or subsequent pregnancy, in a stable relationship and living in comfortable circumstances: 28% of those who died in the most recent enquiry were in professional occupations. She is likely to have had contact with psychiatric services and a history of mental illness, and may be in current treatment. She is likely to die violently, e.g. by hanging, drowning, jumping from a height or in front of a train, causing an intentional road traffic accident, self-immolation or throat cutting. In the most recent enquiry, 33% of the women who died had been referred to child protection services during pregnancy. Fear of their child being removed can lead to women disengaging from services.

## *Self-harm*

A review in 1968 estimated that between 5 and 12% of women attempting suicide were pregnant (Whitlock & Edwards, 1968). In 1984, 0.07% of calls to a US metropolitan poison control centre were from or about pregnant women (Rayburn *et al*, 1984), and the attempt reported was usually the woman's first. Half of the overdoses were taken during the first trimester, most commonly using an over-the-counter analgesic, iron or a vitamin.

Studies in Sweden and the USA have found that issues relating to pregnancy and interpersonal difficulties are often cited as the main provoking factors for self-harm in pregnant women. These may include prior loss of children (through death or adoption), prior termination, desire for a termination or the potential loss of a partner.

Lindahl *et al* (2005) reviewed 27 studies that reported rates of suicidal ideation, intention, attempts and completed suicide in pregnant and postpartum women. Suicidal thoughts (assessed by endorsement of item 10 on the Edinburgh Postnatal Depression Scale: 'the thought of harming myself has occurred to me') occurred in up to 14% of pregnant women. The authors observed lower rates of suicide during pregnancy than that in the general population, but found that when it did occur, violent methods were more likely to be used. Particular groups at risk are teenagers and women from cultures where being unmarried and pregnant is stigmatised. Women with past histories of abuse are more also likely to die by suicide. A USA study of over 2000 women who attempted suicide found that young, single, multiparous, less well educated, and African American women were more likely to harm themselves. Twenty six per cent of them were substance misusers (Gandhi *et al*, 2006). Follow-up found that those who self-harmed were more likely than controls to have a preterm labour, to have a Caesarean delivery and to require a blood transfusion. Their infants showed an increased risk of respiratory distress syndrome and low birth weight. A Hungarian study of 1044 women found that those who overdosed with a hypnotic containing amobarbital, glutethimide and promethazine were more likely to deliver an infant with an intellectual disability (Petik *et al*, 2012). Another report from the same data-set observed an increased risk of congenital abnormalities in infants born to women who had self-harmed with nitrazepam (Gidai *et al*, 2010).

Comtois *et al* (2008) reported a 27.4-fold increased risk of a suicide attempt requiring hospital admission if a woman has a psychiatric disorder, a 6.2-fold increased risk with a substance misuse diagnosis and an 11.1-fold increased risk with a dual diagnosis. A study of referrals to a perinatal mental health team in the UK observed that 58% of women booking for maternity care who had a history of postnatal depression disclosed an episode of self-harm with the intent of killing themselves (Healey *et al*, 2013).

## Infanticide

Although the majority of postpartum women who die by suicide do not also kill their infant, the 2004 CEMD report identified three cases in which the infant was also killed at the time of the suicide. In two cases, an older child was also killed at the same time, and four suicides occurring in pregnancy near term also resulted in the death of a viable fetus. Infanticidal ideas are common in the severely mentally ill postpartum population. In a study by Chandra *et al* (2002), 43% of the mothers reported having infanticidal ideas, 36% reported infanticidal behaviour and 34% reported both. Depression and psychotic ideas predicted infanticidal ideas, whereas the presence of psychotic ideas towards the infant predicted infanticidal behaviour.

Infanticide is a legal term used in the UK to refer to the killing of a child under the age of 12 months. Neonaticide is not a legal term but refers to the killing of a child within 24h of birth. Craig (2004) has reviewed the associated factors and Friedman *et al* (2005a) included infanticide and neonaticide in a wider review of child murder. They found that women who commit neonaticide are usually young, poorly educated and primiparous. They are often living at home with their parents and have often concealed their pregnancy. Most do not have a mental illness at the time of killing their child. Very few of them are psychotic; where a psychiatric diagnosis is found, this is more likely to be a personality disorder or a mild or borderline intellectual disability. Nesca & Dalby (2011) describe a case of neonaticide linked to post-traumatic stress disorder and discuss the legal aspects.

Mothers who commit infanticide are more likely to be older and married or living with a partner. There is more likely to be a mental illness present, and the infant death is often part of an extended suicide or, occasionally, an 'altruistic' act based upon a delusional idea that some terrible fate was about to befall the infant. Schizophrenic mothers who relapse in relation to pregnancy or childbirth may incorporate the infant into their delusional system or be acutely disturbed and carry out the act for no rational reason.

Substance misuse is a factor often associated with infant homicide. Only very rarely is infanticide the consequence of factitious disorder by proxy.

Friedman and colleagues (2005b) examined a case series of mothers who had killed their children and were adjudicated as not guilty by reason of insanity ($n = 39$). Their children's ages varied from birth to 16 years (mean 3.7; one-third were infants). More than 80% of the mothers had a psychotic disorder or mood disorder with psychotic features and many had had recent contact with psychiatric services. Almost half had made previous suicide attempts and 56% had planned suicide along with the death of their child. Half were depressed and the majority were experiencing auditory hallucinations, including command hallucinations to kill their children. Three-quarters were delusional at the time of the killing, and two-thirds of these had delusions that involved their children. These delusions frequently involved a belief that the child was possessed by the devil or demons, that the mother herself was a god or religious figure, and that some terrible thing would happen to the child. More than one-third were pregnant or within the first postpartum year. The most common method used was suffocation.

In England and Wales, women who kill a child under the age of 12 months are usually disposed of by the judiciary by means of Chapter 36 of the Infanticide Act 1938 as amended by Section 57 of the Coroners and Justice Act 2009.

> 'Where a woman by any wilful act or omission causes the death of her child being a child under the age of twelve months, but at the time of the act or omission the balance of her mind was disturbed by reason of her not having fully recovered from the effect of giving birth to the child or by reason of the effect of lactation consequent upon the birth of the child, then, notwithstanding that the circumstances were such that but for this Act the offence would have amounted to murder, she shall be guilty of felony, to wit of infanticide, and may for such offence be dealt with and punished as if she had been guilty of the offence of manslaughter of the child.'

In Northern Ireland, the relevant legislation is the Infanticide Act (Northern Ireland) 1939. In Scotland, despite similar infanticide rates to England and Wales, there is no specific infanticide legislation and mothers are dealt with via the general homicide laws.

Disposal is usually non-custodial and can be tied in with ongoing treatment in a community rehabilitation order with conditions of treatment or a hospital order. However, this law gives rise to anomalies. For example, a women who kills her infant who is a day over a year old, despite clear evidence of her illness being consequent upon childbirth, will be charged with murder and, despite a plea of diminished responsibility, will be much more likely to receive a custodial sentence.

# Management

## Assessment

The assessment of any acutely ill puerperal woman is essentially the standard psychiatric examination (history, mental state examination and physical examination), with the addition of the biopsychosocial context of recent childbirth and the infant's well-being to consider, as well as the mother, her partner, and other children and family members.

It is essential in all women with depression or psychosis to assess suicidal and infanticidal ideas. Delusions should be clearly defined and the content examined carefully for reference to harming herself and/or her infant and/or older children. A mother who believes that her child has changed in some way, looks strange, is not hers, or is, for example, evil, is at risk of harming that child, as is a woman with command hallucinations to harm herself or her child.

Chandra et al (2006) found that 53% of women with a severe postpartum illness and 78% of those with psychotic postpartum disorders had delusional beliefs about their infant. The mothers whose delusions involved believing that the baby was a devil, ill-fated or someone else's baby were more likely to shout at or hit the baby or to have attempted to smother him or her. Caregivers of those women who believed their baby was God were more likely to consider the woman to be unsafe with her baby, and other delusions (more elaborate or bizarre) were associated with the mother being unable to manage chores related to the baby and with talking negatively about him or her.

A number of rating scales have been devised to assess disturbances of the mother–infant relationship. The Bethlem Mother–Infant Interaction Scale has seven subscales and was designed to be used on a weekly basis by nursing staff on an in-patient unit (Kumar & Hipwell, 1996). It can be repeated to monitor progress. There are also scales that assess mother–infant bonding (Brockington et al, 2001; Taylor et al, 2005). These last two have been compared (Wittkowski et al, 2007).

Some patients may superficially appear to have an acute mental disorder but, when an adequate history and examination are performed, are found to have an acute medical or surgical problem. There are case reports of chronic subdural haematoma presenting as puerperal psychosis in which the patient's complaint of persistent headache after epidural anaesthesia was ignored (Campbell & Varma, 1993), and of a woman appearing confused and complaining of auditory hallucinations and *déja vu* the day after a Caesarean delivery, who was found to have a meningioma (Khong *et al*, 2007). The misattribution of physical symptoms to functional psychiatric disorder can cause a delay in making the correct diagnosis or lead to the admission of acutely medically ill women to psychiatric hospitals. Such mistakes led to the deaths of several women reported to the last three CEMD (Lewis & Drife, 2004; Lewis, 2007, 2011). In 2016, the report of The Maternal, Newborn and Infant Clinical Outcome Review Programme noted that the rate of maternal suicide had not reduced since 2003 (Knight *et al*, 2016).

## In-patient care

Most acutely psychotic women will require admission, as will some of those with severe depressive illnesses and other diagnoses. Women who require acute admission for a severe mental illness in the postpartum should be admitted to a specialist mother and baby unit unless there are compelling child protection issues which preclude this. In Scotland, this is enshrined within the Mental Health Care and Treatment Act.

## Drug treatment

Most women with psychotic illnesses will require antipsychotic medication in addition to antidepressants and/or mood stabilisers, depending upon the precise nature of the episode. Care should be taken not to over-sedate a woman caring for an infant, particularly if she is breastfeeding and needs to do night feeds. However, in the early days of an admission, many women will require their baby to be looked after in the nursery at night to allow them to sleep. At other times, even very psychotic women can, with the support of nursery nurses and psychiatric nurses skilled in the care of mothers, undertake a good deal of infant care and maintain a close bond with their baby. Prescribing for breastfeeding mothers is discussed in Chapter 9.

There are case reports of neuroleptic malignant syndrome (NMS) occurring in women with puerperal psychosis (Alexander *et al*, 1998; Price *et al*, 1989), and some authors have postulated that it may be more likely to occur in women with puerperal psychosis. NMS can be difficult to distinguish clinically from the 'organic' features of puerperal psychosis, or from acute sepsis or other physical complications of the postpartum period. However, it should be considered if a patient deteriorates after medication with psychotropics, and the serum creatine phosphokinase level should be checked.

Women in a very retarded or stuperose state may need anticoagulant therapy if they have recently delivered and are inactive, in order to prevent venous thromboembolism. As such women may well need ECT, an anaesthetist's opinion should be sought well in advance. A systematic review of the treatments of puerperal psychosis has been carried out by Doucet *et al* (2011).

## Oestradiol

There are three small case series examining the role that oestradiol might have as an effective treatment for puerperal psychosis. The first two describe women with low oestradiol levels and refractory to antipsychotics being given sublingual 17ß-oestradiol. The rise in serum concentrations is reported as paralleling the improvement in symptoms (Ahokas & Aito, 1999; Ahokas *et al*, 2000*a*). In the third study, 10 women with puerperal psychosis and low oestradiol levels after delivery were given sublingual 17ß-oestradiol 3 to 6 times daily until their serum concentration was 400pmol/L (Ahokas *et al*, 2000*b*). Symptoms measured by the Brief Psychiatric Rating Scale improved by the end of the first week; however, it should be noted that two-thirds of the women had had treatment before starting oestradiol (psychotherapy and antipsychotics), although this is reported as having been ineffective. None of these studies report any safety data, which is important given the potential risks of thromboembolic events and endometrial hyperplasia. Clearly, there is a need for larger, controlled, methodologically sound studies before oestradiol can be declared an effective and safe treatment for puerperal psychosis.

There is a published report of progesterone used as a treatment for puerperal mania (Meakin & Brockington, 1990), but the improvement in the two cases reported in this paper could have been attributed to antipsychotic medication that was also prescribed. There are no controlled data to support the use of progesterone as a treatment for puerperal psychosis.

## *Electroconvulsive therapy*

There has long been a belief that puerperal psychosis is particularly responsive to ECT, and this has been confirmed by Reed *et al* (1999), who reported that women with puerperal illnesses showed greater clinical improvement than those with non-puerperal disorder when given ECT. Babu *et al* (2013) carried out a naturalistic study of ECT in 78 in-patients with puerperal psychosis, most of whom had a mood disorder. He reported few transient side-effects in the women and no adverse effects on breastfed infants. Focht & Kellner (2012) reviewed the literature on ECT in the treatment of puerperal psychosis, concluding that as it may be effective more quickly than medication while avoiding some of the adverse effects of medication, it should be considered as a first-line treatment for puerperal psychosis. The use of ECT in pregnant women is described in Chapter 8.

## Psychological treatment

Although no specific intervention has been trialled in women with puerperal psychotic illnesses, it is clear that many will benefit from psychotherapeutic work, particularly when the acute phase of the disorder is settling. There may be specific issues which need addressing, such as bereavement or coping with stressful life events and marital problems, in addition to coming to terms with having been acutely ill and what that means for the future. A woman with her first psychotic episode and her partner will benefit from education about the disorder, the risk of recurrence after later pregnancies or at other times, and what can be done to prevent it recurring. (The prevention of puerperal psychosis is described in Chapter 7.)

## Contraception

Contraceptive needs must be addressed and in place before a woman begins periods of leave. Do not assume the primary care team will deal with this on discharge. If in doubt, seek advice from the midwife with a responsibility for contraceptive advice or the local family planning clinic. Mother and baby units should keep a stock of condoms to give to patients who have not made any contraceptive plans before going on leave.

# Conclusions

Puerperal psychosis is a serious mental disorder, which can have devastating consequences for sufferers, their children and families. However, early identification, prompt treatment and care not to misattribute serious physical illness to puerperal psychosis can do much to reduce mortality and morbidity.

# References

Agrawal P, Bhatia MS, Malik SC (1990) Postpartum psychosis: a study of indoor cases in a general hospital psychiatric clinic. *Acta Psychiatrica Scandinavica*, **81**: 571–575.

Ahokas A, Aito, M (1999) Role of estradiol in puerperal psychosis. *Psychopharmacology*, **147**: 108–110.

Ahokas A, Aito M, Turiainen S (2000a) Association between oestradiol and puerperal psychosis. *Acta Psychiatrica Scandinavica*, **101**: 167–169.

Ahokas A, Aito M, Rimon R (2000b) Positive treatment effect of estradiol in postpartum psychosis: a pilot study. *Journal of Clinical Psychiatry*, **61**: 166–169.

Alexander PJ, Thomas RM, Das A (1998) Is risk of neuroleptic malignant syndrome increased in the postpartum period? *Journal of Clinical Psychiatry*, **59**: 254–255.

Allwood CW, Berk M, Bodemer W (2000) An investigation into puerperal psychoses in black women admitted to Baragwanath Hospital. *South African Medical Journal*, **90**: 518–520.

Babu GN, Thippeswamy H, Chandra PS (2013) Use of electroconvulsive therapy (ECT) in postpartum psychosis – a naturalistic prospective study. *Archives of Women's Mental Health*, **16**: 247–251.

Bergink V, Lambregste-van den Berg MP, Koorengevel KM, *et al* (2011) First-onset psychosis occurring in the postpartum period: a prospective cohort study. *Journal of Clinical Psychiatry*, **72**: 1531–1537.

Bergink V, Burgerhout KM, Weigelt K, *et al* (2013) Immune system dysregulation in first-onset postpartum psychosis. *Biological Psychiatry*, **73**: 1000–1007.

Blackmore ER, Jones I, Doshi M, *et al* (2006) Obstetric variables associated with bipolar affective puerperal psychosis. *British Journal of Psychiatry*, **188**: 32–36.

Blackmore ER, Rubinow DR, O'Connor TG, *et al* (2013) Reproductive outcomes and risk of subsequent illness in women diagnosed with postpartum psychosis. *Bipolar Disorders*, **15**: 394–404.

Bokhari R, Bhatara VS, Bandettini F, *et al* (1998) Postpartum psychosis and postpartum thyroiditis. *Psychoneuroendocrinology*, **23**: 643–650.

Brockington IF (1996) *Motherhood and Mental Illness*. Oxford University Press.

Brockington IF (2005) Post-abortion psychosis. *Archives of Women's Mental Health*, **8**: 53–54.

Brockington IF, Czernik KF, Schofield EM *et al* (1981) Puerperal psychosis: phenomena and diagnosis. *Archives of General Psychiatry*, **38**: 829–833.

Brockington IF, Winokur G, Dean C (1982) Puerperal psychosis. In *Motherhood and Mental Illness* (eds IF Brockington, R Kumar): pp. 37–59. Academic Press.

Brockington IF, Oates M, Rose G (1990) Prepartum psychosis. *Journal of Affective Disorders*, **19**: 31–35.

Brockington IF, Oates J, George S, *et al* (2001) A screening questionnaire for mother–infant bonding disorders. *Archives of Women's Mental Health*, **3**: 133–140.

Campbell DA, Varma TR (1993) Chronic subdural haematoma following epidural anaesthesia, presenting as puerperal psychosis. *British Journal of Obstetrics and Gynaecology*, **100**: 782–784.

Canterbury RJ, Haskins B, Khan N, *et al* (1987) Postpartum psychosis induced by bromocriptine. *Southern Medical Journal*, **80**: 1463–1464.

Chandra PS, Venkatasubramanian G, Thomas T (2002) Infanticidal ideas and infanticidal behavior in Indian women with severe postpartum psychiatric disorders. *Journal of Nervous and Mental Disease*, **190**: 457–461.

Chandra PS, Bhargavarman RP, Raghunandan VNGP, *et al* (2006) Delusions related to infant and their association with mother–infant interactions. *Archives of Women's Mental Health*, **9**: 285–288.

Chaudron LH, Pies RW (2003) The relationship between postpartum psychosis and bipolar disorder: a review. *Journal of Clinical Psychiatry*, **64**: 1284–1292.

Comtois KA, Schiff MA, Grossman DC (2008) Psychiatric factors associated with postpartum suicide attempt in Washington State, 1992–2001. *American Journal of Obstetrics & Gynecology*, **199**: 120.e1–120e5.

Coyle N, Jones I, Robertson E, *et al* (2000) Variation at the serotonin transporter gene influences susceptibility to bipolar affective puerperal psychosis. *Lancet*, **356**: 1490–1.

Craddock N, Brockington I, Mant R, *et al* (1994) Bipolar affective puerperal psychosis associated with consanguinity. *British Journal of Psychiatry*, **164**: 359–364.

Craig M (2004) Perinatal risk factors for neonaticide and infanticide: can we identify those at risk? *Journal of the Royal Society of Medicine*, **97**: 57–61.

Da Silva L, Johnstone EC (1981) A follow-up study of severe puerperal psychiatric illness. *British Journal of Psychiatry*, **139**: 346–354.

Dean C, Kendell RE (1981) The symptomatology of puerperal illnesses. *British Journal of Psychiatry*, **139**: 128–133.

Dean C, Williams RJ, Brockington IF (1989) Is puerperal psychosis the same as bipolar manic-depressive disorder? A family study. *Psychological Medicine*, **19**: 637–647.

Dhasmana DJ, Brockington IF, Roberts A (2010) Post-partum transverse sinus thrombosis presenting as acute psychosis. *Archives of Women's Mental Health*, **13**: 365–367.

Di Florio A, Jones L, Forty L, *et al* (2014) Mood disorders and parity – a clue to the aetiology of the postpartum trigger. *Journal of Affective Disorders*, **152–154**: 334–339.

Doucet S, Jones I, Letourno N, et al (2011) Interventions for the prevention and treatment of postpartum psychosis: a systematic review. Archives of Women's Mental Health, 14: 89–98.

Doucet S, Letourno N, Blackmore ER (2012) Support needs of mothers who experience postpartum psychosis and their partners. Journal of Obstetric, Gynecological & Neonatal Nursing, 41: 236–245.

Engqvist I, Nilsson K (2013) Experiences of the first days of postpartum psychosis : an interview study with women and next of kin in Sweden. Issues in Mental Health Nursing, 34: 82–89.

Esquirol, E (1838) Des Maladies Mentales considérées sous les rapports Médical, Hygiénique et Médico Légal. Baillière.

Fassier T, Guffon N, Acquaviva C, et al (2011) Misdiagnosed postpartum psychosis revealing a late-onset urea cycle disorder. American Journal of Psychiatry,168: 576–580.

Focht A, Kellner CH (2012) Electroconvulsive therapy (ECT) in the treatment of post partum psychosis. Journal of ECT, 28: 31–33.

Friedman SH, Rosenthal MB (2003) Treatment of perinatal delusional disorder: a case report. International Journal of Psychiatry in Medicine, 33: 391.

Friedman SH, Horwitz SM, Resnick PJ (2005a) Child murder by mothers: a critical analysis of the current state of knowledge and a research agenda. American Journal of Psychiatry, 162: 1578–1587.

Friedman SH, Hrouda DR, Holden CE (2005b) Child murder committed by severely mentally ill mothers: an examination of mothers found not guilty by reason of insanity. Journal of Forensic Science, 50: 1–6.

Gandhi SG, Gilbert WM, McElvy SS, et al (2006) Maternal and neonatal outcomes after attempted suicide. Obstetrics & Gynecology, 107: 984–990.

Ganjekar S, Desai G, Chandra PS (2013) A comparative study of psychopathology, symptom severity, and short-term outcome of postpartum and nonpostpartum mania. Bipolar Disorders, 15: 713–718.

Garfield P, Kent A, Paykel ES, et al (2004) Outcome of postpartum disorders: a 10-year follow-up of hospital admissions. Acta Psychiatrica Scandinavica, 109: 434–439.

Gidai J, Ács N, Bánhidy F, et al (2010) Congenital anomalies in children of 43 pregnant women who attempted suicide with large doses of nitrazepam. Pharmacoepidemiology and Drug Safety, 19: 175–182.

Glaze R, Chapman G, Murray D (1991) Recurrence of puerperal psychosis during late pregnancy. British Journal of Psychiatry, 159: 567–569.

Hanson GD, Brown MJ (1973) Waxy flexibility in a postpartum woman: a case report and review of the catatonic syndrome. Psychiatric Quarterly, 47: 95–103.

Hanzak EA (2005) Eyes Without Sparkle: A Journey Through Postnatal Illness. Radcliffe.

Harlow BL, Vitonis AF, Sparen P, et al (2007) Incidence of hospitalization for postpartum psychotic and bipolar episodes in women with and without prior prepregnancy or prenatal psychiatric hospitalizations. Archives of General Psychiatry, 64: 42–48.

Healey C, Morriss R, Henshaw C, et al (2013) Self-harm in postpartum depression: an audit of referrals to a perinatal mental health team. Archives of Women's Mental Health, 16: 237–245.

Hellerstedt WL, Phelan SM, Cnattingius S, et al (2013) Are prenatal, obstetric and infant complications associated with postpartum psychosis among women with pre-conception psychiatric hospitalisations? BJOG, 120: 446–455.

Heron J, Robertson-Blackmore E, McGuiness M, et al (2007) No 'latent period' in the onset of bipolar affective puerperal psychosis. Archives of Women's Mental Health, 10: 79–81.

Heron J, McGuinness M, Blackmore ER, et al (2008) Early postpartum symptoms in puerperal psychosis. BJOG, 115: 348–353.

Heron J, Gilbert N, Dolman C, et al (2012) Information and support needs during recovery from postpartum psychosis. Archives of Women's Mental Health, 15: 155–165.

Hopker SW, Brockington IF (1991) Psychosis following hydatidiform mole in a patient with recurrent puerperal psychosis. British Journal of Psychiatry, 158: 122–123.

Howe GB, Srinavasan M (1999) A case study on the successful management of Cotard's syndrome in pregnancy. *International Journal of Psychiatry in Clinical Practice*, **3**: 293–295.

Hunt N, Silverstone T (1995) Does puerperal illness distinguish a subgroup of bipolar patients? *Journal of Affective Disorders*, **34**: 101–107.

Jones I, Craddock N (2001) Familiality of the puerperal trigger in bipolar disorder: results of a family study. *American Journal of Psychiatry*, **158**: 913–917.

Jones I, Hamshere M, Nangle J-M, *et al* (2007) Bipolar affective puerperal psychosis: genome-wide significant evidence for linkage to chromosome 16. *American Journal of Psychiatry*, **164**: 1099–1104.

Kane Jr JF (1968) Postpartum psychosis in identical twins. *Psychosomatics*,**9**: 278–281.

Kapfhammer H-P, Reininghaus EZ, Fitz W, *et al* (2014) Clinical course of illness in women with early onset puerperal psychosis: a 12 year follow-up study. *Journal of Clinical Psychiatry*, **75**: 1096–1104.

Kendell R, Wainwright S, Hailey A, *et al* (1976) The influence of childbirth on psychiatric morbidity. *Psychological Medicine*, **6**: 297–302.

Kendell RE, Chalmers JC, Platz C (1987) Epidemiology of puerperal psychoses. *British Journal of Psychiatry*, **150**: 662–673.

Kendell R, Maguire R, Connor Y, *et al* (1981) Mood changes in the first three weeks after childbirth. *Journal of Affective Disorders*, **3**: 317–326.

Khong S-Y, Leach J, Greenwood C (2007) Meningioma mimicking puerperal psychosis. *Obstetrics & Gynecology*, **109**: 515–516.

Kitabayashi Y, Hamamoto Y, Hirosawa R, *et al* (2007) Postpartum catatonia associated with atypical posterior reversible encephalopathy syndrome. *Journal of Neuropsychiatry and Clinical Neuroscience*, **19**: 91–92.

Knight M, Tuffnell D, Kenyon S, *et al* (eds) (2015) *Saving Lives, Improving Mothers' Care*. MBRRACE-UK.

Knight M, Nair M, Tufnell D, *et al* (eds) (2016) *Saving Lives, Improving Mothers' Care*. MBRRACE-UK.

Kumar R, Hipwell AE (1996) Development of a clinical rating scale to assess mother–infant interaction in a psychiatric mother and baby unit. *British Journal of Psychiatry*, **169**: 18–26.

Lai J-Y, Huang T-I (2004) Catatonic features noted in patients with post-partum mental illness. *Psychiatry and Clinical Neuroscience*, **58**: 157–162.

Lewis G (2007) *Saving Mothers' Lives: Reviewing Maternal Deaths to Make Motherhood Safer – 2003–2005*. CEMD.

Lewis G (2011) Saving Mothers' Lives: Reviewing Maternal Deaths to Make Motherhood Safer – 2006–2008. *BJOG*, **118** (Suppl 1): 134–144.

Lewis G, Drife J (2004) *Why Mothers Die 2000–2002. The Sixth Report of the Confidential Enquiries into Maternal Death in the United Kingdom*. RCOG Press.

Lindahl V, Pearson JL, Colpe L (2005) Prevalence of suicidality during pregnancy and the postpartum. *Archives of Women's Mental Health*, **8**: 77–87.

Mallett P, Marshall EJ, Blacker CV (1989) 'Puerperal psychosis' following male-to-female sex reassignment? *British Journal of Psychiatry*, **155**: 257–259.

Martini A (2008) *A Memoir of Madness and Motherhood*. Simon & Schuster.

McCarthy A, Dineen J, McKenna P, *et al* (2012) Anti-NDMA receptor encephalitis with associated catatonia during pregnancy. *Journal of Neurology*, **259**: 2632–2635.

McGrath L, Peters S, Wieck A, *et al* (2013) The process of recovery in women who experienced psychosis following childbirth. *BMC Psychiatry*, **13**: 341.

Meakin C, Brockington IF (1990) Failure of progesterone treatment in puerperal mania. *British Journal of Psychiatry*, **156**: 910.

Meakin CJ, Brockington IF, Lynch S, *et al* (1995) Dopamine supersensitivity and hormonal status in puerperal psychosis. *British Journal of Psychiatry*, **166**: 73–79.

Meltzer ES, Kumar R (1985) Puerperal mental illness, clinical features and classification: a study of 142 mother-and-baby admissions. *British Journal of Psychiatry*, **147**: 647–654.

Menick MDM (2005) Accidents psychiatriques et manifestations psychopathologiques de la gravido-puerpéralité au Cameroun. *Médecine Tropicale*, **65**: 563–569.

Munk-Olsen T, Laursen TM, Pedersen CB, *et al* (2006) New parents and mental disorders: a population-based register study. *JAMA*, **296**: 2582–2589.

Nager A, Johansson L-M, Sundquist K (2005) Are sociodemographic factors and year of delivery associated with hospital admission for postpartum psychosis? A study of 500,000 first-time mothers. *Acta Psychiatrica Scandinavica*, **112**: 47–53.

Nager A, Johansson L-M, Sundquist K (2006) Neighbourhood socioeconomic environment and risk of postpartum psychosis. *Archives of Women's Mental Health*, **9**: 81–86.

Nager A, Szulkin R, Johansson S-E, *et al* (2013) High lifelong relapse rate of psychiatric disorders among women with postpartum psychosis. *Nordic Journal of Psychiatry*, **67**: 53–58.

Ndosi NK, Mtawali ML (2002) The nature of puerperal psychosis at Muhimbili National Hospital: its physical co-morbidity associated main obstetric and social factors. *African Journal of Reproductive Health*, **6**: 41–49.

Nesca M, Dalby JT (2011) Maternal neonaticide following traumatic childbirth: a case study. *International Journal of Offender Therapy and Comparative Criminology*, **55**: 1166–1178.

Oates M (2003) Suicide: the leading cause of maternal death. *British Journal of Psychiatry*, **183**: 279–281.

Oates M, Cantwell R (on behalf of the Centre for Maternal and Child Enquiries) (2011) Deaths from psychiatric causes. *BJOG*, **118** (Suppl 1): 132–142.

Okano T, Nomura J, Kumar R, *et al* (1998) An epidemiological and clinical investigation of postpartum psychiatric illness in Japanese mothers. *Journal of Affective Disorders*, **48**: 233–240.

Oosthuizen P, Russouw H, Roberts M (1995) Is puerperal psychosis bipolar mood disorder a phenomenological comparison. *Comprehensive Psychiatry*, **36**: 77–81.

O'Sullivan D, Dean C (1991) The Fregoli syndrome and puerperal psychosis. *British Journal of Psychiatry*, **159**: 274–277.

Paffenbarger RS (1964) Epidemiological aspects of parapartum mental illness. *British Journal of Preventive and Social Medicine*, **18**: 189–195.

Petik D, Czeizel B, Bánhidy F, *et al* (2012) A study of the risk of mental retardation among children of pregnant women who have attempted suicide by means of a drug overdose. *Journal of Injury and Violence Research*, **4**: 10–19.

Pfuhlmann B, Stober G, Franzek E, *et al* (1998) Cycloid psychoses predominate in severe postpartum psychiatric disorders. *Journal of Affective Disorders*, **50**: 125–134.

Pfuhlmann B, Stober G, Franzek E, *et al* (2000) Differential diagnosis, course and outcome of postpartum psychoses. A catamnestic investigation. *Nervenarzt*, **71**: 386–392.

Pinardo Zabala A, Alberca Munoz ML, Gimenez Garcia JM (2003) Postpartum psychosis associated with bromocriptine. *Anales de Medicina Interna*, **20**: 50–51.

Price DK, Turnbull GJ, Gregory RP, *et al* (1989) Neuroleptic malignant syndrome in a case of post-partum psychosis. *British Journal of Psychiatry*, **155**: 849–852.

Ranzini AC, Vinekar AS, Houlihan C, *et al* (1996) Puerperal psychosis mimicking eclampsia. *Journal of Maternal-Fetal Medicine*, **5**: 36–38.

Rayburn W, Aronow R, DeLancey B, *et al* (1984) Drug overdose during pregnancy: an overview from a metropolitan poison control center. *Obstetrics & Gynecology*, **64**: 611–614.

Reed P, Sermin N, Appleby L, *et al* (1999) A comparison of clinical response to electroconvulsive therapy in puerperal and non-puerperal psychoses. *Journal of Affective Disorders*, **54**: 255–60.

Reeves RR, Pinkofsky HB (1997) Postpartum psychosis induced by bromocriptine and pseudoephedrine. *Journal of Family Practice*, **45**: 164–166.

Robertson E, Lyons A (2003) Living with puerperal psychosis: a qualitative analysis. *Psychology & Psychotherapy: Theory, Research and Practice*, **76**: 411–431.

Robertson E, Jones I, Haque S, *et al* (2005) Risk of puerperal and non-puerperal recurrence of illness following bipolar affective puerperal (post-partum) psychosis. *British Journal of Psychiatry*, **186**: 258–259.

Rohde A, Marneros A (1993) Zur Prognose der Wochenbettpsychosen: Verlauf und Ausgand nach durchschnittlich 26 Jahren. *Nervenarzt*, **64**: 175–180.

Schöpf J, Rust B (1994) Follow-up and family study of postpartum psychoses. Part I: Overview. *European Archives of Psychiatry and Clinical Neuroscience*, **244**: 101–111.

Schwartz AC, Afejuku A, Garlow SJ (2013) Bifrontal meningioma presenting as postpartum depression with psychotic features. *Psychosomatics*, **54**: 187–191.

Shaaban HS, Choo HF, Sensakovic JW (2012) Anti-NMDA receptor encephalitis presenting as postpartum psychosis in a young woman, treated with rituximab. *Annals of Saudi Medicine*, **32**: 421–3.

Sharma V, Mazmanian D (2003) Sleep loss and puerperal psychosis. *Bipolar Disorders*, **5**: 98–105.

Sharma V, Smith A, Khan M (2004) The relationship between duration of labour, time of delivery and puerperal psychosis. *Journal of Affective Disorders*, **83**: 215–20.

Taylor A, Atkins R, Kumar R, *et al* (2005) A new mother-to-infant bonding scale: links with early maternal mood. *Archives of Women's Mental Health*, **8**: 45–51.

Terp I, Mortensen P (1998) Post-partum psychosis. *British Journal of Psychiatry*, **172**: 521–526.

Videbech P, Gouliaev G (1995) First admission with puerperal psychosis: 7-14 years of follow-up. *Acta Psychiatrica Scandinavica*, **91**: 167–173.

Viguera AC, Emmerich AD, Cohen LS (2008) Case 24-2008: A 35-year-old woman with postpartum confusion, agitation and delusions. *New England Journal of Medicine*, **359**: 509–515.

Vinogradov S, Csernansky JG (1990) Postpartum psychosis with abnormal movements: dopamine supersensitivity unmasked by withdrawal of endogenous estrogens? *Journal of Clinical Psychiatry*, **51**: 365–366.

Whitlock FA, Edwards JE (1968) Pregnancy and attempted suicide. *Comprehensive Psychiatry*, **9**: 1–12

Wieck A, Kumar R, Hirst AD, *et al* (1991) Increased sensitivity of dopamine receptors and recurrence of affective psychosis after childbirth. *BMJ*, **303**: 613–616.

Wieck A, Davies RA, Hirst AD, *et al* (2003) Menstrual cycle effects on hypothalamic dopamine receptor function in women with a history of puerperal bipolar disorder. *Journal of Psychopharmacology*, **17**: 204–209.

Wisner KL, Peindl K, Hanusa BH (1994) Symptomatology of affective and psychotic illnesses related to childbearing. *Journal of Affective Disorders*, **30**: 77–87.

Wittkowski A, Wieck A, Mann S (2007) An evaluation of two bonding questionnaires: a comparison of the Mother-to-Infant Bonding Scale with the Postpartum Bonding Questionnaire in a sample of primiparous mothers. *Archives of Women's Mental Health*, **10**: 171–175.

Yu AYX, Moore FGA (2011) Paraneoplastic encephalitis presenting as puerperal psychosis. *Psychosomatics*, **52**: 568–570.

# Further reading

Brockington I (1996) *Motherhood and Mental Health*. Oxford University Press.

Gentile S (2005) The role of oestrogen therapy in postpartum psychiatric disorders: an update. *CNS Spectrums*, **10**: 944–52.

Pariente C, Conroy S, Dazzan P, *et al* (2013) *Perinatal Psychiatry: The Legacy of Channi Kumar*. Oxford University Press.

Sit D, Rothschild AJ, Wisner KL (2006) *A review of postpartum psychosis*. Journal of Women's Health, 15: 352–68.

Spinelli MG (2003) *Infanticide: Psychosocial and Legal Perspectives on Mothers Who Kill*. American Psychiatric Publishing.

# CHAPTER 4

# Childbearing in women with existing mental disorders

It has long been observed that patients with serious mental disorders, particularly schizophrenia, have fewer children than the general population. To a certain extent this is true, especially of men (Power *et al*, 2013). Several studies have shown reduced fertility rates in women with schizophrenia (reviewed by Bundy *et al*, 2011). The lower rate is less marked in women with bipolar disorder and absent in women with unipolar depression (Power *et al*, 2013).

Estimates of the number of women with a psychotic illness who are mothers range from 56 to 63% (McGrath *et al*, 1999; Howard *et al*, 2001), i.e. the majority. Women with bipolar and unipolar affective disorders are more likely to be multiparous than women with schizophrenia (Jablensky *et al*, 2005). For a comprehensive review of fertility and pregnancy in women with psychotic disorders, see Howard (2005).

Unfortunately, many general medical and psychiatric services in primary and secondary care appear to be ignorant of the possibility that their female patients with serious mental illness are current or potential parents. For example, women with psychotic disorders are less likely than matched controls drawn from the General Practice Database to have received contraceptive advice (Howard *et al*, 2004). Despite mental health workers estimating that 49% of their female patients were sexually active and 22% using contraception, they had only discussed this with the patient in one-third of cases (McLennan & Ganguli, 1999). They were more confident in knowing their patients' sexual activity status (in 93.5% of cases) than whether they were using contraception (69% of cases). There was no clinician gender bias. Mental health professionals may lack contraceptive knowledge, have insufficient training or feel uncomfortable discussing the subject.

A small study of mothers with severe mental illness found that only 28.9% had full custody of their children, with the majority being cared for by partners or relatives and 26% fostered or in residential care settings (Sands *et al*, 2004).

Clearly, reduced fertility rates in psychosis are likely to be multifactorial in aetiology, but it appears that some women may be advised by others not to become pregnant. A study of women with bipolar disorder attending a specialist perinatal psychiatry service for advice revealed that 45% had previously been advised not to become pregnant: 69% by a psychiatrist or other mental health professional and 14% by an obstetrician or general practitioner (GP) (Viguera *et al*, 2002*a*). Family members, including spouses, parents and siblings, had also advised against pregnancy in 29% of these cases. After consultation and a full risk–benefit analysis, 63% attempted to conceive and 69% of these were successful within 12 months. The 37% who chose not to pursue a pregnancy most frequently cited as a reason fear of the impact of medication on fetal development, and the possibility of recurrence of illness if maintenance medication was stopped.

Many women with mental disorders also engage in other risky behaviours when pregnant or planning to conceive. They are significantly more likely to smoke or use illicit drugs (Shah & Howard, 2006; Battle *et al*, 2014; Judd *et al*, 2014) and are at increased risk of pregnancy loss (Gold *et al*, 2007; Matevosyan, 2011). The increased risk of preterm birth in an Australian study of women with schizophrenia and bipolar disorder was entirely attributable to smoking (Judd *et al*, 2014). Attempts should be made to reduce or stop smoking, in addition to limiting the intake of alcohol and drugs, tackling obesity and minimising caffeine intake. Some women will require support in attending antenatal care visits. As diet is often poor and medication may increase the risk of neural tube defects (NTD), vitamins and folic acid should be considered for women of reproductive age, especially those intending to conceive. The suggested dose of folic acid is 5 mg daily, and although there is no clear evidence that this prevents NTD, it may reduce the risk (Kjaer *et al*, 2008).

*Saving Mothers' Lives* (Centre for Maternal and Child Enquiries, 2011) recommends that:

> 'Women of childbearing age with pre-existing medical illness, including psychiatric conditions, whose conditions may require a change of medication, worsen or otherwise impact on a pregnancy, should be informed of this at every opportunity. This is particularly important since 50% of pregnancies are not planned. They should be pro-actively offered advice about planning for pregnancy and the need to seek pre-pregnancy counselling whenever possible. Prior to pregnancy, these women should be offered specific counselling and have a prospective plan for the management of their pregnancy developed by clinicians with knowledge of how their condition and pregnancy interact'.

# Schizophrenia

Although women with tightly defined schizophrenia who remain on medication are less likely to relapse after delivery than women with affective illnesses or more broadly defined schizophrenia (Davies *et al*, 1995), a substantial minority (21.72%) of those who have had admissions before pregnancy will relapse postpartum (Harlow *et al*, 2007). There are also many features of the illness and of the women's lives that can lead to poor outcomes for them and their children. For example, they are more likely to have multiple partners or no current partner, to have unplanned pregnancies, to experience coercive sex, to take part in risky sexual behaviour, and to be the victim of violence during pregnancy (for a review, see Matevosyan, 2011). They are also more likely to be single mothers or to have partners who are unemployed or disabled, to be socially disadvantaged and lacking in social support and to be either very young (< 20) or older (>35) mothers (Jablensky *et al*, 2005). Women with psychotic disorders are more likely than controls to use illicit drugs before pregnancy, to drink and/or use illicit drugs during pregnancy, and to experience to a relapse within 3 months of delivery. This is most frequently a nonpsychotic depressive or anxiety disorder (Howard *et al*, 2004). They are less likely to attend antenatal clinics and often receive poorer-quality antenatal care.

Even when smoking and other relevant factors such as maternal age, education and pregnancy-induced hypertension are controlled for, the odds of poor outcomes such as low-birth-weight (LBW) or small for gestational age (SGA) infants, preterm delivery and stillbirth are higher in women with schizophrenia (Bennedson *et al*, 1999; Nilsson *et al*, 2002; Vigod *et al*, 2014). Increased risk of pre-eclampsia, venous thromboembolism, operative delivery, maternal and neonatal intensive care (Vigod *et al*, 2014), and sudden infant death syndrome (Bennedson *et al*, 2001) has also been reported. Being overweight and folate-deficient when pregnant (which may relate to poor diet or weight gain on atypical antipsychotics, or may be a direct metabolic consequence of schizophrenia), increases the risk of NTD (Freeman *et al*, 2002a; Koren *et al*, 2002), as does vitamin B12 deficiency.

A large, well-controlled birth cohort study identified a higher rate of obstetric complications in women with schizophrenia, especially placental abruption and antepartum haemorrhages, a significantly increased odds ratio (OR) of 1.40 for the percentage of offspring with expected birth weight below the 10th centile and an excess of cardiovascular malformations (especially patent ductus arteriosus), whether diagnosed at birth or later (Jablensky *et al*, 2005). A meta-analysis of studies focused on this issue revealed a twofold increase in the relative risk for fetal death or stillbirth in the offspring of parents with psychosis, a magnitude similar to that resulting from smoking (Webb *et al*, 2005). Schizophrenia and schizoaffective disorder have been reported as independent risk factors for congenital anomalies (OR = 2.1) (Hizkiyahu *et al*, 2010). In addition, parental mental disorder involving past admissions doubles the risk of sudden infant death syndrome (King-Hele *et al*, 2007) and raises the risk of child homicide by 5–10 times (Webb *et al*, 2007). Delayed walking, visual dysfunction, language disorders, enuresis and disturbed behaviour are significantly increased in the offspring of mothers with schizophrenia (Henriksson & McNeil, 2004).

Schizophrenic women are also more likely to be separated from their children at birth or during childhood and to have reduced contact with them after their children go into care. This leaves many very traumatised, a fact that some health professionals do not always appear to recognise (Dipple *et al*, 2002). Health professionals are poor at recording information regarding the children of their patients, and this study found a lack of information in the case notes of women who had experienced the trauma of being separated from their children or even the death of a child. The Victoria Climbié inquiry report (Laming, 2003) and other cases have highlighted the potentially disastrous consequences of failing to recognise and communicate information about children who may be at risk. *Working Together to Safeguard Children* (HM Government, 2015*a*) provides statutory guidance, and all health professionals should be able to understand the risk factors relevant to safeguarding issues – including parents' need for support and the risks to unborn children – and should know where to refer for help. They should be prepared to share appropriate information with other agencies. *What to do if you're worried a child is being abused* (HM Government, 2015*b*) provides guidance on action where there are concerns about a child's welfare.

Psychotic denial of pregnancy may occur in a chronically unwell woman, particularly if she has previously had children removed and fears the removal of the current baby (Miller, 1990). There is also a case report of a pregnant woman with schizophrenia (unmedicated at the time) who performed her own Caesarean section at 37 weeks gestation (Yoldas *et al*, 1996). Childless women may have delusions of maternity, i.e. believing that they have children (Hrdlička, 1998).

There are numerous case reports of delusion of pregnancy since Esquirol first reported one in the 19th century. It can occur in both male and female patients, in organic or functional psychoses, depression and dementia. Advances in reproductive technology have influenced the content of the delusions; for example, a case is described where a woman believed herself to have a 'test-tube pregnancy' (Manoj *et al*, 2004). There have also been also cases occurring in the context of antipsychotic-induced hyperprolactinaemia (Ahuja *et al*, 2008*a*, 2008*b*), and one in a drug-naïve woman with hyperprolactinaemia and hypothyroidism (Penta & Lasalvia, 2013), who improved with antipsychotic treatment and cognitive–behavioural therapy (CBT). There may also be delusional interpretations of pregnancy changes, e.g. that the growing fetus is a demon or a parasite. Kornischka and Schneider (2003) stressed that delusions of pregnancy must be distinguished from:

- pseudocyesis, in which a woman believes herself to be pregnant and develops signs and symptoms of pregnancy
- simulated pregnancy: the person is aware that she is not pregnant

- organic pseudo-pregnancy: the symptoms may result from an endocrine tumour
- Couvade syndrome: a father developing symptoms as if he were pregnant or giving birth.

Brockington (1996) provides a comprehensive review of the literature up to the 1990s.

## Management

The aim of treating a woman with schizophrenia who becomes pregnant is to maximise functioning so that she can cope with pregnancy, the delivery and parenting. Ideally, she should be jointly managed by her usual team, with advice and support from a specialist perinatal service. Midwifery and health visiting staff should be invited to care plan reviews, which will need to take place more frequently during pregnancy and postpartum. Pre-birth planning meetings should also involve child protection staff if there are concerns regarding parenting ability and child safety.

By 32 weeks, a care plan for the remainder of the pregnancy, the delivery and the postpartum period should have been devised, agreed by all and copied to all parties concerned, including mental health, maternity services and primary care. There should be a copy in all paper and electronic records and in the hand-held record. If there are significant concerns about the well-being of the child, a social services assessment must be sought.

Although there are interventions aimed at increasing mother–child sensitivity and attachment, the most efficacious being sensitivity-focused behavioural techniques and toddler–parent psychotherapy, no published studies have involved mothers with schizophrenia (Wan *et al*, 2008).

### Medication

A careful individual risk–benefit analysis should be taken with respect to antipsychotic medication. There may be a risk of relapse if medication is discontinued or switched, and there may be potential risks to the pregnancy and/or fetus from a drug. It is not usual to start a patient on clozapine during pregnancy, but most women already taking it will be doing so because they have failed to respond to or tolerate alternatives. Women on depot medication are usually on it because they have not adhered to oral drugs, so stopping may not be advisable. However, as a depot cannot be quickly withdrawn if side-effects do occur, initiating depot medication during pregnancy is not advised.

See Chapter 8 for an outline of the issues regarding rapid tranquilisation of a pregnant or perinatal woman and detail regarding medication and physical treatments during pregnancy.

# Bipolar disorder

Women with bipolar disorder have a high risk of recurrence related to childbirth, with up to 67% experiencing an episode in the immediate postpartum period (Kendell *et al*, 1987; Terp & Mortensen 1998; Freeman *et al*, 2002*b*; Robertson *et al*, 2005). Those with a family history of puerperal relapse are particularly likely to relapse postpartum (Jones & Craddock, 2001). The risk of recurrence appears to be the same in both bipolar I and II patients, but it is more likely in those who have had more than four episodes (Viguera *et al*, 2000). Di Florio *et al* (2013) observed that women with bipolar I disorder had approximately 50% risk of a perinatal major affective episode per pregnancy/postpartum period. Risks were lower in women with recurrent major depression or bipolar II disorder, at approximately 40% per pregnancy/postpartum period. Symptoms tend to onset rapidly, within 48–72 h of delivery in the case of a manic relapse; days or weeks after delivery in the case of a depressive relapse. Mixed affective states may be more common at this time (Wisner *et al*, 1994).

Relapse postpartum is particularly likely if maintenance medication has been discontinued (Viguera *et al*, 2000; Maina *et al*, 2014). The risk is greater with a rapid discontinuation; therefore, if a mood stabiliser must be discontinued, this should be tapered slowly rather than being stopped abruptly, to reduce the risk of recurrence. If there is a history of recurrence of illness following previous discontinuations, discontinuation might not be advised.

Initially, it was thought that women with bipolar disorder were less likely to experience an episode of illness during pregnancy, and this was supported by two studies (Sharma & Persad, 1995; Grof *et al*, 2000). However, it now seems clear that this is not the case. Blehar *et al* (1998) reported that almost one-third experienced worsening of symptoms; Akdeniz *et al* (2003) reported 32% of women with bipolar disorder having pregnancy or postpartum episodes; and Freeman and colleagues (2002*b*) found that 50% experienced symptoms while pregnant. Those who did have symptoms while pregnant were more likely to have a postpartum episode, and such episodes were almost exclusively depressive. The women who had a postpartum episode after the birth of their first child all had a mood episode after subsequent pregnancies; those who did not have an episode after the birth of their first child were still at high risk of having one after subsequent pregnancies. Viguera & Cohen (1998) also found that pregnancy episodes were more likely to be depressive or dysphoric mixed states.

Whether or not mood stabilisers are continued throughout pregnancy seems to be important. If they are discontinued, pregnant women relapse as frequently as non-pregnant women; 57% *v.* 52% (Viguera *et al*, 2000). The time to relapse is shorter, with a rapid (within 2 weeks) rather than a slower (more than 2–4 weeks) discontinuation. Cohen *et al* (1995)

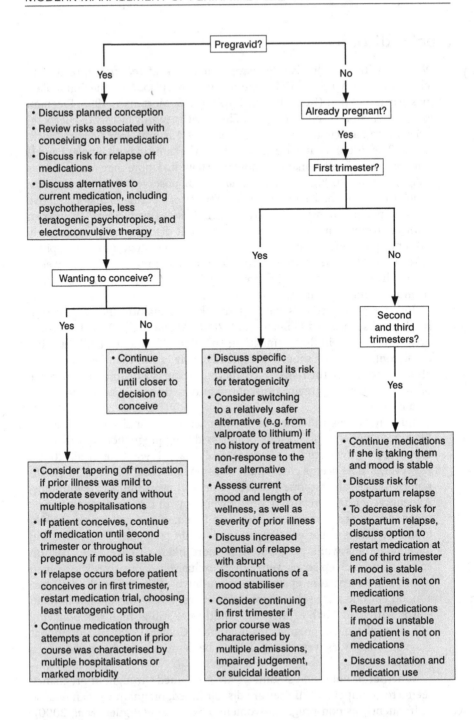

Fig. 4.1 Suggested approach for women with bipolar disorder who wish to conceive or are pregnant. Reproduced with permission from Altshuler *et al*, 2003.

estimated the relative risk of recurrence for women who did not receive maintenance medication as 8.6 times that of women who did. Sodium valproate should be avoided during pregnancy if at all possible, owing to the increased risk of NTD and neurodevelopmental disorders (see Chapter 8 for more detail).

## Prevention of postpartum recurrence

A non-randomised, single-blind study found that divalproex semisodium is no better than monitoring for preventing recurrent episodes (Wisner *et al*, 2004; for detail see Chapter 7), but there are more promising data for olanzapine (Sharma *et al*, 2006). Therefore, current best advice is to provide prophylaxis with the drug a woman has responded to in the past and increase the dose rapidly if symptoms occur. If she intends to breastfeed, the medication must be compatible with this (see Chapter 9). If medication is refused, then close monitoring is essential and all professionals involved in maternity care in the postpartum period (in primary and secondary care) should be aware of the risks. A clear management plan to follow if relapse occurs should be in the woman's handheld record and in all her hospital and GP records (paper and electronic).

## Management

Women with bipolar disorder who are considering a pregnancy must have the opportunity to discuss how their care might be managed before and during pregnancy and in the postpartum in order to minimise the risk of recurrence (Fig. 4.1). Factors to consider are: how severe the illness is; response to previous medications; previous recurrences and their triggers; and what effect previous reductions and discontinuations of medication have had, including the time to recurrence after discontinuation and time to recovery on reintroduction. Take into account the length of time the patient has been euthymic or stable and the reproductive risks of the medication being considered (see Chapter 8).

In reality, 50% of pregnancies in the UK are unplanned, so having to deal with a pregnant woman on medication when the period of greatest risk – the first trimester – is underway is not unusual. In many cases, the woman may have stopped maintenance medication on discovering her pregnancy or may have been advised to do so by someone else (often a health professional).

There should be a comprehensive risk–benefit assessment for each woman, based on her history and current mental state, as well as other risk factors for poor obstetric outcome such as smoking, alcohol and drug consumption and how these might change should she relapse. A detailed discussion of particular medications and their use in pregnancy is to be found in Chapter 8. There should always be a discussion regarding the very high risk of recurrence after subsequent pregnancies, estimated to be 50–90% (Reich & Winokur, 1970; Parry, 1989; Hunt & Silverstone, 1995; Viguera *et al*, 2002*b*; Maina *et al*, 2014) in bipolar I disorder. Women with bipolar II disorder have a lower risk of recurrence, of around 40% (Di Florio *et al*, 2013). Although there is some evidence that women whose first bipolar episode is puerperal have significantly fewer episodes of mood disorder at 5–10-year follow up (Serretti *et al*, 2006), the fact that there are also likely to be non-puerperal episodes must be considered.

Anticonvulsants are increasingly being used as mood stabilisers and anti-manic medication. Clinicians should be aware that they might reduce the efficacy of oral contraceptives via enzyme induction or increased clearance, or by increasing sex hormone-binding globulin levels, thus reducing the availability of the free hormones. Carbamazepine is the most likely drug to act in this way, followed by topiramate. Women on these drugs who are using oral contraceptives will require a preparation with at least 50 mg ethinyloestradiol in order to maintain efficacy, or should consider a second or alternative form of contraception. Lamotrigine levels can be reduced by oral contraceptives, but there does not appear to be any interaction between valproate or gabapentin and oral contraceptives (Kaplan, 2004).

If a woman with bipolar disorder develops a mild to moderate depressive episode while pregnant, the first choice is to offer a psychological treatment such as CBT. However, if her depression is more severe, a selective serotonin reuptake inhibitor (SSRI) antidepressant or an atypical antipsychotic is advised. A woman with bipolar disorder who becomes manic should be prescribed a typical or atypical antipsychotic, with lithium or electroconvulsive therapy (ECT) being reserved for severe and/or unresponsive cases.

## Anxiety disorders

Ding *et al* (2014) conducted a systematic review of studies published up to 2013 and found that maternal anxiety during pregnancy was associated with a significantly increased risk of preterm birth (pooled relative risk (RR) = 1.50, 95% CI 1.33–1.70) and LBW (pooled RR = 1.76, 95% CI 1.32–2.33). Other studies with small sample sizes and potential selection bias owing to the inclusion of potentially higher-risk populations have reported contradictory findings when examining whether or not anxiety disorders during pregnancy predict other poor outcomes. Some of these studies (e.g. Crandon 1979; Schmitz & Reif 1994) report lower Apgar scores in infants, whereas others (Grimm & Venet 1996; McCool *et al*, 1994) contradict these findings. A larger study comparing outcomes in women with anxiety symptoms and those without, recruited from a general population study in Norway and controlling for confounders, confirmed that the presence of anxiety was associated with lower Apgar scores at 1 and 5 min after delivery (Berle *et al*, 2005). Panic disorder is associated with an increased risk of anaemia, shorter gestational age and increased preterm births (Bánhidy *et al*, 2006).

The mechanisms are still uncertain, but anxiety symptoms in pregnancy are associated with increased uterine artery resistance (Teixeira *et al*, 1999), which might lead to poor fetal growth. Other possibilities are changes in the hypothalamic–pituitary–adrenal (HPA) axis and cortisol secretion, increased use of medication during pregnancy or delivery, or other health-related behaviours that might affect fetal well-being, such as smoking, alcohol use or poor nutrition.

## Panic disorder

There is conflicting evidence regarding the impact that pregnancy and the postpartum period have on the course of illness in women with pre-existing panic disorder. Two studies suggest that most women experience no change in their level of symptoms (Cohen *et al*, 1996; Wisner *et al*, 1996). In another study, 43% improved, 33% worsened and 23% reported no change (Northcott & Stein 1994). Even if symptoms improve during pregnancy, they may recur postpartum (Curran *et al*, 1995; Bandelow *et al*, 2006), particularly if the woman has not continued to take prophylactic medication (Cohen *et al*, 1994).

Hendrick & Altshuler (1997) report a case of a woman maintained on nortriptyline and CBT, with lorazepam as required during attacks, who became pregnant. She chose to stop the lorazepam when she attempted to conceive: her symptoms increased and her antidepressant had to be increased in order to gain better control of her attacks.

The authors of a review of studies up to 1999 concluded that of the 215 pregnancies reported in the studies, 41% showed improvement during pregnancy but 38% had onset or recurrence postpartum (Hertzberg & Wahlbeck 1999). All but one of the studies reviewed by Cohen *et al* (1996) are retrospective. Women whose first onset of panic disorder was while pregnant are more likely to experience a recurrence in relation to a later pregnancy than those whose first illness onset was not linked with pregnancy (Dannon *et al*, 2006). A small prospective study observed that most women found their symptoms improved in the early postpartum period (Guler *et al*, 2008). A recent prospective study has reported that women with panic disorder are at increased risk of experiencing a depressive episode postpartum (Rambelli *et al*, 2010).

## Post-traumatic stress disorder

A study in the USA examined 744 pregnant women and found that 7.7% met diagnostic criteria for post-traumatic stress disorder (PTSD). In half, the precipitating event had occurred before the age of 15 and only 12% had had any treatment. Those with PTSD were five times more likely to have a major depressive disorder and three times more likely to have a generalised anxiety disorder (Loveland Cook *et al*, 2004). For women, the majority of traumatic experiences involve physical or sexual abuse, or assault or intimate partner violence. One study of ethnically diverse pregnant women observed that although symptoms of PTSD tended to decline during pregnancy, there was often a peak just prior to delivery (Onoye *et al*, 2013).

Pregnancy complications have been examined in women identified from Michigan Medicaid records as having PTSD, and in those with records showing no mental illness(Seng *et al*, 2001). Twenty two per cent of those with PTSD also had a substance misuse diagnosis. Those with PTSD had higher ORs for:

- ectopic pregnancy (OR = 1.7, 95% CI 1.1–2.8)
- hospital admission for miscarriage (OR = 1.9, 95% CI 1.3–2.9)
- hyperemesis (OR = 3.9, 95% CI 2.0–7.4)
- preterm contractions (OR = 1.4, 95% CI 1.1–1.9)
- macrosomia (OR = 1.5, 95% CI 1.0–2.2).

There were no differences in labour or in the occurrence of other complications such as gestational diabetes and pre-eclampsia. However, it was difficult to determine the chronology of the events in this study. A later study of pregnant women with PTSD observed a non-significant increase in preterm delivery but no association with LBW (Rogal *et al*, 2007). This study may have been underpowered and could not control for all possible confounders. Two more recent studies have explored the relationship with preterm birth. A prospective study of over 2000 women reported that those with PTSD and major depression have a fourfold increased risk of preterm birth, the risk being independent of antidepressant and benzodiazepine use (Yonkers *et al*, 2014), and a large retrospective study that controlled for confounders (Shaw *et al*, 2014) also reported an increased risk of preterm birth (OR = 1.35, 95% CI 1.14–1.61). Others have identified that PTSD subsequent to childbirth is most strongly associated with adverse outcomes (Seng *et al*, 2011).

## Management

Although we may feel intuitively that actively treating anxiety disorders in pregnant women should lead to better neonatal outcomes, this is not borne out by good evidence as yet. One study has shown that low-income US women (of whom up to a quarter reported 'negative mood' – a composite indicator of various symptoms, including anxiety) receiving at least 45 min of psychosocial care were less likely to have a LBW infant (Zimmer-Gembeck & Helfand, 1996). Field *et al* (1985) gave mothers video and verbal feedback during ultrasound scans. The women enjoyed the sessions, anxiety symptoms were reduced and fetal movements reduced. Infants of primiparous mothers appeared to have better outcomes, but there were no biological markers to support the hypothesis that reducing anxiety was causal, and the women did not have anxiety disorders.

# Obsessive–compulsive disorder

Women with pre-existing obsessive–compulsive disorder (OCD) may find that their symptoms worsen during pregnancy, as did 29% of a retrospective study of 57 women (Williams & Koren, 1997). Four women reported symptom improvement during pregnancy, but two of these had postpartum relapses. Miscarriage can also precipitate recurrences (Geller *et al*, 2001). Uguz and colleagues (2007) found a prevalence of 3.5% in the third trimester, and only two of the women had had pregnancy onsets. In the other 13, almost half reported pre-existing symptoms worsening, and 23% found that their symptoms decreased. The most common obsessions were contamination and symmetry/exactness, with cleaning/washing and checking the most common compulsions.

# Eating disorders

The majority of women with eating disorders are of childbearing age. Study of a large population-based birth cohort has reported prevalence estimates in the 6 months before pregnancy as anorexia nervosa 0.1%, bulimia nervosa 1.0%, binge-eating disorder (BED) 3.3% and eating disorder not otherwise specified purging disorder (EDNOS-P) 0.1%. In early pregnancy, the estimates were bulimia nervosa 0.2%, BED 4.8% and EDNOS-P <0.01%. (Watson *et al*, 2013). A recent UK study reported the prevalence in pregnancy of anorexia nervosa as 0.5%, bulimia nervosa 0.1%, BED 1.8%, purging disorder 0.1% and EDNOS 5.0% (Easter *et al*, 2013).

## Consequences

The literature on the consequences of eating disorders in relation to pregnancy and childbirth is mixed, as there are differing samples and sample sizes, varying study designs and differences in how the findings are interpreted. A comprehensive review is provided by Astrachan-Fletcher *et al* (2008).

Several studies report that symptoms improve during pregnancy (Namir *et al*, 1986; Lemberg & Phillips, 1989; Abraham, 1998; Morgan *et al*, 1999; Rocco *et al*, 2005), although women may relapse again after delivery (Blais *et al*, 2000; Koubaa *et al*, 2005). A large Norwegian study (Knoph *et al*, 2013) observed that although many women had remitted 18 and 36 months postpartum, a substantial proportion persisted with disordered eating. There is a case report of a woman who induced abortion by self-imposed starvation and excessive exercising (Bulik *et al*, 1994).

A large-scale community study found recall of parental mental health problems and early unwanted sexual experiences to be independently associated with laxative use, vomiting and marked concern over shape and weight during pregnancy (Senior *et al*, 2005). Hyperemesis appears to be more common in women with eating disorders (Stewart *et al*, 1987;

Abraham, 1998; Conti *et al*, 1998), although it is not clear whether this is actually the case or whether women with bulimia nervosa merely find this a more acceptable explanation for their behaviour.

Whether the eating disorder is treated or not may make a difference. Carter *et al* (2003) found that women with bulimia nervosa who had recently received treatment for their eating disorder were less symptomatic, in the same year as childbirth and for the year following childbirth, than women who had not had a child. However, women with eating disorders do seem to be at increased risk of having a postnatal depressive episode (Abraham, 1998; Morgan *et al*, 1999; Franko *et al* 2001; Morgan *et al*, 2006), particularly if they also have a past history of depression (Micali *et al*, 2011).

Several studies point to poorer outcomes for women with anorexia nervosa or bulimia nervosa who are symptomatic during pregnancy. They appear to have an elevated rate of termination of pregnancy (Abraham, 1998; Blais *et al*, 2000), preterm delivery and perinatal mortality (Brinch *et al*, 1988; Morgan *et al*, 2006), hyperemesis (Koubaa *et al*, 2005) and gestational diabetes (Morgan *et al*, 2006). Several studies have reported that infants born to women with anorexia nervosa have lower birth weights (see systematic review and meta-analysis by Solmi *et al* (2014)), and these women may also be at greater risk of having a Caesarean section (Abraham, 1998; Franko *et al*, 2001). There is an increased risk of delivering an SGA baby or an infant with a smaller head circumference or microcephaly (Koubaa *et al*, 2005). The rate of miscarriage also appears to be increased (Abraham, 1998; Bulik *et al*, 1999; Morgan *et al*, 2006; Micali *et al*, 2007). However, other studies report good outcomes, e.g. Lemberg & Phillips (1989).

Predictors for a LBW preterm infant include vomiting during pregnancy and low maternal pre-pregnancy weight (Conti *et al*, 1998). Poor fetal growth has been observed during the last trimester in women with anorexia nervosa, but their infants demonstrated accelerated postnatal growth (Treasure & Russell, 1988; Koubaa *et al*, 2013). In the latter study, reduced head circumference persisted and was associated with difficulties in language skills at 5 years of age. Mothers with eating disorders seem to have more difficulty maintaining breastfeeding (Waugh & Bulik, 1999).

Large studies include one of 302 women previously hospitalised with eating disorders and controls recruited from Danish population registers (Sollid *et al*, 2004). The Danish study reported the OR in the eating disorder group for a LBW infant as 2.2, for preterm delivery 1.7 and for SGA 1.8. Anorexic women showed lower pregnancy weight gain; eating disordered women were more likely to be anaemic and to experience hyperemesis. LBW was found in anorexia nervosa only, whereas reduced head circumference occurred in bulimia nervosa and anorexia nervosa. A large UK study (Micali *et al*, 2007) reported higher rates of miscarriage in women with a history of bulimia nervosa (RR = 2.0) and significantly higher risk of LBW in women with anorexia nervosa. There were no differences in rates of preterm delivery. However, a large study of women who had recovered from bulimia nervosa found that they did not have a higher rate of birth complications than the general population (Ekéus *et al*, 2006). Krug *et al* (2013) carried out a systematic review reporting non-significant associations between anorexia nervosa and an increased risk of instrumental delivery and preterm delivery.

There are a number of possible mechanisms for these findings: weight-controlling behaviour by restricting food intake, excessive exercise, vomiting, or using diuretics or laxatives may lead to compromised flow of nutrients via the placenta. Under-nourishment can impair the immune system, which could lead to an increased risk of maternal infection with adverse consequences for the fetus. The use of laxatives and diuretics can lead to metabolic disturbances and may also exert a teratogenic effect.

## Management

There is a great deal of shame and secrecy around eating disorders. Pregnant women may be very reluctant to disclose their problem to health professionals, perhaps because they fear being forced to gain weight (Johnson *et al*, 2001; Lemberg & Phillips, 1989). The following may be a useful guide.

- Any woman booking for antenatal care with a body mass index of 19 or less requires further evaluation.

- In anorexia nervosa there may be:
  - hypotension
  - bradycardia
  - intolerance of cold
  - carotenaemia
  - dry skin, brittle hair or lanugo.

- Women with bulimia nervosa may be of normal weight, but self-induced vomiting may cause:
  - oral mucosa damage and dental erosion
  - calluses or abrasions on knuckles (Russell's sign)
  - parotid gland enlargement.

- Laxative or diuretic misuse may lead to:
  - abdominal cramps or diarrhoea
  - metabolic disturbances.

The Eating Disorders Examination (Cooper *et al*, 1989) is too time-consuming for routine clinical use, but questions from it may be used as screening questions. The use of simple questions to detect bulimia nervosa in a primary care setting has been demonstrated: 'Are you satisfied with your eating patterns?' and 'Do you eat in secret?' have been by found to have high specificity and sensitivity in differentiating women with bulimia nervosa from controls (Freund *et al*, 1993). Franko & Spurrell (2000) suggest three warning signs that merit further assessment:

- lack of weight gain over two consecutive visits in the second trimester
- history of an eating disorder
- hyperemesis gravidarum.

Caring for pregnant women with an eating disorder requires a team approach, with regular communication between maternity services, dieticians and mental health professionals. More frequent monitoring will be required during pregnancy. Maternity staff may need to be made aware of the lengths women with eating disorders may go to in order to conceal their true weight when being weighed and take care that this is done in scanty clothing, with nothing in their pockets and, if possible, without them having had the opportunity to 'tank up' by drinking excessive amounts of water before being weighed. However, a critical manner must be avoided. Give information but avoid scare tactics. Systematic enquiry about self-induced vomiting, use of laxatives, diuretics and diet pills and the frequency of these must be carried out. For some women, a desire to protect the fetus can prove motivating, help in improving eating and reduce restricting or other behaviours.

However, pregnancy-related improvement may not persist into the postnatal period. Close postpartum surveillance is required, with attention to eating disorder symptoms and mood owing to the increased likelihood of depression. Video feedback during mealtimes focusing on mother–infant interaction has been shown in a randomised controlled trial to reduce mealtime conflict and increase infant autonomy in mother–infant pairs where the mother suffers from bulimia (Stein *et al*, 2006).

## Assessment and admission of mothers

When an adult requires a mental health assessment (perhaps after self-harm), input from a crisis or home treatment team or admission to hospital, determining whether or not she or he has parental responsibility and the whereabouts of any children is an essential part of the assessment. Whether or not other agencies are involved and whether children are known to social services or are on a Child Protection Plan should be established. Local social services (and out of working hours the Emergency Duty Team) can provide this information if you have the child's full name and date of birth.

The Code of Practice for the Mental Health Act 1983 (Department of Health, 2008) states that if parent and child are separated by admission, the hospital should have a policy about visiting, and children should only visit if, after review, this is deemed to be in their best interests and is safe. If a woman has no partner and no other carer for her child or children, then short-term fostering may be required. Relevant professionals should be involved in care plan reviews and discharge planning. This might include maternity staff if the woman is pregnant, a health visitor if there are children under the age of five, and social services if they are involved.

# Assessing parenting capacity in serious mental illness

Chapter 6 outlines the ways in which parental mental disorder might pose a risk to infants and children. Adult psychiatrists may be asked to provide an opinion regarding the parenting capacity of a woman with severe mental illness, most often for social services or the family law courts. Health professionals must remain aware that a child or children's well-being is paramount and the challenge is to be able to safeguard this while maintaining a therapeutic relationship with their patient (the parent, most often the mother), which includes an awareness of and advocacy for their rights. Other professionals, focusing their attention on the child's needs and parent–child relationships – and perhaps observation of interaction, possible risks and family functioning, including the capacity for change – will need to be apprised of the mother's diagnosis, current treatment and prognosis.

In recent years, some mother and baby units have begun to undertake planned parenting assessments of women with serious mental illness funded by social services. Approximately 50% of such women admitted for such assessments go home without their babies or are subject to social services supervision (Kumar *et al*, 1995; Howard *et al*, 2003), whereas only 12% of mothers admitted with an acute illness require supervision on discharge.

Poor outcomes are associated with a diagnosis of schizophrenia, behavioural disturbance, low social class, psychiatric illness in the woman's partner, a poor relationship with partner (Howard *et al*, 2003; Salmon *et al*, 2003) and single marital status, (Howard *et al*, 2003). The latter study found that the diagnoses most strongly associated with social services supervision on discharge were schizophrenia and personality disorder. Only half of women with schizophrenia are judged as having good parenting outcomes by staff. However, those of higher social class with a mentally well partner and supportive relationships are judged to do better (Abel *et al*, 2005). Legal status on admission and duration of admission do not influence outcome. Mowry & Lennon (1998), studying an Australian sample, found the only predictor of someone other than the mother caring for the baby on discharge was 'maternal hostility' rather than diagnosis or any sociodemographic variable.

Assessing parenting skills involves not only considering the mother's mental illness and the impact it has on her ability to care for and nurture her child, but also the presence or absence of physical illness or disability and substance misuse. The social and physical environment the mother and infant are located in, the presence or absence of a partner, and any difficulties they might have are highly relevant (Nair & Morrison, 2000).

All assessments should be systematic and follow the guidance in the *Framework for Assessing Children in Need and their Families* (Department of Health, 2000). Such assessments should be multidisciplinary and involve direct observation of the mother and infant, plus medical and psychiatric assessment of the parents, occupational therapy assessment of daily living skills, assessment of the social setting, relationships and supports in the family and wider networks, and paediatric assessment of any medical or developmental problems the infant might have.

Referrals for parenting assessments can be triggered by potential risks or follow an incident. Ideally, the possibility of parenting problems should be considered when a woman with serious mental health problems becomes pregnant, so that pre-birth planning can take place – and, if necessary, a child protection case conference can be held and/or referral can be made for residential assessment – as early as possible. Women referred to one UK centre waited on average 6 months for admission (Seneviratne et al, 2003).

## Interventions

There are numerous parenting programmes targeted at the general population or 'at risk' groups such as the socially disadvantaged, but these are unlikely to meet the specific needs of mothers with serious mental illness. There are service descriptions in the literature (reviewed by Craig, 2004) but few outcome data. Brunette & Dean (2002) reviewed seven studies of nurse home visitation models that they thought might be relevant to mothers with serious mental illness. These involved four components: a supportive home visitor; education and training about child development and in parenting skills; modelling and feedback; and links to other services and supports. Longer-term interventions appear to be more successful than those delivered in less than a year. Phelan et al (2006) describe their 'Parenting and Mental Illness Group' programme, which is open to parents of children aged 2–10 years and consists of a 6-week group intervention followed by 4 weekly, individual home visits. The group sessions include:

- positive parenting and the causes of child behaviour problems
- mental health and parenting
- developing positive relationships with children
- promoting children's development
- managing misbehaviour
- implementing routines and strategies.

Two-thirds of the parents (the majority were female) who started the programme completed it, and positive outcomes in children's behaviour and positive parenting were reported by the evaluation. The participants viewed the intervention favourably. Further work is needed to establish how to replicate this in other settings and populations.

## Conclusion

There are many obstacles to good outcomes for mother and infant if the mother suffers from an enduring or recurrent mental illness or learning disability. We have shown in this chapter that proactive management and multidisciplinary and multi-agency working, with an appreciation of the reproductive and parenting needs of women with mental disorder, can reduce the impact of these obstacles.

# References

Abel KM, Webb RT, Salmon MP, et al (2005) Prevalence and predictors of parenting outcomes in a cohort of mothers with schizophrenia admitted for joint mother and baby psychiatric care in England. *Journal of Clinical Psychiatry*, **66**: 781–789.

Abraham S (1998) Sexuality and reproduction in bulimia nervosa patients over 10 years. *Journal of Psychosomatic Research*, **44**: 491–502.

Ahuja N, Moorhead S, Lloyd AJ, et al (2008a) Antipsychotic-induced hyperprolactinemia and delusion of pregnancy. *Psychosomatics*, **49**: 163–167.

Ahuja N, Vasudev K, Lloyd A (2008b) Hyperprolactinemia and delusion of pregnancy. *Psychopathology*, **41**: 65–68.

Akdeniz F, Vahip S, Pirildar S, et al (2003) Risk factors associated with childbearing-related episodes in women with bipolar disorder. *Psychopathology*, **36**: 234–238.

Altshuler L, Richards M, Yonklers K (2003) Treating bipolar disorders during pregnancy. *Current Psychiatry*, **2**: 14–26.

Astrachan-Fletcher E, Veldhus C, Lively N, et al (2008) The reciprocal effects of eating disorders and the postpartum period: a review of the literature and recommendations for clinical care. *Journal of Women's Health*, **17**: 227–239.

Bandelow B, Sojka F, Broocks A, et al (2006) Panic disorder during pregnancy and postpartum period. *European Psychiatry*, **21**: 495–500.

Bánhidy F, Ács N, Puhó E, et al (2006) Association between maternal panic disorders and pregnancy complications and delivery outcomes. *European Journal of Obstetrics & Gynecology and Reproductive Biology*, **124**: 47–52.

Battle CL, Weinstock LM, Howard M (2014) Clinical correlates of perinatal bipolar disorder in an interdisciplinary obstetrical setting. *Journal of Affective Disorders*, **158**: 97–100.

Bennedson BE, Mortensen PB, Olesen AV et al (1999) Preterm birth and intrauterine growth retardation among children of women with schizophrenia. *British Journal of Psychiatry*, **175**: 239–245.

Bennedson BE, Mortensen PB, Olesen AV et al (2001) Congenital malformations, stillbirths and infant deaths among children of women with schizophrenia. *Archives of General Psychiatry*, **58**: 674–679.

Berle JÃ, Mykletun A, Daltveit AK, et al (2005) Neonatal outcomes in offspring of women with anxiety and depression during pregnancy. *Archives of Women's Mental Health*, **8**: 181–189.

Blais MA, Becker AE, Burwell RA, et al (2000) Pregnancy: outcome and impact on symptomatology in a cohort of eating-disordered women. *International Journal of Eating Disorders*, **27**: 140–149.

Blehar MC, DePaulo Jr JR, Gershon ES, et al (1998) Women with bipolar disorder: findings from the NIMH Genetics Initiative sample. *Psychopharmacology Bulletin*, **34**: 239–243.

Brinch M, Isager T, Tolstrup K (1988) Anorexia nervosa and motherhood: reproduction pattern and mothering behaviour of 50 women. *Acta Psychiatrica Scandinavica*, **77**: 611–617.

Brockington I (1996) *Motherhood and Mental Health*. Oxford University Press.

Brunette MF, Dean W (2002) Community mental health care for women with severe mental illness who are parents. *Mental Health Journal*, **38**: 153–165.

Bulik CM, Carter FA, Sullivan PF (1994) Self-induced abortion in a bulimic woman. *International Journal of Eating Disorders*, **15**: 297–299.

Bulik CM, Sullivan PF, Fear JL, et al (1999) Fertility and reproduction in women with anorexia nervosa: a controlled study. *Journal of Clinical Psychiatry*, **60**: 130–135.

Bundy H, Stahl D, MacCabe JH (2011) A systematic review and meta-analysis of the fertility of patients with schizophrenia and their unaffected relatives. *Acta Psychiatrica Scandinavica*, **123**: 98–106.

Carter FA, McIntosh VV, Joyce PR, *et al* (2003) Bulimia nervosa, childbirth, and psychopathology. *Journal of Psychosomatic Research*, **55**: 357–361.

Centre for Maternal and Child Enquiries (2011) Saving Mothers' Lives: reviewing maternal deaths to make motherhood safer: 2006–2008. *BJOG*, **118** (Suppl 1): 132–142.

Cohen LS, Sichel DA, Dimmock JA, *et al* (1994) Postpartum course in women with preexisting panic disorder. *Journal of Clinical Psychiatry*, **55**: 289–292.

Cohen L, Sichel D, Robertson L, *et al* (1995) Postpartum prophylaxis for women with bipolar disorder. *American Journal of Psychiatry*, **152**: 1641–1645.

Cohen LS, Sichel DA, Faraone SV, *et al* (1996) Course of panic disorder during pregnancy and the puerperium: a preliminary study. *Biological Psychiatry*, **39**: 950–954.

Conti J, Abraham S, Taylor A (1998) Eating behavior and pregnancy outcome. *Journal of Psychosomatic Research*, **44**: 465–477.

Cooper Z, Cooper P, Fairburn C (1989) The validity of the eating disorders examination and its subscales. *British Journal of Psychiatry*, **154**: 807–812.

Craig E (2004) Parenting programmes for women with mental illness who have young children: a review. *Australian and New Zealand Journal of Psychiatry*, **38**: 923–938.

Crandon AJ (1979) Maternal anxiety and obstetric complications. *Journal of Psychosomatic Research*, **23**: 109–111.

Curran S, Nelson TE, Rodgers RJ (1995) Resolution of panic disorder on pregnancy. *Irish Journal of Psychological Medicine*, **12**: 107–108.

Dannon PN, Iancu I, Lowengrub K, *et al* (2006) Recurrence of panic disorder during pregnancy: a 7-year naturalistic follow-up study. *Clinical Neuropharmacology*, **29**: 132–137.

Davies A, McIvor RJ, Kumar RC (1995) Impact of childbirth on a series of schizophrenic mothers: a comment on the possible influence of oestrogen on schizophrenia. *Schizophrenia Research*, **16**: 25–31.

Department of Health (2000) *Framework for Assessing Children in Need and their Families*. TSO (The Stationery Office).

Department of Health (2008) *The Code of Practice for the Mental Health Act 1983*. TSO (The Stationery Office).

Di Florio A, Forty L, Gordon-Smith K, *et al* (2013) Perinatal episodes across the mood disorder spectrum. *JAMA Psychiatry*, **70**: 168–175.

Ding XX, Wu YL, Xu SJ, *et al* (2014) Maternal anxiety during pregnancy and adverse birth outcomes: a systematic review and meta-analysis of cohort studies. *Journal of Affective Disorders*, **159**: 103–110.

Dipple H, Smith S, Andrews H, *et al* (2002) The experience of motherhood in women with severe and enduring mental illness. *Social Psychiatry and Psychiatric Epidemiology*, **37**: 336–340.

Easter A, Bye A, Taborelli E, *et al* (2013) Recognising the symptoms: how common are eating disorders in pregnancy? *European Eating Disorders Review*, **21**: 340–344.

Ekéus C, Lindberg L, Lindblad F, *et al* (2006) Birth outcomes and pregnancy complications in women with a history of anorexia nervosa. *BJOG*, **113**: 925–929.

Field T, Sandberg D, Quetel TA, *et al* (1985) Effects of ultrasound feedback on pregnancy anxiety, fetal activity, and neonatal outcome. *Obstetrics & Gynecology*, **66**: 525–528.

Franko DL, Spurrell EB (2000) Detection and management of eating disorders during pregnancy. *Obstetrics & Gynecology*, **95**: 942–946.

Franko DL, Blais MA, Becker E, *et al* (2001) Pregnancy complications and neonatal outcomes in women with eating disorders. *American Journal of Psychiatry*, **158**: 1461–1466.

Freeman MP, Gracious BL, Wisner KL (2002a) Pregnancy outcomes in schizophrenia. *American Journal of Psychiatry*, **159**: 1609.

Freeman MP, Smith KW, Freeman SA, *et al* (2002b) The impact of reproductive events on the course of bipolar disorder in women. *Journal of Clinical Psychiatry*, **63**: 284–287.

Freund KM, Graham SM, Lesky LG (1993) Detection of bulimia in a primary care setting. *Journal of General and Internal Medicine*, **8**: 236–242.

Geller PA, Klier CM, Neugebauer R (2001) Anxiety disorders following miscarriage. *Journal of Clinical Psychiatry*, **62**: 432–438.

Gold KJ, Dalton VK, Schenk TL, *et al* (2007) What causes pregnancy loss? Preexisting mental illness as an independent risk factor. *General Hospital Psychiatry*, **29**: 207–213.

Grimm ER, Venet WR (1966) The relationship of emotional attitudes to the course and outcome of pregnancy. *Psychosomatic Medicine*, **28**: 34–49.

Grof P, Robbins W, Alda M, *et al* (2000) Protective effect of pregnancy in women with lithium-responsive bipolar disorder. *Journal of Affective Disorders*, **61**: 31–39.

Guler O, Koken GN, Emul M, *et al* (2008) Course of panic disorder during the early postpartum period: a prospective analysis. *Comprehensive Psychiatry*, **49**: 30–34.

Harlow BL, Vitonis AF, Sparen P, *et al* (2007) Incidence of hospitalization for postpartum psychotic and bipolar episodes in women with and without prior prepregnancy or prenatal psychiatric hospitalizations. *Archives of General Psychiatry*, **64**: 42–48.

Hendrick VC, Altshuler LL (1997) Management of breakthrough panic disorder symptoms during pregnancy. *Journal of Clinical Psychopharmacology*, **17**: 228–229.

Henriksson KM, McNeil TF (2004) Health and development in the first 4 years of life in offspring of women with schizophrenia and affective psychoses: Well-Baby Clinic information. *Schizophrenia Research*, **70**: 39–48.

Hertzberg T, Wahlbeck K (1999) The impact of pregnancy and puerperium on panic disorder: a review. *Journal of Psychosomatic Obstetrics & Gynaecology*, **20**: 59–64.

Hizkiyahu R, Levy A, Sheiner E (2010) Pregnancy outcome of patients with schizophrenia. *American Journal of Perinatology*, **27**: 19–23.

HM Government (2015a) *Working Together to Safeguard Children: a guide to inter-agency working to safeguard and promote the welfare of children.* Department for Education.

HM Government (2015b) *What to do if you're worried a child is being abused.* Department for Education.

Howard LM (2005) *Fertility and pregnancy in women with psychotic disorders.* European Journal of Obstetrics & Gynecology and Reproductive Biology, 119: 3–10.

Howard LM, Kumar R, Thornicroft G (2001) Psychosocial characteristics and needs of mothers with psychotic disorders. *British Journal of Psychiatry*, **178**: 427–432.

Howard L, Shah N, Salmon M, *et al* (2003) Predictors of social services supervision of babies of mothers with mental illness after admission to a psychiatric mother and baby unit. *Social Psychiatry and Psychiatric Epidemiology*, **38**: 450–455.

Howard LM, Goss C, Leese M *et al* (2004) The psychosocial outcome of pregnancy in women with psychotic disorders. *Schizophrenia Research*, **71**: 49–60.

Hrdlička M (1998) Delusion of maternity. *Psychopathology*, **31**: 270–273.

Hunt N, Silverstone T (1995) Does puerperal illness distinguish a subgroup of bipolar patients? *Journal of Affective Disorders*, **34**: 101–107.

Jablensky AV, Morgan V, Zubrick SR, *et al* (2005) Pregnancy, delivery, and neonatal complications in a population cohort of women with schizophrenia and major affective disorders. *American Journal of Psychiatry*, **162**: 79–91.

Johnson JG, Spitzer RL, Williams JBW (2001) Health problems, impairment and illnesses associated with bulimia nervosa and binge-eating disorder among primary care and obstetric gynecology patients. *Psychological Medicine*, **31**: 1455–1466.

Jones I, Craddock N (2001) Familiality of the puerperal trigger in bipolar disorder: results of a family study. *American Journal of Psychiatry*, **158**: 913–917.

Judd F, Komiti A, Sheehan P, *et al* (2014) Adverse obstetric and neonatal outcomes in women with severe mental illness: to what extent can they be prevented? *Schizophrenia Research*, **157**: 305–309.

Kaplan PW (2004) Reproductive health effects and teratogenicity of antiepileptic drugs. *Neurology*, **63**: S13–S23.

Kendell RE, Chalmers JC, Platz C (1987) Epidemiology of puerperal psychoses. *British Journal of Psychiatry*, **150**: 662–673.

King Hele SA, Abel KM, Webb RT, *et al* (2007) Risk of sudden infant death syndrome with parental mental illness. *Archives of General Psychiatry*, **64**: 1323–1330.

Kjaer D, Horvath-Puho E, Christensen J, *et al* (2008) Antiepileptic drug use, folic acid supplementation, and congenital abnormalities: a population-based case-control study. *BJOG*, **115**: 98–103.

Knoph C, von Holle A, Zerwas S, *et al* (2013) Course and predictors of maternal eating disorders in the postpartum period. *International Journal of Eating Disorders*, **46**: 355–368.

Koren G, Cohn T, Chitayat D, *et al* (2002) Use of atypical antipsychotics during pregnancy and the risk of neural tube defects in infants. *American Journal of Psychiatry*, **159**: 136–137.

Kornischka J, Schneider F (2003) Delusion of pregnancy. A case report and review of the literature. *Psychopathology*, **36**: 276–278.

Koubaa S, Hällström T, Lindholm C, *et al* (2005) Pregnancy and neonatal outcomes in women with eating disorders. *Obstetrics & Gynecology*, **105**: 255–260.

Koubaa S, Hällström T, Hagenäs L, *et al* (2013) Retarded head growth and neurocognitive development in infants of mothers with a history of eating disorders. *BJOG*, **120**: 1413–1422.

Krug I, Taborelli E, Sallis H, *et al* (2013) A systematic review of obstetric complications as risk factors for eating disorders and meta-analysis of delivery method and prematurity. *Physiology & Behavior*, **109**: 51–62.

Kumar R, Marks M, Platz C, *et al* (1995) Clinical survey of a psychiatric mother and baby unit: characteristics of 100 consecutive admissions. *Journal of Affective Disorders*, **33**: 11–22.

Laming WH (2003) *The Victoria Climbié Inquiry: Report of an Inquiry by Lord Laming*. TSO (The Stationery Office).

Lemberg R, Phillips J (1989) The impact of pregnancy on anorexia nervosa and bulimia. *International Journal of Eating Disorders*, **8**: 285–295.

Loveland Cook CA, Flick LH, Homan SM, *et al* (2004) Posttraumatic stress disorder in pregnancy: prevalence, risk factors, and treatment. *Obstetrics & Gynecology*, **103**: 710–717.

Maina G, Rosso G, Aguglia A, *et al* (2014) Recurrence rates of bipolar disorder during the postpartum period: a study on 276 medication-free Italian women. *Archives of Women's Mental Health*, **17**: 367–372.

Manoj PN, John JP, Gandhi A, *et al* (2004) Delusion of test-tube pregnancy in a sexually abused girl. *Psychopathology*, **37**: 152–154.

Matevosyan NR (2011) Pregnancy and postpartum specifics in women with schizophrenia: a meta-study. *Archives of Obstetrics and Gynecology*, **283**: 141–147.

McCool WF, Dorn L, Susman E (1994) The relation of cortisol reactivity and anxiety to perinatal outcome in primiparous adolescents. *Research in Nursing and Health*, **17**: 411–420.

McGrath JJ, Hearle J, Lenner J, *et al* (1999) The fertility and fecundity of patients with psychoses. *Acta Psychiatrica Scandinavica*, **99**: 441–446.

McLennan JD, Ganguli R (1999) Family Planning and parenthood needs of women with severe mental illness: clinicians' perspective. *Community Mental Health Journal*, **35**: 369–380.

Micali N, Simonoff E, Treasure J (2007) Risk of major adverse perinatal outcomes in women with eating disorders. *British Journal of Psychiatry*, **190**: 255–259.

Micali N, Simonoff E, Treasure J (2011) Pregnancy and post-partum depression and anxiety in a longitudinal general population cohort: the effect of eating disorders and past depression. *Journal of Affective Disorders*, **131**: 150–157.

Miller LJ (1990) Psychotic denial of pregnancy: phenomenology and clinical management. *Hospital and Community Psychiatry*, **41**: 1233–1237.

Morgan JF, Lacey JH, Sedgwick PM (1999) Impact of pregnancy on bulimia nervosa. *British Journal of Psychiatry*, **174**: 135–140.

Morgan JF, Lacey JH, Chung E (2006) Risk of postnatal depression, miscarriage, and preterm birth in bulimia nervosa: retrospective controlled study. *Psychosomatic Medicine*, **68**: 487–492.

Mowry BJ, Lennon DP (1998) Puerperal psychosis: associated clinical features in a psychiatric hospital mother–baby unit. *Australian & New Zealand Journal of Psychiatry*, **32**: 287–290.

Nair S, Morrison MF (2000) The evaluation of maternal competency. *Psychosomatics*, **41**: 523–530.

Namir S, Melman KN, Yager J (1986) Pregnancy in restrictor-type anorexia nervosa: a study of six women. *International Journal of Eating Disorders*, **5**: 837–845.

Nilsson E, Lichtenstein P, Cnattingius S, *et al* (2002) Women with schizophrenia: pregnancy outcome and infant death among their offspring. *Schizophrenia Research*, **58**: 221–229.

Northcott CJ, Stein MB (1994) Panic disorder in pregnancy. *Journal of Clinical Psychiatry*, **55**: 539–542.

Onoye JM, Shafer LA, Goebert DA, *et al* (2013) Changes in PTSD symptomatology and mental health during pregnancy and postpartum. *Archives of Women's Mental Health*, **16**: 453–463.

Parry B (1989) Reproductive factors affecting the course of affective illness in women. *Psychiatric Clinics of North America*, **12**: 207–219.

Penta E, Lasalvia A (2013) Delusion of pregnancy in a drug-naïve young woman showing hyperprolactinaemia and hypothyroidism: a case report. *General Hospital Psychiatry*, **35**: 679e1–679e3.

Phelan R, Lee L, Howe D, *et al* (2006) Parenting and mental illness: a pilot group programme for parents. *Australasian Psychiatry*, **14**: 399–402.

Power RA, Kyaga S, Uher R, *et al* (2013) Fecundity of patients with schizophrenia, autism, bipolar disorder, depression, anorexia nervosa, or substance abuse vs their unaffected siblings. *JAMA Psychiatry*, **7**: 22–30.

Rambelli C, Montagnani MS, Oppo A, *et al* (2010) Panic disorder as a risk factor for postpartum depression. Results from the Perinatal Depression-Research & Screening Unit (PND-ReScU) study. *Journal of Affective Disorders*, **122**: 139–143.

Reich T, Winokur G (1970) Postpartum psychosis in patients with manic depressive disease. *Journal of Nervous and Mental Disease*, **151**: 60–68.

Robertson E, Jones I, Haque S, *et al* (2005) Risk of puerperal and non-puerperal recurrence of illness following bipolar affective puerperal (post-partum) psychosis. *British Journal of Psychiatry*, **186**: 258–259

Rocco PL, Orbitello B, Perini L, *et al* (2005) Effects of pregnancy on eating attitudes and disorders: a prospective study. *Journal of Psychosomatic Research*, **59**: 175–179.

Rogal SS, Poschman K, Belanger K, *et al* (2007) Effects of posttraumatic stress disorder on pregnancy outcomes. *Journal of Affective Disorders*, **10**: 137–143.

Salmon M, Abel K, Cordingley L, *et al* (2003) Clinical and parenting skills outcomes following joint mother–baby psychiatric admission. *Australian & New Zealand Journal of Psychiatry*, **37**: 556–562.

Sands RG, Koppelman N, Solomon P (2004) Maternal custody status and living arrangements of children of women with severe mental illness. *Health and Social Work*, **29**: 317–325.

Schmitz K, Reif LA (1994) Reducing prenatal risk and improving birth outcomes: the public health nursing role. *Public Health Nursing*, **11**: 174–180.

Seneviratne G, Conroy S, Marks M (2003) Parenting assessment in a psychiatric mother and baby unit. *British Journal of Social Work*, **33**: 535–555.

Seng JS, Oakley DJ, Sampselle CM, *et al* (2001) Posttraumatic stress disorder and pregnancy complications. *Obstetrics & Gynecology*, **97**: 17–22.

Seng JS, Low LK, Sperlich M, *et al* (2011) Post-traumatic stress disorder, child abuse history, birthweight and gestational age: a prospective cohort study. *BJOG*, **118**: 1329–1339.

Senior R, Barnes J, Emberson JR, et al (2005) Early experiences and their relationship to maternal eating disorder symptoms, both lifetime and during pregnancy. British Journal of Psychiatry, 187: 268–273.

Serretti A, Olgiati P, Colombo C (2006) Influence of postpartum onset on the course of mood disorders. BMC Psychiatry, 6: 4.

Shah N, Howard L (2006) Screening for smoking and substance misuse in pregnant women with mental illness. Psychiatric Bulletin, 30: 294–297.

Sharma V, Persad E (1995) Effect of pregnancy on three patients with bipolar disorder. Annals of Clinical Psychiatry, 7: 39–42.

Sharma V, Smith A, Mazmanian D (2006) Olanzapine in the prevention of postpartum psychosis and mood episodes in bipolar disorder. Bipolar Disorders, 8: 400–404.

Shaw JG, Asch SM, Kimmerling R, et al (2014) Posttraumatic stress disorder and risk of spontaneous preterm birth. Obstetrics & Gynecology, 124: 1111–1119.

Sollid CP, Wisborg K, Hjort J, et al. (2004) Eating disorder that was diagnosed before pregnancy and pregnancy outcome. American Journal of Obstetrics & Gynecology, 190: 206–210.

Solmi F, Sallis H, Stahl D, et al (2014) Low birth weight in the offspring of women with anorexia nervosa. Epidemiologic Reviews, 36: 49–56.

Stein A, Woolley H, Senior R, et al (2006) Treating disturbances in the relationship between mothers with bulimic eating disorders and their infants: a randomized, controlled trial of video feedback. American Journal of Psychiatry, 163: 899–906.

Stewart DE, Raskin J, Garfinkel PE, et al (1987) Anorexia nervosa, bulimia, and pregnancy. American Journal of Obstetrics & Gynecology, 157: 1194–1198.

Teixeira JM, Fisk NM, Glover V (1999) Association between maternal anxiety in pregnancy and increased uterine artery resistance index: cohort based study. BMJ, 318: 153–157.

Terp IM, Mortensen PB (1998) Post-partum psychoses. Clinical diagnoses and relative risk of admission after parturition. British Journal of Psychiatry, 172: 521–526.

Treasure JL, Russell GFM (1988) Intrauterine growth and neonatal weight gain in babies of women with anorexia nervosa. BMJ, 296: 1038.

Uguz F, Gezginc K, Zeytini IE, et al (2007) Obsessive-compulsive disorder in pregnant women during the third trimester. Comprehensive Psychiatry, 48: 441–445.

Vigod SN, Kurdyak PA, Dennis CL, et al (2014) Maternal and newborn outcomes among women with schizophrenia: a retrospective population-based cohort study. BJOG, 121: 566–574.

Viguera AC, Cohen LS (1998) The course and management of bipolar disorder during pregnancy. Psychopharmacology Bulletin, 34: 339–346.

Viguera AC, Nonacs R, Cohen LS, et al (2000) Risk of recurrence of bipolar disorder in pregnant and nonpregnant women after discontinuing lithium maintenance. American Journal of Psychiatry, 157: 179–184.

Viguera AC, Cohen LS, Bouffard S, et al (2002a) Reproductive decisions by women with bipolar disorder after prepregnancy psychiatric consultation. The American Journal of Psychiatry, 159: 2102.

Viguera AC, Cohen LS, Baldessarini R, et al (2002b) Managing bipolar disorder during pregnancy: weighing the risks and benefits. Canadian Journal of Psychiatry, 47: 426–436.

Wan M, Moulton S, Abel K (2008) A review of mother–child relational interventions and their usefulness for mothers with schizophrenia. Archives of Women's Mental Health, 11: 171–179.

Watson HJ, von Holle A, Hamer RM, et al (2013) Remission, continuation and incidence of eating disorders during early pregnancy: a validation study in a population-based cohort. Psychological Medicine, 43: 1723–1734.

Waugh E, Bulik CM (1999) Offspring of women with eating disorders. International Journal of Eating Disorders, 25: 171–179.

Webb R, Able K, Pickle A, et al (2005) Mortality in offspring of parents with psychotic disorders: a critical review and meta-analysis. American Journal of Psychiatry, 162: 1045–1056.

Webb RT, Pickels AR, Appleby L, *et al* (2007) Death by unnatural causes during childhood and early adulthood in offspring of psychiatric inpatients. *Archives of General Psychiatry*, **64**: 345–352.

Williams KE, Koran LM (1997) Obsessive-compulsive disorder in pregnancy, the puerperium, and the premenstruum. *Journal of Clinical Psychiatry*, **58**: 330–334.

Wisner KL, Peindl K, Hanusa BH (1994) Symptomatology of affective and psychotic illnesses related to childbearing. *Journal of Affective Disorders*, **30**: 77–87.

Wisner KL, Peindl KS, Hanusa BH (1996) Effects of childbearing on the natural history of panic disorder with comorbid mood disorder. *Journal of Affective Disorders*, **41**: 173–180.

Wisner KL, Hanusa BH, Peindl KS, *et al* (2004) Prevention of postpartum episodes in women with bipolar disorder. *Biological Psychiatry*, **56**: 592–596.

Yoldas Z, Iscan A, Yoldas T, *et al* (1996) A woman who did her own Caesarean section. *Lancet*, **348**: 13.

Yonkers KA, Smith MV, Forray A, *et al* (2014) Pregnant women with post-traumatic stress disorder and risk of preterm birth. *JAMA Psychiatry*, **71**: 897–904.

Zimmer-Gembeck MJ, Helfand M (1996) Low birthweight in a public prenatal care program: behavioral and psychosocial risk factors and psychosocial intervention. *Social Science & Medicine*, **43**:187–197.

# Further reading

Dolman C, Jones I, Howard LM (2013) Pre-conception to parenting: a systematic review and meta-synthesis of the qualitative literature on motherhood for women with severe mental illness. *Archives of Women's Mental Health*, **16**: 173–196.

Ostler T (2008) *Assessment of Parenting Competency in Mothers with Mental Illness*. Brookes.

Reder P, Duncan S, Lucey C (2003) *Studies in the Assessment of Parenting*. Brunner-Routledge.

Sharma V, Pope CJ (2012) Pregnancy and bipolar disorder: a systematic review. *Journal of Clinical Psychiatry*, **73**: 1447–1455.

Solari H, Dickson KE, Miller L (2009) Understanding and treating women with schizophrenia during pregnancy and postpartum. *Canadian Journal of Clinical Pharmacology*, **16**: e23–e32.

Wolfe BE (2005) Reproductive health in women with eating disorders. *Journal of Obstetric, Gynecologic & Neonatal Nursing*, **34**: 255–263.

## *Guidelines and policy*

Refer to the appropriate clinical guidelines for the management of the specific mental disorder in question (www.nice.org.uk; www.sign.ac.uk) and read it in conjunction with this chapter.

- Management of Women with Mental Health Issues in Pregnancy and the Postpartum Period (Good Practice Guide No 14) (www.rcog.org. uk/en/guidelines-research-services/guidelines/good-practice-14).

- Parents as Patients: Supporting the Needs of Patients who are Parents and their Children (CR164) (www.rcpsych.ac.uk/usefulresources/ publications/collegereports/cr/cr164.aspx).

- www.everychildmatters.gov.uk/safeguarding/ has all the latest guidance and policy relating to safeguarding children.

# CHAPTER 5

# Substance misuse

This chapter will address use, misuse and harmful use of, and dependence on drugs (including nicotine) and alcohol in relation to pregnancy, childbirth and the postpartum period. This is particularly pertinent as the number of young women of reproductive age smoking, drinking alcohol and using illicit drugs has increased (Crome & Kumar, 2007). The Confidential Enquiry into Maternal Deaths (CEMD) in the UK from 2011 to 2013 found that 7% of all maternal deaths and 25% of maternal suicides from 2009 to 2013 were in substance misusers (Knight *et al*, 2015).

## Definitions

- 'Harmful use' refers to a pattern of substance use which is causing physical or mental damage to health.
- 'Dependence syndrome' (or 'addiction') refers to substance use where three of the following are present:
  - a strong desire or compulsion to take the substance
  - difficulties in controlling use
  - a withdrawal state if use of the substance ceases, which is relieved by the substance
  - evidence of tolerance
  - neglect of alternative activities
  - persistent use despite adverse consequences.

Women who are dependent on drugs or alcohol are likely to have additional problems arising from the need to maintain their supply and often turn to crime, particularly theft and prostitution, to finance it. Self-neglect is common and leads to undernutrition and neglect of health, well-being and social networks. A chaotic lifestyle often leads to poor antenatal care and late presentations. Women who are experiencing violence from their partner have more severe social and psychiatric problems.

# Screening and assessment

Most pregnancies in substance-misusing women are unplanned. In addition to the direct physical effects of maternal substance misuse on the fetus, it is important to consider the disruption to the process of pregnancy caused by addiction. Screening usually takes place when a woman books for antenatal care. However, women may book late because services may be too difficult to attend owing to their location, or because usual referral procedures (which may rely on general practitioner (GP) initiation) are not possible if a woman does not have a GP, is being moved on from practice to practice every few weeks, or is homeless. Lifestyles can be very chaotic, with multiple competing demands, and women who are substance misusers may perceive services to be judgemental or hostile, and that losing their children may be a risk. Addiction diverts attention away from preparing for the arrival of a child. Substance-misusing women often neglect themselves and do not attend for antenatal care, putting the unborn child at risk.

Hence, specialised services for drug-misusing women have been developed which have easier access and are staffed by non-judgemental staff, who are skilled in the management of substance misuse and can deal with the multiple needs that pregnant substance misusers often have in one consultation, offering easy referral to other services where appropriate.

Detailed questions regarding smoking, alcohol and drug use during pregnancy are more likely to yield accurate reporting than yes/no tickbox-style assessments (Clark *et al*, 1999), although a structured interview is more reliable at detecting cannabis exposure than opiate or cocaine use (Ostrea *et al*, 2001).

If a woman discloses substance misuse, a full assessment of which substance she uses and the pattern of use – how long, by which route, how much the substances cost and how this is financed – is required, in addition to information about a partner if she has one and other supports, including professional agencies she is involved with. If she already has children, their details and information about their care arrangements must be sought, as well as a full social history, including housing, income, debt and benefits, any outstanding charges or prosecutions, and whether or not she is involved in prostitution. As with any other pregnant woman, information regarding the pregnancy – including whether it was planned or unplanned, wanted or unwanted – and her relationship with the expected baby's father should be obtained. An assessment of physical health is required, with particular care devoted to the detection of problems related to drug or alcohol use.

# Nicotine

In the USA and Western Europe, the prevalence of smoking in young women has declined in recent decades, particularly in highly educated women. However, there are variations within Europe, as rates appear to be increasing in the former Eastern bloc countries, and the rates among different ethnic minority communities within countries also vary (Cnattingius, 2004). Women with schizophrenia or an affective psychosis are more likely to smoke during pregnancy than well controls (31% and 24% compared with 12% in controls) (Henriksson & McNeil, 2006).

Estimating the prevalence of smoking during pregnancy can be difficult. Most estimates are based on self-report and, when compared with biochemical markers, it has been found – in most but not all studies – that some women conceal their smoking. Hence, reported prevalences are likely to be underestimates. Recent data from the UK reported that around a quarter (26%) of mothers smoked before or during pregnancy (McAndrew et al, 2012). Rates are lowest in England and highest in Wales. Those who smoke before or during pregnancy tend to be younger, less well educated white women without partners and with no employment outside the home.

Women who stop smoking during pregnancy (54% of smokers) usually cite fears for the health of their baby as the reason. They tend to stop early in pregnancy, but around half will recommence smoking at some point before delivery and most will start again within 6 months afterwards (Colman & Joyce, 2003). Several studies have found that having a partner who also smokes is associated with failure to stop.

It is abundantly clear from the literature that smoking during pregnancy leads to significant adverse outcomes for both mother and infant (Box 5.1). In addition, there are a host of studies reporting other adverse outcomes, such as increased rates of gestational diabetes, Caesarean section (Urato et al, 2005), poor maternal weight gain (Albuquerque et al, 2001), autonomic dysfunction in infants (Browne et al, 2000), bilateral cryptorchidism (Thorup et al, 2006), neonatal excitability and hypertonia (Law et al, 2003), increased blood pressure in early childhood (Blake et al, 2000), a variety of childhood behavioural disorders, and poor school performance. A systematic review including nine studies of nicotine during pregnancy found a greater risk of attention-deficit hyperactivity symptoms in the 4–7-year-old children of mothers who smoked during pregnancy (Linnet et al, 2003), while a systematic review by Williams & Ross (2007) concluded that nicotine exposure is associated with poor academic performance, and heavy use with a diminished IQ. There are also data linking maternal smoking with conduct disorder in late adolescence (Fergusson et al, 1998) and criminal behaviour in adult males (Brennan et al, 1999).

Studies suggesting links between maternal smoking and various childhood cancers have produced conflicting results, as did early studies examining the relationship between smoking and miscarriage. However, a recent systematic review and meta-analysis has reported an increased risk of miscarriage with smoking in pregnancy (Pineless et al, 2014).

A good review of studies on how low-to-moderate exposure to nicotine, alcohol or cannabis relates to inattention, impulsivity, increased externalising behaviour, reduced cognitive functioning and learning and

**Box 5.1 Maternal and infant outcomes following smoking during pregnancy**

*Maternal*
- Placenta previa
- Ectopic pregnancy
- Premature rupture of membranes (Castles *et al*, 1999)
- Miscarriage (Pineless *et al*, 2014)
- Stillbirth (Gold *et al*, 2007)
- Reduced risk of pre-eclampsia (Castles *et al*, 1999; Conde-Aguelo *et al*, 1999)
- Increased risk of pre-eclampsia (Hammoud *et al*, 2005; England & Zhang, 2007)
- Placental abruption (Ananth *et al*, 1999; Castles *et al*, 1999)
- Preterm delivery (Shah *et al*, 2000; Hammoud *et al*, 2005; Raatikainen *et al*, 2007; Malik *et al*, 2008)
- Sudden intrauterine unexplained death (Froen *et al*, 2002)
- Perinatal death (Raatikainen *et al*, 2007)

*Infant*
- Low birth weight (Okah *et al*, 2005; Steyn *et al*, 2006; Malik *et al*, 2008; Murphy *et al*, 2013; Erickson & Arbour, 2012)
- Small for gestational age (Raatikainen *et al*, 2007; Erickson & Arbour, 2012; Murphy *et al* 2013)
- Small head circumference for gestational age (Källen, 2000)
- Craniosynostosis (Hackshaw *et al*, 2011)
- Intrauterine growth retardation (Hammoud *et al*, 2005; Erickson & Arbour, 2012)
- Cardiovascular defects (Hackshaw *et al*, 2011; Lee & Lupo, 2013)
- Facial clefts (Wyszynski *et al*, 1997; Hackshaw *et al*, 2011)
- Digital anomalies (Man & Chang, 2006; Hackshaw *et al*, 2011)
- Parental reports of cyanotic episodes (Ponsonby *et al*, 1997)
- Admitted to hospital for more days over first 5 years of life and greater health costs (Petrou *et al*, 2005)
- Musculoskeletal and limb reduction defects, club foot, eye defects, gastrointestinal defects, gastroschisis, anal atresia, hernia and undescended testes (Hackshaw *et al*, 2011)
- Sudden infant death syndrome (Mitchell, 1995; Blair *et al*, 1996; Froen *et al*, 2002; Chong *et al*, 2004; Smith & White, 2006; Zhang & Wang, 2013)

memory deficits on tasks has been undertaken by Huizink & Mulder (2006). Using a smokeless tobacco alternative to cigarettes (e.g. snuff) is not considered to be safe, as it is associated with adverse outcomes, including preterm delivery and pre-eclampsia (England, *et al*, 2010).

Possible mechanisms for some of these adverse events are suggested by reports of increased resistance in uterine, umbilical and middle cerebral arteries (Albuqueruqe *et al*, 2004) and changes in the placentas of smokers, which might provide a route to impaired fetal growth (Zdravkovic *et al*, 2005). Impaired arousal from sleep and co-sleeping may contribute to the strong relationship between sudden infant death syndrome and maternal smoking (Horne *et al*, 2004; Zhang & Wang, 2013).

## Smoking cessation interventions

Smoking is one of the few potentially modifiable predictors of some of the adverse events described above, and pregnancy is a motivating factor for many women to stop; hence, there have been numerous strategies devised aiming at cessation. These include giving information about the risks, advice to stop, individual or group counselling, more specific therapies sometimes using rewards, peer support, nicotine replacement therapy (NRT) and a host of leaflets, books and computer-based programmes. There have also been public education programmes. Much of the early research on these interventions was conducted in private healthcare settings and therefore could not necessarily be generalised to public healthcare settings. Now, there are more studies in public healthcare and disadvantaged populations. For example, telephone counselling, when compared with usual cessation advice in a publicly funded antenatal clinic with an ethnically diverse population, was superior in achieving cessation (Dornelas et al, 2006); and a randomised controlled trial (RCT) of a tailored leaflet supported with SMS text messaging was superior in achieving cessation in a UK pregnant population (Naughton et al, 2012).

A Cochrane review (Chamberlain et al, 2013) found a significant reduction in smoking following the interventions in the 87 included trials and a reduction in low-birth-weight (LBW) infants and preterm births. Counselling interventions demonstrated a significant effect compared to usual care, and incentive-based interventions had larger effect sizes. Social support appeared effective when provided by peers. Effects were mixed when the smoking cessation support was provided as part of a broader intervention aimed at improving maternal health, rather than as a specific targeted intervention.

However, more than half of all smokers do not manage to stop smoking completely during pregnancy (Schneider et al, 2010), and even if they do, the effects may not persist postpartum (e.g. Lawrence et al, 2005). A Cochrane review of trials of relapse prevention in pregnant and postpartum ex-smokers did not find evidence of effectiveness for any intervention (Hajek et al, 2013).

### Pharmacological interventions

NRT is widely used in smoking cessation, and exposure to nicotine via replacement therapy is less than through continued smoking, although pregnant women metabolise nicotine more quickly. The aim should be to use the lowest effective dose for the shortest possible time and as early in pregnancy as possible. A recent large population study in Denmark found no increase in congenital malformations in the infants of mothers who smoked during pregnancy, but there was a 60% increased risk (relative prevalence ratio 1.61) of malformations (particularly skeletal) in infants of non-smoking mothers using NRT (Morales-Suarez-Varela et al, 2006). A systematic review and meta-analysis of seven trials (six of NRT and one of bupropion) reported that pharmacotherapy had a significant effect on smoking cessation (relative risk (RR) = 1.80, 95 % CI 1.32–2.44) and that most of the adverse effects were minor (Myung et al, 2012). Some more serious adverse events were reported, including preterm birth, small for gestational age (SGA) infants, neonatal intensive care unit (NICU) admission, placental abruption and fetal demise, miscarriage and neonatal death; however, there was no evidence that these were linked to the pharmacotherapy used. There was no significant difference in mean birth weight, gestational age and preterm delivery rates between the intervention and control groups.

A Cochrane review (Coleman et al, 2012) included 6 trials of NRT involving 1745 pregnant smokers. No statistically significant difference was seen for smoking cessation in later pregnancy after using NRT as compared to control (RR = 1.33, CI 0.93–1.91). There were no statistically significant differences in rates of miscarriage, stillbirth, premature birth, LBW, admissions to NICU or neonatal death between the NRT and control groups.

The clinical and cost-effectiveness of bupropion in smoking cessation has been established, and there are studies in pregnant populations (e.g. Miller et al, 2003). However, reported side-effects include seizures; about 0.1% of smokers suffer severe hypersensitivity reactions (e.g. angioedema, dyspnoea/bronchospasm and anaphylactic shock); and a further 3% suffer milder reactions such as rash, urticaria or pruritus. The most common adverse events are insomnia and dry mouth. There are fewer data available on varenicline, although the data that are available include a case report of first-trimester exposure resulting in a normal delivery of a healthy infant (Kaplan et al, 2014) and 23 pregnancy exposures in a New Zealand study (Harrison-Woolrych et al, 2013). The duration of exposure during pregnancy ranged from 1 day to 16 weeks. Adverse outcomes were identified in 5 of 17 live births: one baby had birth asphyxia and recurrent chest infections, one had gastro-oesophageal reflux, one was diagnosed with ankyloglossia and two had feeding difficulties. Therefore, the National Institute for Health and Care Excellence (NICE) currently states that 'neither varenicline or bupropion should be offered to pregnant or breastfeeding women' but advises the use of NRT if smoking cessation without it has failed (NICE, 2010).

### Why are women reluctant to engage in cessation?

Ussher et al (2004) surveyed 206 women who had been identified as smokers at their antenatal booking visit. The majority (87%) said they wanted to stop smoking and expressed a preference for face-to-face behavioural support and self-help materials. Around half were interested in telephone support, half in having an exercise plan and one-third of the total sample in having a 'buddy'. Most preferred individual rather than group appointments, and interest was highest among those in professional or managerial professions and in the heaviest smokers. The same group explored barriers to interventions in a group of 491 pregnant smokers or ex-smokers (Ussher *et al*, 2006). The most frequently endorsed barriers were:

- 'Being afraid of disappointing myself if I failed' (54%)
- not tending to seek help for 'this sort of thing' (41%).

The women did also, however, perceive benefits:

- advice about cravings (71%)
- praise and encouragement about quitting (71%).

An Australian study identified addiction to nicotine, scepticism about the claims of NRT and smoking behaviour of partners as barriers. Some women were concerned about the safety of patches and preferred to continue smoking (Hotham *et al*, 2002). A pilot study of nicotine patches by the same group found low interest in participation and a high withdrawal rate, which the participations attributed to 'too much hassle' and it not being 'a good time to quit' (Hotham *et al*, 2006).

There appears to be a high prevalence of depressive disorders in pregnant women seeking smoking cessation (Blalock *et al*, 2005). Untreated depression may be one factor making it hard for women to stop or increasing the likelihood of relapse if they do stop. Mood should be assessed in those requesting smoking cessation.

### Who should provide the intervention?

Health professionals providing maternity care vary in their attitudes towards smoking cessation and how much they are personally involved. Almost all US obstetrician/gynaecologists surveyed perceived that smoking had negative consequences for the fetus and would ask pregnant patients about smoking when assessing them (Jordan *et al*, 2006). However, only 62% always documented smoking status in the medical record, and 66% always advised their patient to stop smoking. Less than half reported always assessing whether their patients were willing to stop, and only 29% suggested using problem-solving methods for cessation as indicated in national guidelines. Only 2% reported always prescribing NRT, and 6% always provided a referral to a smoking cessation service. In Jordan, a high proportion of obstetricians and gynaecologists are smokers and only 54.3% provide any cessation counselling. Those who do not smoke are more likely to record their patients smoking habits (Amarin, 2005). In the UK, delivery of smoking cessation advice by GPs has increased from 2000 to 2009 and is more likely to be given to younger pregnant women, the most deprived, and those with asthma or other medical comorbidities (Hardy *et al*, 2014).

In many countries, including the UK, midwives have the primary role in maternity care and the most frequent contact with pregnant women. There is documented evidence that interventions given by them can be effective in stopping smoking (e.g. Heggard *et al*, 2003; McLeod *et al*,

2004), and many will agree that it is an important part of the midwife's role. However, the literature indicates that many were reluctant or unable to engage in this work (e.g. Condliffe *et al*, 2005). Possible reasons are lack of time, concern about interfering with the therapeutic relationship, lack of expertise and lack of knowledge (for example, about NRT or where to refer women to for specialist services). Specific training and agreed procedures are likely to be required before staff will regularly deliver smoking cessation interventions. Midwives and doctors appear to respond differently to training; midwives are more likely to take it up and provide more smoking cessation interventions at follow-up (Cooke *et al*, 2001). Health professionals are now required by NICE (2010) to assess smoking at the first antenatal contact and to assess whether a referral to a smoking cessation service has been taken up at subsequent appointments.

# Alcohol

Alcohol has long been recognised to have a detrimental effect on pregnancy and fetal development. One of the earliest studies was that of Lemoine and colleagues (1968), who observed unusual facial characteristics, short stature, frequent malformations and what they referred to as 'psychomotor disturbance' in 127 children of alcoholic parents. Ulleland (1972) reported LBW occurring more frequently in alcoholic mothers than in controls. Jones *et al* (1973) described the morphological features of the children of alcoholic mothers as fetal alcohol syndrome. This is now well documented as the most severe consequence of maternal drinking during pregnancy and occurs in 0.5 to 3 per thousand births (higher in some indigenous populations where heavy drinking occurs). Exposed children may lack the classical triad of poor growth (evidenced by small height and small head size), central nervous system (CNS) disorders (including cognitive deficits) and abnormal facial features (Box 5.2); however, they may exhibit a lifelong condition characterised by distinct facial features, physical health problems affecting the heart, kidneys and bones, intellectual disability, speech and language delay, co-ordination difficulties and behavioural problems known as fetal alcohol spectrum disorder (FASD; Esper & Furtado, 2014).

The probability of FASD depends on the level of alcohol exposure, and there are other associated factors such as advanced maternal age, high gravity and parity, smoking, drug misuse, low socioeconomic status and having a partner with alcohol problems. Alcohol-related neurodevelopmental disorder refers to CNS dysfunction without facial or growth abnormalities. Useful reviews of the disorders and their sequelae include O'Leary (2004), Riley & McGee (2005), Mukherjee *et al* (2006) and Pruett *et al* (2013).

Recent statistics for England show a decrease between 2006 and 2012 both in the proportion of the population consuming more than three units on the heaviest day's drinking in the previous week (from 33 to 28%), and in the proportion drinking more than twice the recommended amount (from

---

**Box 5.2 Diagnostic criteria for fetal alcohol syndrome**

A. Confirmed maternal alcohol exposure

B. Evidence of a characteristic pattern of facial anomalies that includes features such as short palpebral fissures and abnormalities in the premaxillary zone (e.g. flat upper lip, flattened philtrum and flat midface)

C. Evidence of growth retardation, as in at least one of the following:
- low birth weight for gestational age
- decelerating weight over time not owing to nutrition
- disproportional low weight to height

D. Evidence of CNS neurodevelopmental abnormalities, as in at least one of the following:
- decreased cranial size at birth
- structural brain abnormalities (e.g. microcephaly, partial or complete agenesis of the corpus callosum, cerebellar hypoplasia)
- neurological hard or soft signs (as age appropriate) such as impaired fine motor skills, neurosensory hearing loss, poor tandem gait, poor eye–hand coordination

Reproduced with permission from Stratton *et al*, 1996.

---

16 to 13%). Both these proportions have remained the same for the past 2 years (Health and Social Care Information Centre, 2013).

Between a quarter and half of all pregnant women will drink some alcohol while pregnant, with 27% drinking not more than once a month and 15% drinking two to four times per month (Göransson *et al*, 2003). Estimates of the prevalence of drinking above safe limits for pregnancy range from 15.3 to 33.2% (Göransson *et al*, 2003; Houet *et al*, 2005; Alvik *et al*, 2006; Chambers *et al*, 2006), depending on the definition of safe limits used and the population studied.

Data from a large, representative US population study found 2.3% of pregnant women to be alcohol dependent, while 1.3% were defined as misusing alcohol, 16.7% as binge drinking and 38.8% as drinkers without binges (Caetano *et al*, 2006). Other US data indicate that 10% of pregnant women drink and 1.9–4.0% binge drink (Anderson *et al*, 2006). A review (Zelner & Koren, 2013) noted that rates of drinking in pregnancy in Canada and the USA range from 5 to 15% and are declining, but that rates were higher in western Europe, Australia, Russia and Chile.

The NICE guideline on antenatal care for the healthy pregnant woman states:

'Pregnant women and women planning to become pregnant should be advised to avoid drinking alcohol in the first 3 months of pregnancy, because there may be an increased risk of miscarriage. Women should be advised that if they choose to drink alcohol while they are pregnant they should drink no more than 1–2 units once or twice a week [...] women should be advised not to get drunk or binge drink (drinking more than 7.5 units of alcohol on a single occasion) while they are pregnant because this can harm their unborn baby' (NICE, 2008).

A survey of over 4000 pregnant women in the US found that younger, less-well-educated, single and unemployed women were more likely to use alcohol while pregnant, and that those who had a past history of sexual abuse, current or past physical abuse, smoked or used drugs, or lived with or had partners or friends who were substance misusers were at particularly high risk (Leonardson & Loudenberg, 2003). Women who are older (> 30), those who report a history of physical abuse and those who use drugs have also been reported as being more likely to use and misuse alcohol during pregnancy (Haynes *et al*, 2003). Those who misuse alcohol while pregnant are more to smoke, and to smoke heavily (Burns *et al*, 2006*a*).

---

### Box 5.3  Maternal and infant outcomes following alcohol consumption during pregnancy

*Maternal*

- First trimester miscarriage (Kesmodel *et al*, 2002*a*; Rasch, 2003; Henriksen *et al*, 2004; Nielsen *et al*, 2006; Gold *et al*, 2007)
- Seek antenatal care later in pregnancy
- Arrive for delivery unbooked (Burns *et al*, 2006*a*)
- Induction of labour for intrauterine growth retardation or premature rupture of membranes
- Caesarean section for fetal distress
- Epidural pain relief
- General anaesthesia (Burns *et al*, 2006*a*)
- Preterm delivery (Albertsen *et al*, 2004)
- Stillbirth (Kesmodel *et al*, 2002*b*; Gold *et al*, 2007)

*Infant*

- Low birth weight (Burns *et al*, 2006*a*; Mariscal *et al*, 2006)
- Small for gestational age (Whitehead & Lipscomb, 2003; Burns *et al*, 2006*a*)
- Lower Apgar scores (Burns *et al*, 2006*a*)
- Neonatal intensive care admission (Burns *et al*, 2006*a*)
- Congenital anomalies (Baumann *et al*, 2006)
- Orofacial clefts (Munger *et al*,1997)
- Poor visual acuity (Carter *et al*, 2005)
- Early-onset atopic dermatitis (Linneberg *et al*, 2004)
- Greater activity of stress response systems (cortisol, heart rate and affect) (Haley *et al*, 2006)
- Lower scores on MDI of the Bayley Infant Development Scale at 12–13 months (Testa *et al*, 2003)
- Hyperactivity & inattention in girls at 47 months and both genders at 81 months (Sayal *et al*, 2009)
- Deficits in gross & fine motor function (Bay & Kesmodel, 2010)
- Gross motor deficits 0–18 years (Lucas *et al*, 2014)

Alcohol may impair fertility in both men and women and both male and female alcohol intake during the week of conception increase the risk of a miscarriage (Henriksen et al, 2004). Maternal and infant sequelae of drinking during pregnancy are listed in Box 5.3.

Testa et al (2003) undertook a meta-analysis of the effects of fetal alcohol exposure and infant mental development. There appeared to be no effect on 6–8- or 18–24-month-old children, but there was a linear association with scores on the Mental Development Index (MDI) of the Bayley Scales of Infant Development in 12–13-month-old children. There may of course, also be more subtle or specific cognitive effects not detected by global measures like the MDI, and several studies report increased behavioural problems in children exposed in utero. One has identified that binge drinking in early pregnancy, even when not followed by continued drinking, led to children at 7–9 months of age who showed more social disinhibition than the infants of control mothers (Nulman et al, 2004).

For many of the outcomes, there is a dose–response association, with the risk of sequelae increasing with increased alcohol consumption, e.g. for LBW, preterm birth and SGA (Patra et al, 2011). For outcomes such as stillbirth this is related to increased feto-placental dysfunction with increased alcohol intake. It is also related to reduced transfer of essential fatty acids across the placenta to the fetus; these precursors of prostacyclins, prostaglandins, thromboxanes and leukotrienes are important for fetal development (Haggarty et al, 2002). Animal studies have shown that fetal exposure to alcohol increases hypothalamic–pituitary axis activity and impairs immune system functioning (Zhang et al, 2005).

Cognitive deficits in 7-year-old (Burden et al, 2005) and 10-year-old children (Richardson et al, 2002; Wilford et al, 2006) have been found to be related to maternal drinking during pregnancy, but studies which examine the relationship between fetal alcohol exposure and attention-deficit hyperactivity disorder (ADHD) have produced conflicting results (Linnet et al, 2003). A systematic review (Latino-Martel et al, 2010) reported that alcohol intake during pregnancy was associated with childhood acute myeloid leukaemia (odds ratio (OR) = 1.95, CI 1.13–2.15) but not acute lymphoblastic leukaemia.

Young adults whose mothers took part in a large prospective study and who were exposed to one or more binge episodes during fetal life had double the odds of somatoform disorders, substance misuse or dependence, and of paranoid, passive aggressive and antisocial personality disorders (Barr et al, 2006). Drinking during pregnancy is also associated with alcohol disorders in the adult offspring (Alati et al, 2006). Binge drinking, rather than the total amount of exposure, was associated with IQ scores in the intellectual disability range and clinically significant behavioural problems in 7-year-olds (Bailey et al, 2004). Postnatal heavy alcohol consumption is associated with sudden infant death syndrome (Alm et al, 1999).

## Breastfeeding

Alcohol can have effects on the breastfeeding mother and her infant. It diffuses passively into breast milk and within 30–60 min of ingestion reflects levels in maternal blood. The latter is affected by maternal weight, body fat percentage, stomach contents when the alcohol was consumed, the rate at which it was consumed and the strength of the alcoholic drink. Alcohol can suppress lactation via its inhibitory action on oxytocin, and there appears to be a reduction in milk yield in both animals and humans.

Clearly, infants exposed to alcohol via breast milk will absorb it. Human research data on the impact of alcohol on infants' growth, development, sleep–wake cycles and behaviour are limited for ethical reasons, but there is sufficient evidence which, when reviewed systematically, suggests that consumption even within limits regarded as 'safe' for non-lactating women may have adverse effects (Giglia & Binns, 2006).

## Screening and detection

As with smoking, routine antenatal assessment is unlikely to detect all problem drinkers, as women who are drinking may not easily admit to it owing to social pressure, embarrassment or anxiety. An adequate assessment should be undertaken in all pregnant women. There is no laboratory test for chronic, persistent drinking, as blood, urine and breath tests mainly test recent consumption. Although there is interest in developing biomarkers, this remains experimental.

Hence, various brief screening instruments developed for the detection of problem alcohol consumption in other settings could be used in antenatal care settings. A review in 1997 identified CAGE (cut down, annoyed, guilty, eye-opener), the Alcohol Use Disorder Identification Test (AUDIT) and TWEAK (tolerance, worried, eye-opener, amnesia, cut down) as being the optimal questionnaires to use in women, with lower cut-off scores being used than when screening men (Bradley et al, 1998). A modified version of the AUDIT, the AUDIT-C, focuses solely on consumption and asks the following questions.

- During the past 12 months about how often do you drink ANY alcoholic beverage?
- Counting all types of alcohol combined, how many drinks did you usually have on days when you drank during the past 12 months?
- During the past 12 months, about how often did you drink FIVE OR MORE drinks in a single day?

Scores range from 0 to 4 on each question, and the cut-off for identifying problem drinking is 3 or more. This has demonstrated good sensitivity and specificity in US samples of pregnant and non-pregnant women from a variety of racial and ethnic groups. The T-ACE (Box 5.4), a four-item antenatal, self-administered screening questionnaire that asks about

---

**Box 5.4 The T-ACE questionnaire**

T  Tolerance: how many drinks does it take to make you feel high?

A  Annoyed: have people annoyed you by criticising your drinking?

C  Cut down: have you ever felt you ought to cut down on your drinking?

E  Eye-opener: have you ever had a drink first thing in the morning to steady your nerves or get rid of a hangover

---

tolerance to alcohol, being annoyed by other's comments about drinking, attempts to cut down, and having a drink first thing in the morning ('eye-opener') has also been found to outperform clinician questioning about consumption (Chang *et al*, 1998). Burns *et al* (2010) evaluated seven instruments in a systematic review and reported that TWEAK, T-ACE and the AUDIT-C had the highest sensitivity for identifying risky drinking in pregnancy, with CAGE performing less well. NICE (2014) recommends using the AUDIT.

Whether or not a screening questionnaire is used, the actual number of units of alcohol consumed, the drinking pattern, associated problems and presence or absence of dependence should be ascertained. Most women spontaneously reduce or stop drinking once they discover they are pregnant (Tough *et al*, 2006), but others will need help to do so. Those who continue drinking are more likely also to smoke.

## Interventions

Psychosocial interventions with the aim of reducing alcohol intake during pregnancy are usually brief and often based on education and motivational interviewing. They can be a one-off or consist of several contacts, either face-to-face or by telephone, and may involve the use of manuals or workbooks. Interventions involving multiple contacts are more likely to achieve reduction in consumption and can be incorporated into the antenatal care schedule. There is a good evidence base for this approach in women of childbearing age and a growing body of data to support the approach in pregnant women.

Chang *et al* (1999) reported on a RCT of a brief intervention addressing alcohol use during pregnancy. Women in the intervention and control arms received the same assessment. The intervention involved the following.

- Review of general health and pregnancy course to date
- Review of lifestyle changes made since pregnancy
- Participant asked to articulate drinking goals while pregnant
- Participant asked to identify situations and triggers which might lead to drinking.

- Participant asked to identify alternatives to drinking.
- Summary of the session and participant given manual to take home.

Women in both groups reduced their alcohol intake, but there was no significant difference between the groups. Those who were abstinent before assessment were more likely to remain abstinent if they had received the intervention.

Handmaker & Wilbourne (2001) reviewed motivational interviewing in antenatal care settings. They advocated a stepped approach in which women are screened and assessed to determine whether alcohol appears to be a problem. The assessment categorises women into low-risk or high-risk groups, and advice is offered to the low-risk women, whereas those in the high-risk group are offered intervention.

The Protecting the Next Pregnancy project involved intervening with women who identified as drinking during their previous pregnancy. The goal of this approach is to reduce alcohol use during the women's future pregnancies. Following the intervention, these women not only drank significantly less than those in a control group during their later pregnancies, they also had fewer LBW babies and fewer premature deliveries (Hankin & Sokol 1995; Hankin et al, 2000). Moreover, children born to women in the brief intervention group had better neurobehavioural performance at 13 months when compared with control group children (Hankin et al, 2000). Similarly, initial results of an RCT using a motivational intervention in women exposed to alcohol at risk of pregnancy were promising, although follow-up was only for 1 month (Ingersoll et al, 2004). There is also evidence for the efficacy of cognitive–behavioural therapy (Peterson & Lowe, 1992).

As women with alcohol problems are likely to face other difficulties such as trauma and abuse, and to smoke and suffer from depression or anxiety, there is a need for interventions aimed at reducing alcohol intake to be integrated with other health and social care strategies.

## Detoxification

If a pregnant woman with alcohol dependence has to be withdrawn from alcohol, it must be remembered that the fetus will also be withdrawing. The British Association for Psychopharmacology (Lingford-Hughes et al, 2012) advise that if withdrawal symptoms are present, a short reducing course of diazepam (or chlordiazepoxide) will prevent maternal convulsions, which carry a great risk of fetal anoxia. For example, an initial dose of 10 mg diazepam 3 times daily may be reduced by 5 mg each day, rotating the dose to be reduced. Vitamin replacement should also be given. Withdrawal should be carried out in parallel with the interventions described above, under close medical supervision and preferably as an in-patient.

There are no safety data for the use of acamprosate or naltrexone, and very little on disulfiram in pregnant or lactating women. These drugs should be avoided and the focus should be on psychosocial interventions.

# Drug misuse and dependence

## Prevalence

Sherwood et al (1999) demonstrated by testing urine samples positive for pregnancy in a UK inner-city population that around 16% of pregnant women had taken one or more illicit substances, with cannabis accounting for the majority. Meconium sampling revealed 7.9% positive for drugs (mostly opiates and cocaine) in a study carried out in Barcelona, Spain (Pichini et al, 2005). In a nationally representative sample of pregnant women surveyed in the US, 2.8% reported that they had used drugs in the past month, the most commonly used being cannabis (Ebrahim & Gfroerer, 2003), whereas when the drug and alcohol CAGE questionnaires were used to screen pregnant women, 6% scored positive for drug use in the year before they knew they were pregnant (Kelly et al, 2001).

Cannabis is the most common illicit drug in use by women, with 57% of young Australian women reporting ever having used it, 17% using it currently and 31% using it in addition to other drugs (Turner et al, 2003). More than 12000 pregnant women in the Avon Longitudinal Study of Pregnancy and Childhood (ALSPAC) were asked whether they consumed cannabis before and during pregnancy. Five per cent reported doing so, and were also more likely to smoke and to use alcohol and other drugs (Fergusson et al, 2002).

The incidence of methamphetamine use has risen in the past two decades in the UK and USA, and this inevitably raises concerns regarding pregnancy exposures. A USA study estimated that 5.2% of women used methamphetamine at some point during their pregnancy, often in addition to alcohol and tobacco (Arria et al, 2006).

Volatile substances or solvents are a wide group of substances that can be sniffed or ingested orally and which cause CNS stimulation and disinhibitions similar to those seen with alcohol. Volatile substance misuse is commonly referred to as 'glue sniffing' and has been problematic in the UK since the 1980s. Substances misused in this way are often easily accessible and cheap. They include deodorant, antifreeze, pain relief, air freshener and hairspray aerosols; as well as cigarette lighter fuel, gas for mobile homes (butane or propane) and petrol (more commonly used in the US and in indigenous populations in Australia where alternatives are less easily available). Adhesives containing toluene are responsible for most of the UK deaths due to volatile substance misuse. Fire extinguishers, typewriter correction fluid, solvents and degreasing agents also have all been implicated in deaths. Less often used are alkyl nitrites and volatile anaesthetic drugs or propellants.

Most drug-using women come from disadvantaged backgrounds. Polydrug use is common, as is alcohol use, smoking and mental illness such as depression, anxiety and post-traumatic stress disorder. Lifetime and current rates of physical, emotional and sexual abuse are high (Horrigan et *al*, 2000; Velez *et al*, 2006), and poor nutrition and infection are common, all of which have an adverse effect on the pregnancy and fetus.

# Pregnancy and infant outcomes

It is clear that several adverse outcomes are associated with illicit drug use during pregnancy (Table 5.1), and drug use which continues into the postpartum leads to worse developmental outcomes in infants (Schuler *et al*, 2003). However, it is extremely difficult, if not impossible, to isolate specific drug effects from the multiple risk factors to which pregnant drug users and their infants are exposed, including stress, poor nutrition and deprivation.

Women who are homeless and misuse substances are particularly vulnerable. A Canadian study identified that being homeless was associated with an OR of 2.9 for preterm delivery, 6.9 for having a LBW infant and 3.3 for having an infant SGA. The odds were increased if the woman was both homeless and a substance misuser (Little *et al*, 2005).

The neonatal abstinence syndrome (NAS) consists of:

- gastrointestinal disturbances
- high-pitched cry
- irritability
- hyperactivity and hyperreflexia
- feeding and sleeping disturbances
- autonomic hyperactivity
- seizures (rarely).

**Table 5.1 Adverse outcomes associated with pregnancy exposure to illicit drugs**

| Outcome | Odds ratio[1] |
|---|---|
| Placental abruption | 2.53 |
| Antepartum haemorrhage | 1.41 |
| Preterm birth | 2.63 |
| Small for gestational age | 1.79 |
| Congenital anomalies | 1.52 |
| Neonatal nursery care >7 days | 4.07 |
| Stillbirth | 2.54 |
| Neonatal death | 2.92 |
| Polyhydramnios | 28.6% *v.* 3.9%*[2] |

*$P<0.005$.
1. Kennare *et al*, 2005.
2. Panting-Kemp *et al*, 2002.

The timing of NAS onset depends on the drug. Alcohol withdrawal can start within 2 days of birth, heroin within 48–72 h, and methadone around 7–14 days as it has a longer half-life.

## Opiates

Opiate use during pregnancy increases the risk of neonatal mortality, with a relative risk of 3.27 for heroin and 6.37 for methadone when used together, although risks approach unity if either drug is considered in isolation (Hulse *et al*, 1998*a*). There is also an increased risk of antepartum haemorrhage (OR = 2.33) (Hulse *et al*, 1998*b*) and a decrease in birth weight with heroin compared to methadone (RR = 4.61) (Hulse *et al*, 1997*a*). Preterm delivery also seems to be more likely. However, confounding variables are likely to be responsible for at least some of these effects.

## Stimulants

### Amphetamines

Amphetamines are CNS stimulants that can be injected, snorted or ingested orally. Some women use them to control weight. There is no evidence that they are linked with an increase in congenital anomalies, but there are reports of a withdrawal syndrome in exposed infants. An expert panel concluded that although animal studies showed some evidence of developmental toxicity in rats, there are insufficient data in humans. However, the animal work raises concern about the neurobehavioural consequences of prenatal exposure to amphetamines (Golub *et al*, 2005).

### Methamphetamine and methylenedioxymethamphetamine

Methamphetamine can be taken orally, snorted or – in the crystal form (crystal meth) – smoked or injected. A systematic review of 10 studies of infants exposed *in utero* to methamphetamine reported increased risks of preterm birth, LBW and SGA (Ladhani *et al* 2011). This might be due to the vasoconstrictive effect of amphetamines, appetite suppression in the mother or the cluster of risks factors associated with methamphetamine use, such as being young, single and misusing alcohol, tobacco and other drugs. There are also reports of a possible association with ventricular septal defect (Bateman *et al*, 2004). A study of children exposed *in utero* to methamphetamine reported poorer performance on the Personal-Social Ability Subscale and on the Hand and Eye Co-ordination Subscale of the Griffiths Mental Developmental Scales (van Dyk *et al*, 2014), and a study of children exposed to methylenedioxymethamphetamine (MDMA; also known as ecstasy) reported a dose-dependent increased risk of poorer mental and motor development at 12 months (Singer *et al*, 2012).

The use of amphetamines during pregnancy and lactation and the effect on the infant has been reviewed by Oei *et al* (2012).

## Cocaine

A systematic review controlling for confounders appeared to rebut the notion that cocaine is associated with any specific adverse developmental outcomes that cannot be accounted for by other risk factors (Frank *et al*, 2001), but other meta-analyses have confirmed an association with premature rupture of membranes and abruptio placentae (Hulse *et al*, 1997b; Addis *et al*, 2001) and with preterm birth and LBW (Gouin *et al*, 2011). A prospective controlled study confirmed no effect on full-scale, verbal or performance IQ but found an increased risk of specific cognitive impairments (Singer *et al*, 2004). Cone-Wesson (2005) reviewed the literature relating to children's speech and hearing, in addition to cognition. She concluded that exposed children might be liable to language delay or disorder – although cocaine did not appear to increase the risk of sensorineural hearing impairment – but that newborns at least might have some central auditory processing problems. However, LBW cocaine-exposed infants seem to be at risk of poorer developmental outcomes (Frank *et al*, 2002), and mothers who smoke in addition to using cocaine might be particularly liable to having growth-retarded infants. Impairment of growth appears to persist into later childhood, and the effect is more marked in children born to mothers over the age of 30 (Covington *et al*, 2002).

Cocaine intoxication can cause cardiac dysrhythmias and ischaemia, and its toxic effects are enhanced by pregnancy. Hence, there must be a high index of suspicion in any woman known to be using cocaine, as toxicity can mimic pregnancy-induced hypertension. Studies have linked cocaine with thrombocytopenia, which can lead to excessive bleeding (e.g. Kain *et al*, 1995), although a more recent case–control study disputed this (Miller & Nolan, 2001).

Infants exposed to cocaine *in utero* have been reported to exhibit more central and autonomic nervous system symptoms, high-pitched cries, irritability, excessive suck, hyper-alertness and autonomic instability, suggesting NAS. They also appear to have more infections, including hepatitis and syphilis, and are at higher risk of HIV exposure (Bauer *et al*, 2005). Cain *et al* (2013) have reviewed the maternal, fetal and neonatal consequences of cocaine use in pregnancy.

## *Hallucinogens*

Lysergic acid diethylamide (LSD) is a hallucinogen and is often mixed with amphetamines. High doses can provoke psychotic episodes. There have been a variety of congenital anomalies associated with LSD use in the literature, including skeletal dysplasia, hydrocephaly, ocular abnormalities and anophthalmia, neuroblastoma and Fallot's tetralogy. However, the small numbers and confounding factors involved mean that larger studies are required to substantiate a link between LSD and any specific anomalies.

## Benzodiazepines

As reducing the dose of benzodiazepines (BDZ) rapidly or stopping them can cause seizures, this is not advisable during pregnancy. Therefore, either low-dose maintenance or very gradual withdrawal and discontinuation should be negotiated. Women taking very-short-acting drugs should be transferred to the equivalent dose of diazepam. Gopalan *et al* (2014) describe the detoxification of two pregnant women with chronic BDZ use. They used chlordiazepoxide in one case and lorazepam in the other to assist in the management of withdrawal symptoms. The impact of BDZ exposure on the fetus is discussed in Chapter 8.

## Cannabis

The ALSPAC study found no association with increased perinatal morbidity or mortality, but regular cannabis use may be associated with a small reduction in birth weight (Fergusson *et al*, 2002). However, a systematic review in 1997 did not find any evidence to support an association between cannabis and birth weight (English *et al*, 1997). Since then, a large Australian study, which controlled for confounders such as tobacco smoking, alcohol and other illicit drug use, reported an increased risk of LBW (OR = 1.7, CI 1.3–2-2), preterm labour (OR = 1.5, CI 1–1.9), SGA (OR = 2.2, CI 1.8–2.7) and admission to NICU (OR = 2.0, CI 1.7–2.4) (Hayatbakhsh *et al* 2012).

Maternal cannabis use pre-conception, during pregnancy or in the postpartum is not associated with sudden infant death syndrome when smoking and other relevant variables are accounted for, but paternal cannabis use at all these time periods is (Klonoff-Cohen & Lam-Kruglick, 2001). Maternal cannabis use during pregnancy has been shown in several studies to have adverse effects on children's sleep, cognitive development, and behaviour, and performance on memory, attention and executive functioning tests, and it is associated with increased depression and anxiety. It is also a predictor of cannabis use in the offspring at age 14 (Day *et al*, 2006). Jutras-Aswad *et al* (2009) provide an overview of the neurobiological consequences of cannabis for the fetal brain and possible mechanisms for the neuropsychiatric outcomes.

## Volatile substance misuse

Several of the compounds used in volatile substance misuse have been implicated in animal studies as behavioural and developmental teratogens. The first reports of a syndrome similar to FAS emerged in the late 1970s and have continued.

There is a case report of ethylene glycol intoxication in a woman who was 26 weeks pregnant, presenting with symptoms very similar to those of eclampsia, including convulsions, hyperventilation and coma. Both mother and infant experienced a severe metabolic acidosis, but both survived

(Kralova *et al*, 2006). The diagnosis was made by osmolality gap analysis and the detection of oxalate crystals in the urine. Another case report describes a 32-week pregnant woman found lying almost suffocated by a plastic bag containing 'household solvents'. She was successfully delivered by Caesarean section and later disclosed regular volatile substance misuse (Kuczkowski, 2003).

A comprehensive review of the reproductive toxicology and teratology of misused toluene is provided by Hannigan & Bowen (2010), including pregnancy problems, developmental delay and neurobehavioral problems in infants exposed *in utero* to high levels of toluene.

## Ketamine, mephedrone and gamma-hydroxybutyrate (GBH)

There are no published data on the safety of these drugs in human pregnancy.

## Screening and detection

Self-report as a measure of drug use is unreliable and leads to underestimation of substance misuse. Biological markers are more reliable (Markovic *et al*, 2000), with the most accurate test being analysis of meconium, but this is not routinely used in the UK. Urine analysis can lead to false negatives as it is dependent upon the time the sample is taken in relation to the most recent drug use. Hair analysis has a high sensitivity for opiates and cocaine but low sensitivity for cannabis, and a 13% false positive rate for cocaine and opiates, which may be owing to passive exposure (Ostrea *et al*, 2001).

There are increased risks of infection in drug users, including bacterial endocarditis, abscesses and tuberculosis, as well blood-borne viruses such as hepatitis B and C and HIV, and other sexually transmitted diseases (Bauer *et al*, 2002). Conditions such as endocarditis and deep vein thrombosis must be identified, as these may indicate the need for antibiotic cover in labour or anticoagulation. The presence of HIV infection and hepatitis have implications for delivery and aftercare. Dentition may be poor and anaemia present.

## Management during pregnancy

This depends on the drug being used. For example, if there is no substitution therapy (e.g. cocaine, cannabis) or substitution therapy is not yet established (amphetamines), the aim is to stop use.

Aiming for greater stability is more important in those dependent upon opiates, to avoid the cycle of intoxication and withdrawal, which can have a greater adverse impact on the fetus. Insistence upon abstinence may also drive women away from services, and several studies have now shown that maintaining women on methadone enables them to receive more antenatal care and achieve better outcomes (e.g. Burns *et al*, 2006*b*).

### Detoxification

If women do not wish to take methadone throughout pregnancy (for example, to avoid neonatal withdrawal) it is recommended that detoxification is undertaken in the second trimester at a rate of 1 mg methadone per day, or 2–5 ml weekly or every 2 weeks, or whatever is manageable for the patient (Kendall *et al*, 1999). If gradual, this can be carried out on an out-patient basis, or it can be done more rapidly as in-patient treatment. Detoxification in the first trimester may be associated with increased risk of spontaneous abortion, and in the third trimester there may be increased risk of premature labour and fetal death. If possible, detoxification should be avoided in the first trimester and carried out very cautiously in the third.

### Substitution and maintenance

Methadone maintenance treatment decreases illicit opioid use, maternal mortality and morbidity, criminality, drug-seeking behaviour and prostitution, sexually transmitted diseases and the incidence of obstetric complications. It increases fetal stability and improves women's cooperation with obstetric care. Methadone can be taken orally, is difficult to inject, has a low street value, and has a long half-life so it can be taken daily, although it may be helpful in some cases to split the daily dose. It reduces withdrawal in the fetus. A retrospective study of babies born to women already on methadone and those who commenced it during pregnancy reported that higher gestational and birth weight were associated with a longer duration of methadone adherence and substance abstinence (Peles *et al*, 2012).

Disadvantages of methadone include that it is an addictive opiate, it is associated with neonatal withdrawal and it (rarely) causes neonatal thrombocytopenia.

Methadone dose does not always correlate with severity of NAS. Some early studies reported a relationship between maternal methadone dosage and neonatal withdrawal, but a more recent systematic review (Cleary *et al*, 2010) of 29 studies failed to find a significant relationship between maternal methadone dosage and neonatal withdrawal.

A daily dose may vary between 50 and 150 mg, but clearance increases from the first to the third trimester (Wolff *et al*, 2005); a higher dose may be required in the third trimester. Methadone dosage needs to be taken into account when pain relief is assessed during labour. Clearance will decline rapidly after delivery and the mother may become over-sedated if the dose is not adjusted downwards. Neonatal withdrawal may not emerge until 48 h after delivery. Data suggest that methadone-exposed infants function normally at 1–2-year cognitive evaluation (Kaltenbach & Finnegan, 1989).

### Buprenorphine

Buprenorphine is an established medication for the treatment of opiate dependence. Maternal and neonatal outcomes are similar to those seen with methadone maintenance. It therefore seems sensible to leave a woman on the maintenance therapy she is taking when she becomes pregnant rather than switching. Soyka (2013) provides a comprehensive review of the use of buprenorphine in pregnant opiate users.

A high level of suspicion of acute toxicity is required if a pregnant woman known to use drugs presents with altered perception of sensory stimuli, loss of coordination, headache, nausea or vomiting, or reduced respiration. However, clinicians must also be aware of medical disorders which might present in a similar way, especially eclampsia, and seek an urgent obstetric opinion.

## Postnatal care

After delivery, mothers and babies should go to the postnatal ward. Some infants with severe NAS may require admission to a neonatal unit for treatment.

Methadone is excreted in breast milk in small amounts, and this seems to relate to the amount the mother is receiving. It appears insufficient to prevent NAS, despite reports that it can ameliorate NAS, so an infant might still require specific treatment. Small amounts of buprenorphine are also excreted into breast milk, but there are only a few case reports available. A mother who is HIV positive or at high risk of becoming so should not breastfeed; others can be encouraged to do so, but will require considerable support if they have an irritable baby who has difficulty latching on. A good review of the issues relating to methadone and lactation is provided by Jansson and colleagues (2004).

Management should include consideration of contraception during pregnancy, and probably starting it before postnatal discharge. Long-acting progestogen delivered by depot injection, implant or intrauterine system is suitable and can be commenced in the postpartum period.

# Conclusions

Substance misuse in pregnant and postpartum women is an issue of growing concern, being associated with significant morbidity and mortality – both acute and chronic – for the mother and her baby and family. Interventions for substance misuse in the general population are likely to be beneficial, and there is accumulating evidence for some specific treatments.

There is a need for easily accessible comprehensive services, with trained staff, where proper detection and assessment, efficacious and cost-effective management and follow up can be provided. Such services should be a focus for continued research in this priority field.

# References

Addis A, Moretti ME, Ahmed Syed F, et al (2001) Fetal effects of cocaine: an updated meta-analysis. *Reproductive Toxicology*, **15**: 341–369

Alati R, Al Mamum A, Williams GM, *et al* (2006) *In utero* alcohol exposure and prediction of alcohol disorders in early adulthood: a birth cohort study. *Archives of General Psychiatry,* **63**: 1009–1016.

Albertsen K, Andersen A-MN, Olsen J, *et al* (2004) Alcohol consumption during pregnancy and the risk of preterm delivery. *American Journal of Epidemiology,* **159**: 155–161.

Albuquerque CA, Doyle W, Hales K, *et al* (2001) Influence of cigarette smoking on maternal body mass index and fetal growth. *Obstetrics and Gynecology,* **97**: S70–S71.

Albuquerque CA, Smith KR, Johnson C, *et al* (2004) Influence of maternal tobacco smoking during pregnancy on uterine, umbilical and fetal cerebral artery blood flows. *Early Human Development,* **80**: 31–42.

Alm B, Wennergren G, Norvenius G, *et al* (1999) Caffeine and alcohol as risk factors for sudden infant death syndrome. *Archives of Disease in Childhood,* **81**: 107–111.

Alvik A, Heyerdahl S, Haldorsen T, *et al* (2006) Alcohol use before and during pregnancy. *Acta Obstetricia et Gynecologica Scandinavica,* **85**: 1292–1298.

Amarin ZO (2005) Obstetricians, gynecologists and the anti-smoking campaign: a national survey. *European Journal of Obstetrics and Gynecology and Reproductive Biology,* **119**: 156–160.

Ananth CV, Smulian JC, Vintzileos AM (1999) Incidence of placental abruption in relation to cigarette smoking and hypertensive disorders during pregnancy: a meta-analysis of observational studies. *Obstetrics & Gynecology,* **93**: 622–628.

Anderson JE, Ebrahim S, Floyd L (2006) Prevalence of risk factors for adverse pregnancy outcomes during pregnancy and the preconception period — United States, 2002–2004. *Maternal & Child Health Journal,* **10**: S101–S106.

Arria AM, Derauf C, LaGasse LL, *et al* (2006) Methamphetamine and other substance use during pregnancy: preliminary estimates from the infant development, environment, and lifestyle (IDEAL) study. *Maternal and Child Health Journal,* **10**: 293–302.

Bailey BN, Delaney-Black V, Covington CY, *et al* (2004) Prenatal exposure to binge drinking and cognitive and behavioral outcomes at age 7 years. *American Journal of Obstetrics & Gynecology,* **191**: 1037–1043.

Barr H, Bookstein FL, O'Malley KD, *et al* (2006) Binge drinking during pregnancy as a predictor of psychiatric disorders on the structured clinical interview for DSM-IV in young adult offspring. *American Journal of Psychiatry,* **163**: 1061–1065.

Bateman DN, McElhatton PR, Dickinson D, *et al* (2004) A case control study to examine the pharmacological factors underlying ventricular septal defects in the North of England. *European Journal of Clinical Pharmacology,* **60**: 635–641.

Bauer CR, Shankaran S, Bada HS, *et al* (2002) The maternal lifestyle study: drug exposure during pregnancy and short-term maternal outcomes. *American Journal of Obstetrics and Gynecology,* **186**: 487–495.˙

Bauer CR, Langer JC, Shankaran S, *et al* (2005) Acute neonatal effects of cocaine exposure during pregnancy. *Archives of Pediatrics & Adolescent Medicine,* **159**: 824–834.

Baumann P, Schild C, Hume RF, *et al* (2006) Alcohol abuse – a persistent and preventable risk for congenital anomalies. *International Journal of Gynecology & Obstetrics,* **95**: 66–72.

Bay B, Kesmodel US (2010) Prenatal alcohol exposure – a systematic review of the effects on child motor function. *Acta Obstetricia et Gynecologica Scandinavica,* **90**: 210–226.

Blair PS, Fleming PJ, Bensley D, *et al* (1996) Smoking and the sudden infant death syndrome: results from 1993–5 case-control study for confidential inquiry into stillbirths and deaths in infancy. Confidential Enquiry into Stillbirths and Deaths Regional Coordinators and Researchers. *BMJ,* **313**: 195–198.

Blake KV, Gurrin LC, Evans SF, *et al* (2000) Maternal cigarette smoking during pregnancy, low birth weight and subsequent blood pressure in early childhood. *Early Human Development,* **57**: 137–147.

Blalock JA, Fouladi RT, Wetter DW, *et al* (2005) Depression in pregnant women seeking smoking cessation. *Addictive Behaviours,* **30**: 1195–1208.

Bradley KA, Boyd-Wickizer J, Powell SH, *et al* (1998) Alcohol screening questionnaires in women: a critical review. *JAMA*, **280**: 166–171.

Brennan PA, Grekin ER, Mednick SA (1999) Maternal smoking during pregnancy and adult male criminal outcomes. *Archives of General Psychiatry*, **56**: 215–219.

Browne CA, Colditz PB, Dunster KR (2000) Infant autonomic function is altered by maternal smoking during pregnancy. *Early Human Development*, **59**: 209–218.

Burden MJ, Jacobson SW, Jacobson JL (2005) Relation of prenatal alcohol exposure to cognitive processing speed and efficiency in childhood. *Alcoholism: Clinical & Experimental Research*, **29**: 1473–1483.

Burns L, Mattick RP, Cooke M (2006a) Use of record linkage to examine alcohol use in pregnancy. *Alcoholism: Clinical and Experimental Research*, **30**: 642–648.

Burns L, Mattick RP, Lim K, *et al* (2006b) Methadone in pregnancy: treatment retention and neonatal outcomes. *Addiction*, **102**: 264–270.

Burns E, Gray R, Smith LA (2010) Brief screening questionnaires to identify problem drinking during pregnancy: a systematic review. *Addiction*, **105**: 601–614.

Caetano R, Ramisetty-Mikler S, Floyd LR, *et al* (2006) The epidemiology of drinking among women of child-bearing age. *Alcoholism: Clinical and Experimental Research*, **30**: 1023–1030.

Cain MA, Bornick P, Whiteman V (2013) The maternal, fetal and neonatal effects of cocaine exposure in pregnancy. *Clinical Obstetrics and Gynaecology*, **56**: 124–132.

Carter RC, Jacobson SW, Molteno CD, *et al* (2005) Effects of prenatal alcohol exposure on infant visual acuity. *Journal of Pediatrics*, **147**: 473–479.

Castles A, Adams EK, Melvin CL, *et al* (1999) Effects of smoking during pregnancy: five meta-analyses. *American Journal of Preventive Medicine*, **16**: 208–215.

Chamberlain C, O'Mara-Eves A, Oliver S, *et al* (2013) Psychosocial interventions for supporting women to stop smoking in pregnancy. *Cochrane Database of Systematic Reviews*, **10**: CD001055.

Chambers CD, Kavteladze L, Joutchenko L, *et al* (2006) Alcohol consumption patterns among pregnant women in the Moscow region of the Russian Federation. *Alcohol*, **54**: 133–137.

Chang G, Wilkins-Haug L, Berman S, *et al* (1998) Alcohol use and pregnancy: improving identification. *Obstetrics & Gynecology*, **91**: 892–898.

Chang G, Wilkins-Haug L, Berman S, *et al* (1999) Brief intervention for alcohol use in pregnancy: a randomized trial. *Addiction*, **94**: 1499–1508.

Chong DS, Yip PS, Karlberg J (2004) Maternal smoking: an increasing unique risk factor for sudden infant death syndrome in Sweden. *Acta Paediatrica*, **93**: 471–478.

Clark KA, Dawson S, Martin SL (1999) The effect of implementing a more comprehensive screening for substance use among pregnant women in North Carolina. *Maternal and Child Health Journal*, **3**: 161–166.

Cleary BJ, Donnelly J, Strawbridge J, *et al* (2010) Methadone dose and neonatal abstinence syndrome—systematic review and meta-analysis. *Addiction*, **105**: 2071–2084.

Cnattingius S (2004) The epidemiology of smoking during pregnancy: smoking prevalence, maternal characteristics, and pregnancy outcomes. *Nicotine & Tobacco Research*, **6**: S125–S140.

Coleman T, Chamberlain C, Davey MA, *et al* (2012) Pharmacological interventions for promoting smoking cessation during pregnancy. *Cochrane Database of Systematic Reviews*, **9**: CD010078.

Colman GJ, Joyce T (2003) Trends in smoking before, during, and after pregnancy in ten states. *American Journal of Preventive Medicine*, **24**: 29–35.

Conde-Agudelo A, Althabe F, Belizàn JM, *et al* (1999) Cigarette smoking during pregnancy and risk of preeclampsia: a systematic review. *American Journal of Obstetrics & Gynecology*, **181**: 1026–1035.

Condliffe L, McEwen A, West R (2005) The attitude of maternity staff to, and smoking cessations with, childbearing women in London. *Midwifery*, **21**: 233–240.

Cone-Wesson B (2005) Prenatal alcohol and cocaine exposure: Influences on cognition, speech, language, and hearing. *Journal of Communication Disorders*, **38**: 279–302.

Cooke M, Mattick RP, Walsh RA (2001) Differential uptake of a smoking cessation programme disseminated to doctors and midwives in antenatal clinics. *Addiction*, **96**: 495–505.

Covington CY, Nordstrom-Klee B, Ager J, et al (2002) Birth to age 7 growth of children prenatally exposed to drugs: a prospective cohort study. *Neurotoxicology and Teratology*, **24**: 489–496.

Crome I, Ismail KMK, Ghetau E, et al (2005) Opiate misuse in pregnancy: findings of a retrospective case note series. *Drugs: Education, Prevention and Policy*, **12**: 431–436.

Crome IB, Kumar MJ (2007) Epidemiology of drug and alcohol use in young women. *Seminars in Fetal and Neonatal Medicine*, **12**: 98–105.

Day NL, Goldschmidt L, Thomas CA (2006) Prenatal marijuana exposure contributes to the prediction of marijuana use at age 14. *Addiction*, **101**: 1313–1322.

Dornelas EA, Magnavita J, Beazoglu T, et al (2006) Efficacy and cost-effectiveness of a clinic-based counselling intervention tested in an ethnically diverse sample of pregnant smokers. *Patient Education and Counseling*, **64**: 342–349.

van Dyk J, Ramanjam V, Church P, et al (2014) Maternal methamphetamine use in pregnancy and long-term neurodevelopmental and behavioral deficits in children. *Journal of Population Therapeutics and Clinical Pharmacology*, **21**: e185–e196.

Ebrahim SH, Gfroerer J (2003) Pregnancy-related substance use in the United States during 1996–1998. *Obstetrics & Gynecology*, **101**: 374–379.

England L, Zhang J (2007) Smoking and risk of pre-eclampsia: a systematic review. *Frontiers in Bioscience*, **12**: 2471–83.

England LJ, Kim SY, Tomar SL, et al (2010) Non-cigarette tobacco use among women and adverse pregnancy outcomes. *Acta Obstetricia et Gynecologica*, **89**: 454–464.

English DR, Hulse GK, Milne E, et al (1997) Maternal cannabis use and birth weight: a meta-analysis. *Addiction*, **92**: 1553–1560.

Erickson AC, Arbour LT (2012) Heavy smoking during pregnancy as a marker for other risk factors of adverse birth outcomes: a population-based study in British Columbia, Canada. *BMC Public Health*, **12**: 102.

Esper LH, Furtado EF (2014) Identifying maternal risk factors associated with fetal alcohol spectrum disorders: a systematic review. *European Child and Adolescent Psychiatry*, **23**: 877–889.

Fergusson DM, Woodward LJ, Horwood LJ (1998) Maternal smoking during pregnancy and psychiatric adjustment in late adolescence. *Archives of General Psychiatry*, **55**: 721–727.

Fergusson DM, Horwood LJ, Northstone K (2002) Maternal use of cannabis and pregnancy outcome. *BJOG*, **109**: 21–27.

Frank DA, Augustyn M, Knight WG, et al (2001) Growth, development, and behaviour in early childhood following prenatal cocaine exposure: a systematic review. *JAMA*, **285**: 1613–1625.

Frank DA, Jacobs RR, Beeghly M, et al (2002) Level of prenatal cocaine exposure and scores on the Bayley Scales of Infant Development: modifying effects of caregiver, early intervention, and birth weight. *Pediatrics*, **110**: 1143–1152.

Froen JF, Arnestad M, Vege A, et al (2002) Comparative epidemiology of sudden infant death syndrome and sudden intrauterine unexplained death. *Archives of Disease in Childhood. Fetal and Neonatal Edition*, **87**: 118–121.

Giglia R, Binns C (2006) Alcohol and lactation: a systematic review. *Nutrition and Dietetics*, **63**: 103–116.

Gold KJ, Dalton VK, Schwenk TL, et al (2007) What causes pregnancy loss? Preexisting mental illness as an independent risk factor. *General Hospital Psychiatry*, **29**: 207–213.

Golub M, Costa L, Crofton K, et al (2005) NTP-CERHR Expert Panel Report on the reproductive and developmental toxicity of amphetamine and methamphetamine. *Birth Defects Research. Part B, Developmental and Reproductive Toxicology*, **74**: 471–584.

Gopalan P, Glance JB, Azzam PM (2014) Managing benzodiazepine withdrawal during pregnancy: case-based guidelines. *Archives of Women's Mental Health*, **17**: 161–170.

Göransson M, Magnusson A, Bergman H, *et al* (2003) Fetus at risk: prevalence of alcohol consumption during pregnancy estimated with a simple screening method in Swedish antenatal clinics. *Addiction*, **98**: 1513–1520.

Gouin K, Murphy K, Shah PS, *et al* (2011) Effects of cocaine use during pregnancy on low birthweight and preterm birth: systematic review and metaanalyses. *American Journal of Obstetrics & Gynecology*, **204**: 340.e1–340.e12.

Hackshaw A, Rodek C, Boniface S (2011) Maternal smoking in pregnancy and birth defects: a systematic review based on 173 687 malformed cases and 11.7 million controls. *Human Reproduction Update*, **17**: 589–604.

Haggarty P, Abramovich DR, Page K (2002) The effect of maternal smoking and ethanol on fatty acid transport by the human placenta. *British Journal of Nutrition*, **87**: 247–252.

Hajek P, Stead LF, West R, *et al* (2013) Relapse prevention interventions for smoking cessation. *Cochrane Database of Systematic Reviews*, **8**: CD003999.

Haley DW, Handmaker NS, Lowe J (2006) Infant stress reactivity and prenatal alcohol exposure. *Alcoholism, Clinical and Experimental Research*, **30**: 2055–2064.

Hammoud AO, Bujold E, Sorokin Y, *et al* (2005) Smoking in pregnancy revisited: findings from a large population-based study. *American Journal of Obstetrics & Gynaecology*, **192**: 1856–1862.

Handmaker NS, Wilbourne P (2001) Motivational interventions in prenatal clinics. *Alcohol Research and Health*, **25**: 219–229.

Hankin J, McCaul ME, Heussner J (2000) Pregnant, alcohol abusing women. *Alcoholism: Clinical and Experimental Research*, **24**: 1276–1286.

Hankin JR, Sokol RJ (1995) Identification and care of problems associated with alcohol ingestion in pregnancy. *Seminars in Perinatology*, **19**: 286–292.

Hannigan JH, Bowen SG (2010) Reproductive toxicology and teratology of abused toluene. *Systems Biology in Reproductive Medicine*, **56**: 184–200.

Hardy B, Szatkowski L, Tata LJ, *et al* (2014) Smoking cessation advice recorded during pregnancy in United Kingdom primary care. *BMC Family Practice*, **15**: 21.

Harrison-Woolrych M, Paterson H, Tan M (2013) Exposure to the smoking cessation medicine varenicline during pregnancy: a prospective nationwide cohort study. *Pharmacoepidemiology and Drug Safety*, **22**: 1086–1092.

Hayatbakhsh MR, Flenady VJ, Gibbons KS, *et al* (2012) Birth outcomes associated with cannabis use before and during pregnancy. *Pediatric Research*, **71**: 215–219.

Haynes G, Dunnagan T, Christpher S (2003) Determinants of alcohol use in pregnant women at risk for alcohol consumption. *Neurotoxicology and Teratology*, **25**: 659–666.

Health and Social Care Information Centre (2013) *Health Survey for England – 2012, Trend Tables*. HSCIC.

Heggard H, Kjærgaard H, Møller L, *et al* (2003) Multimodal intervention raises smoking cessation rates during pregnancy. *Acta Obstetricia et Gynecologica Scandinavica*, **82**: 813–819.

Henriksen TB, Hjollund NH, Jensen TK, *et al* (2004) Alcohol consumption at the time of conception and spontaneous abortion. *American Journal of Epidemiology Baltimore*, **160**: 661–667.

Henriksson KM, McNeil TF (2006) Smoking in pregnancy and its correlates among women with a history of schizophrenia and affective psychosis. *Schizophrenia Research*, **81**: 121–123.

Horrigan TJ, Schroeder AV, Schaffer RM (2000) The triad of substance abuse, violence, and depression are interrelated in pregnancy. *Journal of Substance Abuse Treatment*, **18**: 55–58.

Horne RSC, Franco P, Adamson TM, *et al* (2004) Influences of maternal cigarette smoking on infant arousability. *Early Human Development*, **79**: 49–58.

Hotham ED, Atkinson ER, Gilbert AL (2002) Focus groups with pregnant smokers; barriers to cessation, attitudes to nicotine patch use and perceptions of counselling by care providers. *Drug and Alcohol Review*, **21**: 163–168.

Hotham ED, Gilbert AL, Atkinson ER (2006) A randomised controlled trial of nicotine patches in pregnant women. *Addictive Behaviours*, **31**: 641–648.

Houet T, Vabret F, Herlicoviez M, *et al* (2005) Comparison of women's alcohol consumption before and during pregnancy. *Journal de Gynecologie, Obstetrique et Biologie de la Reproduction*, **34**: 687–693.

Huiznik AC, Mulder EJH (2006) Maternal smoking, drinking or cannabis use during pregnancy and neurobehavioural and cognitive functioning in human offspring. *Neuroscience and Behavioral Reviews*, **30**: 24–41.

Hulse GK, Milne E, English DR, *et al* (1997*a*) The relationship between maternal use of heroin and methadone and birth weight. *Addiction*, **92**: 1571–1579.

Hulse GK, Milne E, English DR, *et al* (1997*b*) Assessing the relationship between maternal cocaine use and abruption placentae. *Addiction*, **92**: 1547–1551.

Hulse GK, Milne E, English DR, *et al* (1998*a*) Assessing the relationship between maternal opiate use and neonatal mortality. *Addiction*, **93**: 1033–1042.

Hulse GK, Milne E, English DR, *et al* (1998*b*) Assessing the relationship between maternal opiate use and antepartum haemorrhage. *Addiction*, **93**: 1533–1558.

Ingersoll KS, Knisely JS, Dawson KS, *et al* (2004) Psychopathology and treatment outcome of drug dependent women in a perinatal program. *Addictive Behaviours*, **29**: 731–741.

Jansson LM, Velez M, Harrow C (2004) Methadone maintenance and lactation: a review of the literature and current management guidelines. *Journal of Human Lactation*, **20**: 62–71.

Jones KL, Smith DW, Ulleland CN, *et al* (1973) Pattern of malformation in offspring of chronic alcoholic mothers. *Lancet*, **1**: 1267–1271.

Jordan TR, Dake JA, Price JH (2006) Best practices for smoking cessation in pregnancy: do obstetrician/gynecologists use them in practice? *Journal of Women's Health*, **15**: 400–441.

Jutras-Aswad D, DiNieri JA, Harkany T, *et al* (2009) Neurobiological consequences of maternal cannabis on human fetal development and its neuropsychiatric outcome. *European Archives of Psychiatry and Clinical Neuroscience*, **259**: 395–412.

Kain Z, Mayes L, Pakes J, *et al* (1995) Thrombocytopenia in pregnant women who use cocaine. *American Journal of Obstetrics & Gynecology*, **173**: 885–890.

Källen K (2000) Maternal smoking during pregnancy and infant head circumference at birth. *Early Human Development*, **58**: 197–204.

Kaltenbach KA, Finnegan LP (1989) Prenatal narcotic exposure: perinatal and developmental effects. *Neurotoxicology*, **10**: 597–604.

Kaplan YC, Dündar ON, Kasap B, *et al* (2014) Pregnancy outcome after varenicline exposure in the first pregnancy. *Case Reports in Obstetrics and Gynaecology*, **2014**: 263981.

Kelly RH, Zatick D, Anders TF (2001) The detection and treatment of psychiatric disorders and substance use among pregnant women cared for in obstetrics. *American Journal of Psychiatry*, **158**: 213–219.

Kendall SR, Doberczak TM, Jantumen M, *et al* (1999) The methadone maintained pregnancy. *Clinics in Perinatology*, **26**: 173–183.

Kennare R, Heard A, Chan A (2005) Substance use during pregnancy: risk factors and obstetric and perinatal outcomes in South Australia. *Australian and New Zealand Journal of Obstetrics & Gynaecology*, **45**: 220–225.

Kesmodel U, Wisborg K, Olsen S, *et al* (2002*a*) Moderate alcohol intake in pregnancy and the risk of spontaneous abortion. *Alcohol and Alcoholism*, **37**: 87–92.

Kesmodel U, Wisborg K, Olsen SF, *et al* (2002*b*) Moderate alcohol intake during pregnancy and the risk of stillbirth and death in the first year of life. *American Journal of Epidemiology*, **155**: 305–312.

Klonoff-Cohen H, Lam-Kruglick P (2001) Maternal and paternal recreational drug use and sudden infant death syndrome. *Archives of Pediatric and Adolescent Medicine*, **155**: 765–770.

Knight M, Tufnell D, Kenyon S, *et al* (2015) *Saving Lives, Improving Mothers' Care: Lessons learned to inform future maternity care from the UK and Ireland Confidential Enquiries into Maternal Deaths and Morbidity 2009–2012*. National Perinatal Epidemiology Unit, Oxford.

Kralova I, Stepanak Z, Dusek J (2006) Ethylene glycol intoxication misdiagnosed as eclampsia. *Acta Anaesthesiologica Scandinavica*, **50**: 385–387.

Kuczkowski KM (2003) Solvents in pregnancy: an emerging problem in obstetrics and obstetric anaesthesia. *Anaesthesia*, **58**: 1036–1037.

Ladhani NNN, Shah PS, Murphy K, *et al* (2011) Prenatal amphetamine exposure and birth outcomes: a systematic review and metaanalysis. *American Journal of Obstetrics & Gynecology*, **205**: 219.e1–219.e7.

Latino-Martel P, Chan DSM, Druesne-Pecello N, *et al* (2010) Maternal alcohol consumption during pregnancy and risk of childhood leukemia: systematic review and meta-analysis. *Cancer Epidemiology, Biomarkers & Prevention*, **19**: 1238–1260.

Law KL, Stroud LR, LaGasse LL, *et al* (2003) Smoking during pregnancy and newborn neurobehavior. *Pediatrics*, **111**: 1318–1323.

Lawrence T, Aveyard P, Cheng KK, *et al* (2005) Does stage-based smoking cessation advice in pregnancy result in long-term quitters? 18-month postpartum follow-up of a randomized controlled trial. *Addiction*, **100**: 107–116.

Lee LJ, Lupo PJ (2013) Maternal smoking during pregnancy and the risk of congenital heart defects in offspring: a systematic review and metaanalysis. *Pediatric Cardiology*, **34**: 398–407.

Lemoine P, Harousseau H, Borteyru JP, *et al* (1968) Les enfants des parents alcooliques: anomalies observées à propos de 127 cas. *Ouest Medical*, **21**: 476–482.

Leonardson GR, Loudenburg R (2003) Risk factors for alcohol use during pregnancy in a multistate area. *Neurotoxicology and Teratology*, **25**: 651–658.

Lingford-Hughes AR, Welch S, Peters L, *et al* (2012) British Association for Psychopharmacology updated guidelines: evidence-based guidelines for the pharmacological management of substance abuse, harmful use, addiction and comorbidity: recommendations from British Association for Psychopharmacology. *Journal of Psychopharmacology*, **26**: 899–952.

Linneberg A, Petersen J, Gronbaek M, *et al* (2004) Alcohol during pregnancy and atopic dermatitis in the offspring. *Journal of Allergy and Clinical Immunology*, **34**: 1678–1683.

Linnet KM, Dalsgaard S, Obel C, *et al* (2003) Maternal lifestyle factors in pregnancy risk of attention deficit hyperactivity disorder and associated behaviors: review of the current evidence. *American Journal of Psychiatry*, **160**: 1028–1040.

Little M, Shah R, Vermeulen MJ, *et al* (2005) Adverse perinatal outcomes associated with homelessness and substance misuse in pregnancy. *Canadian Medical Association Journal*, **173**: 615–618.

Lucas BR, Latimer J, Pinto RZ, *et al* (2014) Gross motor deficits in children prenatally exposed to alcohol: a meta-analysis. *Pediatrics*, **134**: e192–e209.

Malik S, Cleves MA, Honein MA, *et al* (2008) Maternal smoking and congenital heart defects. *Pediatrics*, **121**: e810–e816.

Man L-X, Chang B (2006) Maternal cigarette smoking during pregnancy increases the risk of having a child with a congenital digital anomaly. *Plastic & Reconstructive Surgery*, **117**: 301–308.

Mariscal M, Palma S, Llorca J, *et al* (2006) Pattern of alcohol consumption during pregnancy and risk for low birth weight. *Annals of Epidemiology*, **16**: 432–438.

Markovic N, Ness R, Cefilli D (2000) Substance use measures among women in early pregnancy. *American Journal of Obstetrics & Gynecology*, **183**: 627–632.

McAndrew F, Thompson J, Fellows L, *et al* (2012) *Infant Feeding Survey 2010*. HSCIC.

McLeod D, Pullon S, Benn C, *et al* (2004) Can support and education for smoking cessation and reduction be provided effectively by midwives within primary maternity care? *Midwifery*, **20**: 37–50.

Miller H, Ranger-Moore J, Hingten M (2003) Bupropion SR for smoking cessation in pregnancy: a pilot study. *American Journal of Obstetrics & Gynecology*, **189**: S133.

Miller J, Nolan T (2001) Case–control study of antenatal cocaine use and platelet levels. *American Journal of Obstetrics & Gynecology*, **184**: 434–437.

Mitchell EA (1995) Smoking: the next major modifiable risk factor. In *Sudden Infant Death Syndrome: New Trends in the Nineties* (ed TO Rognum): pp. 114–118. Scandinavian University Press.

Morales-Suarez-Varela MM, Bille M, Christensen K, *et al* (2006) Smoking habits, nicotine use and congenital malformations. *Obstetrics & Gynecology*, **107**: 51–57.

Mukherjee RAS, Hollins S, Turk J (2006) Fetal alcohol spectrum disorder: an overview. *Journal of the Royal Society of Medicine*, **99**: 298–302.

Munger RG, Romitti PA, Daack-Hirsch S, *et al* (1997) Maternal alcohol use and risk of orofacial birth defects. *International Journal of Pediatric Otorhinolaryngology*, **40**: 217–225.

Murphy DJ, Dunney C, Mullally A, *et al* (2013) Population-based study of smoking behaviour throughout pregnancy and adverse perinatal outcomes. *International Journal of Environmental Research & Public Health*, **10**: 3855–3867.

Myung S-K, Ju W, Jung H-S, *et al* (2012) Efficacy and safety of pharmacotherapy for smoking cessation among pregnant smokers: a meta-analysis. *BJOG*, **119**: 1029–1039.

National Institute for Health and Care Excellence (2008) *Antenatal Care: Routine Care for the Healthy Pregnant Woman*. NICE.

National Institute for Health and Care Excellence (2010) *Quitting Smoking in Pregnancy and Following Childbirth*. NICE.

National Institute for Health and Care Excellence (2014) *Antenatal and Postnatal Mental Health*. NICE.

Naughton F, Prevost AT, Gilbert H, *et al* (2012) Randomized controlled trial evaluation of a tailored leaflet and SMS text message self-help intervention for pregnant smokers (MiQuit). *Nicotine & Tobacco Research*, **14**: 567–577.

Nielsen A, Hannibal CG, Linekilde BE, *et al* (2006) Maternal smoking predicts the risk of spontaneous abortion. *Acta Obstetricia et Gynecologica Scandinavica*, **85**: 1057–1065.

Nulman I, Rovet J, Kennedy D, *et al* (2004) Binge alcohol consumption by non-alcohol-dependent women during pregnancy affects child behaviour, but not general intellectual functioning; a prospective controlled study. *Archives of Women's Mental Health*, **7**: 173–181.

Oei JL, Kingsbury A, Dhawan A, *et al* (2012) Amphetamines, the pregnant woman and her children: a review. *Journal of Perinatology*, **32**: 737–747.

Okah FA, Cai J, Hoff GL (2005) Term-gestation low birth weight and health-compromising behaviors during pregnancy. *Obstetrics & Gynecology*, **105**: 543–550.

O'Leary CM (2004) Fetal alcohol syndrome: diagnosis, epidemiology, and developmental outcomes. *Journal of Paediatrics and Child Health*, **40**: 2–7.

Ostrea J, Enrique M, Knapp DK, *et al* (2001) Estimates of illicit drug use during pregnancy by maternal interview, hair analysis, and meconium analysis. *The Journal of Pediatrics*, **138**: 344–348.

Panting-Kemp A, Nguyen T, Castro L (2002) Substance abuse and polyhydramnios. *American Journal of Obstetrics & Gynecology*, **187**: 602–605.

Patra J, Bakker R, Jaddoe VWV, *et al* (2011) Dose–response relationship between alcohol consumption before and during pregnancy and the risks of low birthweight, preterm birth and small for gestational age (SGA) – a systematic review and meta-analyses. *BJOG*, **118**: 1411–1421.

Peles E, Schrieber S, Bloch M, *et al* (2012) Duration of methadone maintenance treatment in pregnancy and pregnancy outcome parameters in women with opiate addiction. *Journal of Addiction Medicine*, **6**: 18–23.

Peterson PL, Lowe JB (1992) Preventing fetal alcohol exposure: a cognitive behavioral approach. *International Journal of the Addictions*, **27**: 613–626.

Petrou S, Hockley C, Mehta Z, *et al* (2005) The association between smoking during pregnancy and hospital inpatient costs in childhood. *Social Science and Medicine*, **60**: 1071–1085.

Pichini S, Puig C, Zuccaro P, *et al* (2005) Assessment of exposure to opiates and cocaine during pregnancy in a Mediterranean city: preliminary results of the 'Meconium Project'. *Forensic Science International*, **153**: 59–65.

Pineless BL, Park E, Samet JM (2014) Systematic review and meta-analysis of miscarriage and maternal exposure to tobacco smoke among pregnant women. *American Journal of Epidemiology*, **179**: 807–823.

Ponsonby A-L, Dwyer T, Couper D (1997) Factors related to infant apnoea and cyanosis: A population-based study. *Journal of Paediatrics and Child Health*, **33**: 317–323.

Pruett D, Waterman EH, Caughey AB (2013) Fetal alcohol exposure: consequences, diagnosis, and treatment. *Obstetrical & Gynecological Survey*, **68**: 62–69.

Raatikainen K, Huurinainen P, Heinonen S (2007) Smoking in early gestation or through pregnancy: A decision crucial to pregnancy outcome. *Preventive Medicine*, **44**: 59–63.

Rasch V (2003) Cigarette, alcohol, and caffeine consumption: risk factors for spontaneous abortion. *Acta Obstetricia et Gynecologica Scandinavica*, **82**: 182–188.

Richardson GA, Ryan C, Willford J, *et al* (2002) Prenatal alcohol and marijuana exposure: Effects on neuropsychological outcomes at 10 years. *Neurotoxicology and Teratology*, **24**: 309–320.

Riley EP, McGee CL (2005) Fetal alcohol spectrum disorders: an overview with emphasis on changes in brain and behavior. *Experimental Biology and Medicine*, **230**: 357–365.

Sayal K, Heron J, Golding J, *et al* (2009) Binge pattern of alcohol consumption during pregnancy and childhood mental health outcomes: longitudinal population-based study. *Pediatrics*, **123**: e289–e296.

Schneider S, Huy C, Schütz J, *et al* (2010) Smoking cessation during pregnancy: a systematic literature review. *Drug and Alcohol Review*, **29**: 81–90.

Schuler ME, Nair P, Kettinger L (2003) Drug-exposed infants and developmental outcome. *Archives of Pediatrics and Adolescent Medicine*, **157**: 133–138.

Shah NR, Bracken MB (2000) A systematic review and meta-analysis of prospective studies on the association between maternal cigarette smoking and preterm delivery. *American Journal of Obstetrics & Gynecology*, **182**: 465–472.

Sherwood RA, Keating V, Kavvadia A, *et al* (1999) Substance misuse in early pregnancy and relationship to fetal outcome. *European Journal of Pediatrics*, **158**: 488–492.

Singer LT, Minnes S, Short E (2004) Cognitive outcomes of preschool children with prenatal cocaine exposure. *JAMA*, **291**: 2448–2456.

Singer LT, Moore DG, Min MO, *et al* (2012) One-year outcomes of prenatal exposure to MDMA and other recreational drugs. *Pediatrics*, **130**: 407–413.

Smith GC, White IR (2006) Predicting the risk for sudden infant death syndrome from obstetric characteristics: a retrospective cohort study of 505,011 live births. *Pediatrics*, **117**: 60–66.

Soyka M (2013) Buprenorphine use in pregnant opioid users: a critical review. *CNS Drugs*, **27**: 653–662.

Steyn K, de Wet T, Salooje Y, *et al* (2006) The influence of maternal smoking, snuff use and passive smoking on pregnancy outcomes: the Birth to Ten Study. *Paediatric and Perinatal Epidemiology*, **20**: 90–99.

Stratton K, Howe C, Frederick Battaglia F (eds) (1996) *Fetal Alcohol Syndrome: Diagnosis, Epidemiology, Prevention, and Treatment*. National Academy Press.

Testa M, Quigley BM, Eiden RD (2003) The effects of prenatal alcohol exposure on infant mental development: a meta-analytical review. *Alcohol and Alcoholism*, **38**: 295–304.

Thorup J, Cortes D, Petersen BL (2006) The incidence of bilateral cryptorchidism is increased and the fertility potential is reduced in sons born to mothers who have smoked during pregnancy. *Journal of Urology*, **176**: 734–737.

Tough S, Tofflemire K, Clarke M, *et al* (2006) Do women change their drinking behaviors while trying to conceive? An opportunity for preconception counseling. *Clinical Medicine and Research*, **4**: 97–105.

Turner C, Russell A, Brown W (2003) Prevalence of illicit drug use in young Australian women, patterns of use and associated risk factors. *Addiction*, **98**: 1419–1426.

Ulleland CN (1972) The offspring of alcoholic mothers. *Annals of the New York Academy of Sciences*, **197**: 167–169.

Urato A, Craigo S, Collins J, et al (2005) Maternal smoking and pregnancy outcomes. *American Journal of Obstetrics & Gynecology*, **193**: S121.

Ussher M, West R, Hibbs N (2004) A survey of pregnant smokers' interest in different types of smoking cessation support. *Patient Education and Counselling*, **54**: 67–72.

Ussher M, Etter J-F, West R (2006) Perceived barriers to and benefits of attending a stop smoking course during pregnancy. *Patient Education and Counselling*, **61**: 467–472.

Velez ML, Montoya ID, Jansson LM, et al (2006) Exposure to violence among substance-dependent pregnant women and their children. *Journal of Substance Abuse Treatment*, **30**: 31–38.

Whitehead N, Lipscomb L (2003) Patterns of alcohol use before and during pregnancy and the risk of small-for-gestational-age birth. *American Journal of Epidemiology*, **158**: 654–662.

Willford J, Leech S, Day N (2006) Moderate prenatal alcohol exposure and cognitive status of children at age 10. *Alcoholism, Clinical and Experimental Research*, **30**: 1051–1059.

Williams JHG, Ross L (2007) Consequences of prenatal toxin exposure for mental health in children and adolescents: systematic review. *European Child & Adolescent Psychiatry*, **16**: 243–253.

Wolff K, Boys A, Rostami-Hodjegan A, et al (2005) Changes to methadone clearance during pregnancy. *European Journal of Clinical Pharmacology*, **61**: 763–768.

Wyszynski DF, Duffy DL, Beatty TH (1997) Maternal cigarette smoking and oral clefts: a meta-analysis. *The Cleft Palate-Craniofacial Journal*, **34**: 206–210.

Zdravkovic T, Genbacev O, McMaster MT, et al (2005) The adverse effects of maternal smoking on the human placenta: a review. *Placenta*, **26**: S81–S86.

Zelner I, Koren G (2013) Alcohol consumption among women. *Journal of Population Therapeutics & Clinical Pharmacology*, **20**: e201–e206.

Zhang K, Wang X (2013) Maternal smoking and increased risk of sudden infant death syndrome: a meta-analysis. *Legal Medicine*, **15**: 115–121.

Zhang X, Sliwowska JH, Weinberg J (2005) Prenatal alcohol exposure and fetal programming: effects on neuroendocrine and immune function. *Experimental Biology and Medicine*, **230**: 376–388.

# CHAPTER 6

# Perinatal mental illness, children and the family

Since the publication of the first edition of this book, research and clinical practice have continued to inform our understanding of mental illness in parents during the perinatal period. Equally, our knowledge of the impact of perinatal mental illness on the fetus and infant has increased. The evidence suggests that perinatal mental illness is associated with adverse effects on the health and development of children, and that early life experiences may influence the health of an individual across their lifespan (Hogg, 2013). It is therefore important to pay attention to infant mental health (Carter *et al*, 2004). We are increasing our understanding of the mechanisms underlying the associations between perinatal mental illness and child outcome. Our knowledge of how to treat perinatal mental illness has also improved, but there remain questions about how to intervene to modify the effects on children. There is increasing evidence that it is not enough just to treat the parent's illness, and that management should include consideration of how to offset potential adverse child outcomes. Perinatal mental illness often occurs in the context of a multiplicity of adverse psychosocial factors, and determining which of these also contribute to child outcome, and to what extent, is complex. The availability of specialist perinatal mental health services remains limited, particularly services which include both adult and infant/child mental health specialists. Evidence about how best to deliver such services requires further investigation.

'But babies do demonstrate through, for example, poor sleep patterns, difficulties with feeding, restlessness and gastric disturbance, that they are anxious and tense, distressed and fearful. These emotions need to be responded to with love and empathy by those on whom they depend for survival. Supporting families to provide this response is essential, in order to reduce the incidence of mental health problems and their consequences in later life' (Young Minds, 2004).

It is important to note that although perinatal mental illness can be associated with adverse outcomes for the child, this is not always the case. In fact, some children faced with significant adversity achieve good outcomes and healthy lives. Resilience is an important consideration in any assessment of risk and protective factors (Skala & Bruckner, 2014).

Fundamental to child outcome is the relationship between the child and his/her primary caregivers. These relationships are bidirectional, and it is important to explore the nature of parent–child interaction from both the child's and the parent's perspective. Disruption in either direction may potentially affect outcome (Main, 1996; Brockington *et al*, 2006).

Any illness which disrupts the physical and psychological processes of pregnancy has implications for the physical and psychological well-being of the fetus and infant. There are therefore some illness effects that can be generalised across the range of mental health problems. In addition, particular diagnoses are associated with particular risks and effects.

The inclusion of a chapter on the impact of perinatal mental illness on children and families in this book therefore remains relevant. National Institute for Health and Care Excellence (NICE) guidance on the management of perinatal mental illness includes evidence about the impact of mental illness and treatment on child outcomes (NICE, 2014). Whereas the bulk of this book explores the parent's experience of mental illness, the focus of this chapter is on the experience of the fetus and infant. The aim is to highlight the potential risks posed by perinatal mental illness. The existing evidence for the effects of perinatal mental illness on the main indicators of child outcome will be considered and the role of intervention reviewed. The emphasis will be on the management of perinatal mental illness in routine clinical practice.

# Pregnancy

## *Parental psychological adjustment*

The birth of a child represents a significant life event, particularly if it is a first child. In the main, it is expected that this will be a joyful time, but nevertheless it represents a time of enormous transition for all concerned. It is not surprising, therefore, that for some it is overwhelming and associated with increased levels of stress and anxiety. It is important to consider the effects of this, as well as the impact of formal mental illness on the preparedness of parents for the birth of their infant and on the infant. Severe mental health problems in parents will usually be detected and treated. It is likely, however, that there is a significant body of subclinical parental psychopathology that, although not severe enough to necessitate referral to specialist mental health services, nevertheless has the potential to adversely affect developing parent–child relationships and the well-being of the child. It is not uncommon for parents presenting with their children at child and adolescent mental health services to describe parental (most usually maternal) mental health problems in the perinatal period.

The process of pregnancy involves both physical and psychological aspects. Thus, while the mother progresses through the physical changes of pregnancy, both the mother and the father are also undergoing psychological changes in preparation for the arrival of their baby and their new role as parents (Stern, 1999). This 'psychological pregnancy' may be influenced by a range of factors, including normal fears and anxieties, physical and mental illness, and environmental stressors such as financial and housing worries and domestic violence. Previous perinatal loss is a risk factor in that it is associated with increased levels of pregnancy-specific anxiety and depression (Blackmore *et al*, 2011), with mothers having more symptoms than fathers. That is, parents who have lost a baby are understandably more concerned during a subsequent pregnancy.

Parents' previous experiences of being parented are also important in this process. A conflicted past may have a significant effect on a parent's emerging relationship with their child, both *in utero* and postnatally. Fraiberg *et al* (1987) describe maternal negative recollections of childhood relationships with parents as 'ghosts in the nursery' which may adversely affect parent–infant relationships. The ghosts vary in their tenacity, some being transient intruders, while others become more firmly established. It is important to note, however, that many parents who have experienced neglect, cruelty and abuse do not revisit this on their own children.

Parents form expectations (which may include both positive and negative expectations) about what their baby will be like in terms of temperament, personality and abilities, and about their future. In addition, there are cultural expectations and beliefs about babies and how they should behave. Babies may be conceived for specific reasons, e.g. to replace a lost child, to save a marriage, to be a boy or a girl, or so that a parent might feel loved by someone (Maldonano-Duran *et al*, 2000). Stern (1999) describes the 'imagined' baby and the conflicts which may arise after birth if the real and imagined babies do not match up. Factors such as preterm delivery or physical handicaps may immediately raise 'conflicts'. Research into the effects of invasive antenatal screening procedures on prenatal attachment has produced conflicting results (Allison, *et al*, 2011). In the case of preterm delivery, it is important to remember that the parents are also 'preterm' in their preparation for the arrival of their child. Conflicts may arise because of discrepancies between the real and imagined babies in terms of their temperament and behaviour. The psychoanalytic literature describes unconscious and developmental transformations in the perinatal period, which may provide insights into vulnerability to mental health problems and attachment difficulties during this time (Deutsch, 1947; Breen, 1975; Raphael-Leff, 1985; Trad, 1991).

This process of psychological adjustment therefore includes the development of an attachment to and a relationship with the fetus. Various factors potentially influence this. Factors such as supportive family relationships and being psychologically well (which in general are associated with higher socioeconomic status) are associated with higher levels of maternal–fetal attachment, whereas mental health problems such as depression or anxiety and substance misuse are associated with poorer attachment. There is, however, a lack of robust research in this area (Alhusen, 2008; Pisoni *et al*, 2014). Although it might have been expected that previous perinatal loss would affect prenatal attachment, this does not appear to be the case (Armstrong, 2002).

Feeling the baby move and seeing ultrasound pictures enhance parental attachment and parents' developing image of their baby (Sedgman *et al*, 2006). It is interesting that three- or four-dimensional ultrasound scans do not add any additional emotional impact or affect prenatal attachment compared with two-dimensional scans (de Jong-Pleij *et al*, 2013).

Psychological adjustment to pregnancy may not always be positive. In such cases, there must be immediate concerns about the well-being of the expected child. Having an unwanted pregnancy or being ambivalent about pregnancy for whatever reason is associated with some risk to the fetus in terms of preterm delivery and low birth weight (for a review, see Shah *et al*, 2011). Knowing both parents' attitude to the pregnancy is important (Korenman *et al*, 2002). Having an unwanted pregnancy may be associated with later rejection of the baby (Brockington *et al*, 2006).

## Denial of pregnancy and fetal abuse

Denial of pregnancy and concealed pregnancies are associated with risks to the fetus related to lack of antenatal care. Denial of pregnancy may result from inexperience and a lack of awareness of the physical changes of pregnancy. Denial of pregnancy may also occur in the context of psychological conflict, stress, trauma, dissociative states, psychotic illness and intellectual disability. The immediate physical risks to the baby associated with pregnancy denial result from inadequate antenatal care and the sudden unexpected arrival of the baby. There is also an association with neonaticide (Jenkins *et al*, 2011).

Concealment of pregnancy may occur where a mother wishes to have a baby but is worried that the baby may be taken away because of concerns about her ability to look after the child. The available evidence suggests that there be some association between concealed pregnancy and increased risk of preterm delivery (Nirmal *et al*, 2006). Babies born to mothers who have not had any prenatal care are at risk of adverse outcome, including out-of-home placement (Friedman *et al*, 2009). However, it seems that these women are often able to care for their babies following delivery (Friedman *et al*, 2007).

There is a paucity of information about the occurrence of and factors associated with fetal abuse (Kent *et al*, 1997). The concept of fetal abuse encompasses a range of potential insults, from physical assault to misuse of alcohol and drugs (Condon, 1986). Maternal fetal attachment may be important in fetal abuse (Pollock & Percy, 1999), and further investigation is required to improve understanding and to identify mothers and fathers who present a risk for fetal abuse.

Intimate partner violence (IPV) during pregnancy is associated with adverse fetal outcomes, including preterm delivery, low birth weight and maternal and neonatal death. Women are at risk of poor prenatal care, substance misuse and depression. Mechanisms mediating these associations include maternal behaviours such as smoking, and alcohol and substance misuse. In addition, there is evidence of an effect of stress on the hypothalamic–pituitary–adrenal axis (Alhusen *et al*, 2015). Ultimately, women who are victims of IPV are at risk of being murdered (Chambliss, 2008). There is also an association between IPV and unintended pregnancy (Pallitto *et al*, 2013). In the longer term, there is the risk to the child of being born into a violent home. There are associations between exposure to IPV and adverse developmental (language, social and motor) (Gilbert *et al*, 2013) and mental health outcomes (Bauer *et al*, 2013).

## Fetal experiences

It is important to remember that as parents are progressing through the psychological and physical changes of pregnancy, the fetus continues to grow and develop. Maldonano-Duran *et al* (2000) describe the fetus as a 'real presence' and a 'contributor' to the pregnancy who is 'immersed [...] in an emotional field that may be more or less conducive to healthy development'. For this reason, we are interested in fetal experiences *in utero* and to what extent these influence later development (Lecanuet & Schaal, 1996). With modern imaging/scanning techniques we are able to observe the fetus in some detail. Studies have examined fetal neurobehavioural development, as well as fetal response to various maternal states and stimuli. Most of the evidence in relation to fetal perception is from the third trimester of pregnancy. There is evidence that the fetus experiences taste and that these experiences may influence the enjoyment of flavours postnatally (Mennella *et al*, 2001). There is also evidence that the fetus responds to sound and, with increasing maturity, can discriminate the mother's voice (Voegtline *et al*, 2013). There is also evidence that fetal experience of sound may be important in shaping auditory development and the development of the 'musical mind' (Ullal-Gupta *et al*, 2013).

Fetal experience of pain is of particular interest in view of the developing fields of fetal medicine and surgery, with interventions for medical and surgical conditions being performed *in utero*. It is thought that the fetus cannot recognise pain as a noxious stimulus until functional thalamocortical fibres are in place. Our current knowledge suggests that the fetus does not experience pain until after the 26th week of gestation (Rokyta, 2008). An important aspect of fetal pain perception is the potential impact of the physiological response to pain on the developing brain and subsequent neurological outcome.

An association has been demonstrated between maternal psychological state during pregnancy and fetal neurobehavioural function (DiPietro *et al*, 2002; DiPietro, 2012). Measuring the immediate effects of parental mental

**143**

illness on the fetus is challenging and usually confined to physical effects (DiPietro, 2005). Pregnant women who describe their lives as stressful and who experience more 'hassles' in relation to their pregnancy have fetuses that are more active throughout pregnancy. By contrast, women who are more positive and perceive their pregnancy as 'uplifting' have less active fetuses. It is not clear what such findings mean in terms of the postnatal development of the fetus, although some studies have examined the associations between fetal neurobehavioural functioning and infant temperament (DiPietro *et al*, 1996). Pregnancies with more active fetuses tend to result in more difficult and unpredictable infants. This suggests that fetal neurobehavioural functioning may predict differences in infant regulation and reactivity.

Perhaps the most widely explored maternal psychological state in relation to fetal experience is maternal stress. There is a significant body of evidence describing the adverse effects of maternal stress in terms of pregnancy complications (e.g. pre-eclampsia, preterm delivery, miscarriage and fetal distress). In addition, there is evidence that maternal stress during pregnancy is associated with adverse physical and mental health outcomes for the fetus and infant, and indeed throughout life (for a review, see Talge *et al*, 2007). There is evidence that maternal stress during pregnancy is associated with temperamental and behavioural effects in the infant, with an increased risk of adverse mental health outcomes such as attention-deficit hyperactivity disorder (ADHD), anxiety, and cognitive and language problems. The mechanism by which maternal stress leads to these adverse outcomes is complex and still to be clearly elucidated. However, the evidence suggests that the effects are mediated through a mechanism of fetal programming (Knackstedt *et al*, 2005) via the hypothalamic–pituitary–adrenal axis and cortisol.

Pregnancy is a time of great change and great challenges for the expectant parents and for the developing fetus. Even in the best of circumstances this can be difficult, but it is more so when there are other problems such as parental mental illness or psychosocial stressors, all of which potentially affect the baby either directly or indirectly.

## Attachment

From the above, it is clear that a relationship emerges between the fetus and parents antenatally, and that this may be compromised by a range of factors, including parental mental illness and stressors such as worry and anxiety. This emerging relationship can be considered to be part of the attachment process (Main, 1996).

The term 'attachment' has entered common parlance. The term was first used by Sears to describe children's relationships with their parents (Sears 1943). Bowlby later used the term in relation to the affectional ties described in animals by ethologists (Bowlby, 1958). Bowlby considered the attachment of human infants to their mother to be largely biologically based and to represent a biological safety mechanism in which the infant stays close to the mother for protection. The mother, in turn, provides a secure base from which the infant can explore the world. Bowlby considered that the relationship between parent and child formed the basis for the child's later psychological development (Bowlby, 1982). The relationship between parent and child is the context in which the child develops a sense of themselves and of what happens in relationships (Winnicott, 1965; Bowlby, 1982; Stern, 2002).

Ainsworth (1963) further developed Bowlby's ideas, and much of our current understanding of attachment behaviour is based on her seminal work. The first studies of attachment involved examining infants' reactions to separation from their mother. Ainsworth identified three stages of attachment during infancy: undiscriminating social responsiveness, discriminating social responsiveness and active initiation. Ainsworth and Wittig (1969) developed a laboratory experiment to examine children's response to separation from their parents (the 'strange situation') and described different styles of attachment as a result: securely attached, anxiously attached and anxious avoidant. A fourth category of attachment, disorganised attachment (in which the infant shows attachment behaviour that is confused or incomplete) was identified by Main & Solomon (1986).

Psychoanalytic theory emphasises the importance of early parent–child relationships in an individual's development, including their personality and their future relationships (Freud, 1963). Anna Freud described the importance of a mother recognising and responding sensitively to her infant in relation to the child's further psychological development (Freud, 1970). The emphasis is on 'emotional reciprocity', a theme further explored by the object relations theorists, who discuss the importance of parent–infant relationships in the child's future interpersonal relationships (Winnicott, 1970).

Most of the research to date has focused on the role of mothers in attachment, although the evidence base describing attachment to fathers and other figures is developing. Infants do demonstrate attachment behaviours to their fathers; for example, they cry on separation from their fathers and greet them on return. Increasingly research is exploring domains of paternal parenting and the relationship between fathers' behaviour and attachment security between them and their children (Brown et al, 2012). There may, however, be differences in attachment behaviour. For example, there is evidence that in stressful situations the infant is more likely to prefer the mother (Lamb, 1976). Attachment behaviours are also seen with other caregivers such as grandparents (Sands et al, 2009).

Attachment requires maternal and paternal responsiveness. Anything that gets in the way of this can adversely affect attachment, with implications for the infant particularly, in respect of future relationships. In this way, perinatal mental illness may pose a threat to the development of attachment by impairing or limiting the extent of the relationship and bonding. A mother or father affected by mental illness may be less available for or less able to meet the needs of the developing infant. This, in turn, will affect the attachment relationship and, in extreme cases, may lead to the development of attachment disorders. Disorders of attachment (reactive attachment disorder, disinhibited social engagement disorder and disinhibited attachment disorder) are described in ICD-10 (World Health Organization, 1992) and DSM-V (American Psychiatric Association, 2013).

The role of attachment in the development and maintenance of child and adolescent mental health problems is widely recognised. At the extreme of disrupted attachment are those children and young people who have been removed from the care of their parents. Levels of psychopathology are so high in this group of children that specialist mental health services have been developed to address their needs. Any child who has experienced a compromised attachment relationship will be vulnerable to mental health problems. The English and Romanian Adoptees (ERA) Study Team have examined the experiences and outcomes of children adopted into British families following profoundly deprived early life experiences in Romanian institutions (Rutter *et al*, 2004). Their studies have confirmed the validity of the attachment disorder construct (O'Connor & Rutter, 2000) and have highlighted the vulnerability of children deprived in this way to developmental impairment (O'Connor *et al*, 2000). Kochanska & Kim (2013) describe an increased risk of behavioural problems in children who are insecurely attached to both parents. Being securely attached to one parent is protective, although being securely attached to both confers no additional benefit. 'Looked after' children and young people are seen as a vulnerable group in terms of their risks for relationship and mental health problems; however, there is evidence that children who have been maltreated by their parents and removed to foster care can develop secure relationships in adolescence (Joseph *et al*, 2014).

## Impact of parental mental illness on attachment

Any parental mental health problem may interfere with the capacity of the parent to form and maintain an attachment to their infant. Thus, parents with substance misuse disorder who continue to misuse drugs or alcohol following the birth of their child may not be available for the infant. There is, however, experience of substance-misusing mothers being highly motivated during pregnancy and postnatally to reduce and stop their substance misuse in the interests of their child (Pajulo *et al*, 1999). This is in keeping with a commonly expressed desire on the part of parents who have endured adverse experiences themselves: 'I want something better for my child than I have had' (Fraiberg *et al*, 1987).

Depression is most commonly identified in the postnatal period, but a significant number of women date the onset of their depression to the antenatal period. Depression at this time may have an effect on parental psychological adjustment and preparation for the arrival of the new baby. Pregnancy may be perceived as a dark, miserable time, which may affect the developing relationship with the expected child. Expectant parents may also feel guilty about being depressed, recognising the incongruity of their mood with the anticipated joyful event. Here, again, the risk to the infant is the potential impact on bonding and attachment.

Schizophrenic and psychotic illnesses are potentially highly disruptive to the psychological aspects of pregnancy and are associated with risks and poor outcome for the child (Bosanac *et al*, 2003). Both pregnancy occurring during the course of an established psychotic illness and new onset of psychosis during the perinatal period may disrupt the attachment process.

Pre-existing anxiety disorders (e.g. generalised anxiety disorder, post-traumatic stress disorder or obsessive–compulsive disorder (OCD)) may be exacerbated during pregnancy, and concerns may focus on the baby's well-being and outcome. It is easy to imagine how mothers and fathers preoccupied by their own anxieties might be unavailable for their infants, thus putting the attachment relationship is at risk. In acute onset of OCD symptoms during pregnancy or within the first few weeks, postpartum obsessional thoughts are usually about harming the baby. This results in avoidance of situations that evoke the thoughts, which may have implications for family life and attachment (Abramowitz *et al*, 2001).

Personality disorder has been associated with adverse effects on child outcome. The impact during the antenatal period will be on the individual's conceptualisation of their role as a parent, and on their ability to manage the pregnancy and prepare physically and psychologically for the arrival of their child. Postnatally, the risk to the child is in terms of the parents' inability to parent and of impaired attachment relationships (Hobson *et al*, 2005). In borderline personality disorder (BPD), the role of the fluctuating tone of parenting from hostile to aloof has been described (Stepp *et al*, 2011). Macfie & Swan (2009), in a study of children of mothers with BPD compared to normative controls, found more role reversal, fear of abandonment, negative parent–child interactions and shameful representations of themselves in the children of mothers with BPD. Mothers with BPD are less good at recognising their infants' emotions, which may in turn affect their ability to sensitively respond to their babies (Elliot *et al*, 2014). The presence of depression and personality disorder is reported to have independent detrimental effects on early infant care practices (Conroy *et al*, 2010). Personality disorder is one of the predictors of discharge from a mother and baby unit under some form of social services supervision (Howard *et al*, 2003).

There has been considerable debate about parenting in the intellectual disability population. A number of court cases in the past 20 years focusing on the sterilisation of young women with intellectual disability brought to public attention issues such as the right to – and the ability to consent to – sexual relationships, contraception and being a parent, whereas previously it had often been assumed that such things were not important for people with intellectual disability. However, there is a balance to be found between normalisation and the protection of vulnerable adults from potential abuse. As women with moderate to severe intellectual disability are less likely to become pregnant, most of the issues relate to those with mild or borderline intellectual disability.

According to Campion (1995), parental IQ (unless this is < 55–60) does not significantly influence parenting ability in intellectual disability. Instead, the relevant factors are child characteristics such as: age, birth order, sex and temperament; the size of the family (three children or more is more stressful); the quality of the relationship and whether or not the partner has mental health problems; what support is available; and whether or not criticism and conflict are present. These are much the same factors that pertain in parents without intellectual disability.

Problems may not be due to the intellectual disability *per se*, but to poverty, poor housing, discrimination and lack of support – or these factors may magnify any difficulties in parenting competence arising from intellectual disability. The main risks to the child are of maltreatment, developmental delay and behaviour disorders. Abuse is rare and, if present, is often perpetrated by another person associated with the mother, rather than by the mother herself. Where abuse does occur, neglect is the most common form.

### Interventions

Feldman (1994) reviewed 20 studies of educational input for parents with intellectual disability. He found that the most effective interventions were performance rather than knowledge-based and used practice, modelling, feedback and praise. He also pointed out that if training is not carried out in the home, it should be provided in an environment as 'home-like' as possible. Interventions should focus on supervision of children, positive-based child behaviour management, stress and anger management, non-corporal punishment and age-appropriate cognitive stimulation. The school-age or adolescent children of parents with intellectual disability might need specific counselling or tutoring themselves. However, the professionals providing such interventions should have been appropriately trained, and it should not be assumed that community nurses working with parents with intellectual disability have the necessary skills (Culley & Genders, 1999).

## Parental attachment

In the preceding section, the emphasis was on the child's relationship with and attachment to the parent, in particular the detrimental effects on the child when this process is compromised. However, it is also important to explore parent–child relationships from the perspective of the parent. Here, again, we consider mother–infant interaction primarily, because this has been the focus of most research.

Brockington (1996, 2004) describes the crucial psychological process of the development of the mother's relationship with her infant. Disorders of this process are relatively common and may be extreme, involving the mother rejecting her child. There are risks of child abuse and neglect and, later, of adverse effects on child cognitive functioning (Murray *et al*, 1996*a*). Interventions are aimed at helping the mother to enjoy her child.

The neurobiology of parent–infant relationships and behaviour is being elucidated, with studies exploring the neurohormonal and neuroanatomical basis of parents' responses to children (Swain *et al*, 2007). The study of brain systems involved in parental responses to infants using functional magnetic resonance imaging (fMRI) suggests a role for cortico-limbic networks. Mental illness affects these networks (for a review, see Swain *et al* 2014). Oxytocin has been shown to be linked to sensitive caregiving and to enhance the neural circuits implicated in parental attachment behaviours (Rilling, 2013).

## Resilience

It is important to note that the child is not passive in their relationship with their parent or caregiver. There is an increasing awareness that children's responses to parental mental illness and their outcomes vary, with some children doing well (Kim-Cohen, 2007). It is also recognised that, from birth, children have different temperamental styles. This may be important in how the infant responds to adverse factors such as parental mental illness, and also in the development of attachment, as described above.

The most notable research into infant temperament was undertaken by Thomas *et al* (1968) in the New York Longitudinal Study. They described nine characteristics of infant temperament, including activity level, rhythmicity of biological functions, quality of mood, approach or withdrawal in response to new experiences, persistence, and ease of adaptability. On analysing these characteristics, they found that some clustered together and identified three patterns of infant temperament: difficult (irregular eating and sleeping patterns, withdraw from new situations, adapt poorly, have negative mood and intense reactions); easy (positive mood, biological regularity, mild intensity, adaptable and react positively to new situations) and slow to warm up (initial withdrawal, slow adaptation and mild intensity). Not surprisingly, the infants with the easy temperament had the best outcomes and were least likely to develop mental health problems.

From the above, it is apparent how infant temperament may compromise developing attachments in the perinatal period. Attachment is a reciprocal process: the infant's response to their parent has an effect on the parent's subsequent behaviour. For example, infants who are difficult to soothe and who do not feed or sleep well may undermine parental self-confidence, which in turn affects the way the parent feels towards the child. In this way, a negative spiral of a deteriorating attachment relationship may develop. It is not uncommon in clinical practice for parents of children with emotional and behavioural problems to say that their child was a 'difficult baby' who did not feed well or settle easily to sleep, and to be hostile and critical towards their child. The role of expressed emotion in child emotional and behavioural problems has been described (Sonuga-Barke *et al*, 2013; Richards *et al*, 2014).

The concept of resilience is increasingly acknowledged as important in child outcome. Although child temperament may be a component of resilience, it is likely that it is more complex than this. Various authors have attempted to operationalise resilience, measuring it in terms of achievement against a range of global markers of outcome (Daniel, 2006; Skala & Bruckner, 2014). An awareness of resilience is important in day-to-day clinical practice, recognising that some children will do well despite adverse circumstances (e.g. having a parent with mental illness). Intervention must include an assessment of resilience factors and strategies to promote these, as well as treating risk factors.

# Child outcome

Parental mental illness is associated with adverse outcomes in all aspects of child development and mental health. In addition, children of parents with mental illness are at increased risk of abuse and neglect. The mechanisms underpinning these associations are complex and include genetic and environmental factors. There is an increasing body of evidence that demonstrates the genetic basis of mental illness, and that such children are at increased risk of developing problems in their own right. Factors associated with parental mental illness may further compromise child outcome. Women with mental health problems are more at risk of having unplanned pregnancies, of being single parents, of being socially disadvantaged, of misusing substances, of having poorer antenatal care and of relapsing following the birth of their child (Kent, 2011). Women with mental health problems are also more likely to have their children removed. All of these factors are associated with poor child outcome.

## Antenatal mental illness

There is now a considerable body of evidence that shows an association between maternal mental health problems during pregnancy and adverse outcomes for the child, including effects on their emotional, cognitive and physical health and development. Women are just as likely to become mentally unwell during pregnancy as at any other time; they are also at risk of deterioration of an established illness during pregnancy, and some expectant mothers kill themselves in the context of mental illness (Knight et al, 2015). Much less information is available about paternal antenatal mental health problems.

Although maternal depression was at one time thought to be primarily a postnatal phenomenon, it is now widely recognised that in some cases depression begins in the antenatal period. Also, some women have established mood disorders when they become pregnant. There is evidence of an increased risk of complications during pregnancy and delivery in women with major affective disorders, and of early neonatal problems, including fetal distress (Jablensky et al, 2005). Antenatal depression has been shown to increase the risk of preterm delivery, low birth weight and intrauterine growth retardation (Grote et al, 2010). There are also risks associated with self-harm and suicide (Lindahl et al, 2005; Knight et al, 2015). The mechanism for this link between antenatal depression and adverse outcome is unclear, as depression occurs against a background of other risk and protective factors (Alder et al, 2007).

Antenatal anxiety and psychosocial stress are associated with greater levels of fetal activity and higher rates of preterm birth and low birth weight (Ding, et al, 2014). A range of stressors have been implicated, including pregnancy denial, getting back with a partner, being unhappy about the pregnancy and having an unplanned pregnancy (Sable & Wilkinson, 2000). The effects of maternal stress on the developing fetal brain, modifying hypothalamic–pituitary–adrenal function and neurotransmitter systems (Kapoor et al, 2006) are described earlier in this chapter.

Maternal starvation or bingeing and vomiting as part of an eating disorder can potentially threaten the physical well-being of the developing fetus. Reported risks linked to anorexia nervosa include low infant birth weight together with prematurity, and antepartum haemorrhage (Eagles et al, 2012; Solmi et al, 2014). Binge eating is linked with intra-uterine growth impairment, preterm delivery (Micali et al, 2007) and babies that are large for gestational age (Bulik et al, 2009).

Mothers with a diagnosis of schizophrenia or bipolar disorder are at increased risk of complications such as antepartum haemorrhage, pre-eclampsia, preterm delivery and babies who have either high or low birth weight (Jablensky et al 2005; Vigod et al, 2014). There is also an association with an increased risk of stillbirth and neonatal death (King-Hele, 2009).

The effects of the misuse of various substances on the developing fetus are well described in the literature and are summarised in Chapter 5 of this book (for a review, see Keegan et al, 2010). The harmful effects of maternal substance misuse on fetal development are widely accepted (Connery & Rayburn, 2014). Substance misuse is associated with a range of fetal effects, including growth retardation, physical abnormalities and neurobehavioural changes. It is noteworthy that the two most commonly available substances of misuse, nicotine and alcohol, are associated most clearly with adverse fetal outcomes: nicotine with the highest risk of fetal growth retardation, and alcohol with fetal alcohol spectrum disorder (FASD), which represents a spectrum of physical and psychological difficulties. The direct fetal effects of other substances of misuse are less clear. Neonatal abstinence syndrome is increasingly recognised and treated, but there is less information about the long-term effects (Jansson & Velez, 2012; Kocherlakota, 2014).

In addition to these immediate effects, there is increasing evidence that antenatal mental illness is associated with longer-term adverse effects beyond the immediate perinatal period. Antenatal mental illness may continue into the postnatal period, and new illnesses may develop during this time. Postnatal mental illness is associated with adverse effects on all aspects of child development and represents a risk factor for child mental health. In addition, there are the implications for parenting and attachment, described earlier in this chapter. Children whose parents have mental health problems are at increased risk of abuse and neglect, and mothers with mental illness are at increased risk of having their babies taken into care (Howard *et al*, 2004).

## Child development

Parental mental illness is known to potentially adversely affect child physical, social, emotional, behavioural and cognitive development. The risks lie in the effects of illness on a parent's ability to meet their child's emerging developmental needs. Children require different things of their parents at different stages in their development. In the immediate neonatal period, the most apparent needs are physical and relate to the child being fed and kept warm and safe. In addition, the parent has a role in responding to the child's emotional state and, for example, soothing the child when they are distressed as a result of being hungry or uncomfortable. The parent has an important role here in helping the child differentiate between different arousal states, which is important in the early development of higher-order executive functions (Kopp, 1982, 1989). Thus, parent–child interaction in infancy is important to the child's later cognitive development.

There is some evidence that compromised or poor interaction between mother and child, as in the case of perinatal mental illness, is associated with poor physical health outcomes for children (Mantymaa *et al*, 2003). Antenatal and postnatal screening programmes in the UK are designed to alert healthcare professionals to any child at risk. Thus, any child who is failing to thrive should be identified and appropriate interventions put in place through child protection and safeguarding processes (Hall & Williams, 2008).

The longer-term effects of maternal substance misuse on child outcome have focused on nicotine, alcohol, opiates, methamphetamine and cocaine. Prenatal exposure to nicotine is associated with lower IQ, and with attention and conduct problems. Maternal cannabis use during pregnancy is associated with mild withdrawal symptoms. Longer-term outcomes include difficulties with reading and spelling, and with higher-order executive function. Studies of the association between maternal cocaine use during pregnancy and longer-term child outcome produce conflicting results but suggest subtle central nervous system (CNS) abnormalities. There is some evidence for lower weight-to-height ratios, and problems with perceptual reasoning and attention. In addition, there are associations with behavioural problems. Longer-term follow-up studies of prenatal opiate exposure have also produced conflicting results. Some studies have shown some evidence for general cognitive delays and associations with disruptive behavioural problems (for reviews, see Bandstra *et al*, 2010; Lester & Lagasse, 2010; and Minnes *et al*, 2011).

Animal models have demonstrated a link between maternal antenatal stress and later behavioural problems. The effect of excessive maternal stress on the development and functioning of the fetal stress system may have a longer-term effect on aspects of child psychological well-being (Charmandari *et al*, 2003). Talge *et al* (2007) review the evidence linking antenatal maternal stress and later risk of emotional, behavioural, cognitive and language problems.

Postnatally, mothers with eating disorders may have a distorted image or perception of their baby and may worry that he/she is too fat. This puts the baby at risk of feeding difficulties and failure to thrive (Waugh & Bulik, 1999; Cooper *et al*, 2004). In their review of the children of mothers with eating disorders, Park *et al* (2003) explore the effect on feeding in infancy and childhood, together with the effects on growth. They describe the lack of systematic controlled studies of mothers with eating disorders and a relative absence of information about the effects of paternal eating problems. Overall, the evidence suggests that children of mothers with eating disorders are at risk of eating problems, but that other factors are important in the expression of these problems. Eating disturbances are present from birth, with mothers finding that feeding infants and children can be difficult. Mothers with eating disorders are more irregular in their feeding patterns and more inclined to feed their baby as a way of comforting them. As children get older, mothers with eating disorders are more likely to be negative to their infants and mealtimes are often tense. Maternal eating disorder and disturbed eating patterns are associated with child feeding disorders, problems regulating food intake and eating difficulties. There are also effects on growth, with infants of mothers with eating disorders weighing less than controls. Mothers with eating disorders worry that their children will become fat and are more concerned about their children's weight. Later in life, mothers are concerned that their children will develop eating disorders. It is likely that the development of eating disorders in adolescent girls is influenced by other factors such as sociocultural pressures (Sanftner *et al*, 1996).

Maternal postnatal depression has been linked with poor infant outcomes, including problems with attachment, and cognitive, social and emotional development. Children are most at risk where maternal depression is severe and long-standing. It is likely that the mechanism for this involves impaired mother–infant interaction. Murray et al (1996b), in a study examining the longer-term influence of postnatal depression on child cognitive function, found that at 5 years of age there was no evidence for an adverse effect on child cognitive function. Insensitive mother–child interaction did, however, predict the persistence of poorer cognitive function. Other risk factors may be important in longer-term cognitive outcome, particularly the chronicity of maternal depression, gender (boys are more at risk than girls) and other socioeconomic risks (Kurstjens & Wolke, 2001). In general, however, exposure to maternal depression (pre- and postnatally) is a risk factor for child cognitive and language delays (Sohr-Preston & Scaramella, 2006).

# Child mental health problems

We know that the children of parents affected by mental illness are themselves at increased risk of mental health problems. The explanation for this is likely to be multifactorial, including genetic predisposition and environmental influences (in terms of both the environmental effects of parental mental illness and associated risk factors). There is increasing evidence for a genetic contribution to many of the major psychiatric illnesses seen in adulthood; as a result, being born to a parent with a mental health problem is itself a risk factor. At this stage, however, we do not understand the complexity of the interaction between a child's genetic predisposition and their experience of the environment in which they live, and how this affects the later expression of mental illness. Further work is needed to explore this. It is important to recognise that not every child whose parent has a mental illness will become mentally ill or present with emotional or behavioural problems. Protective or resiliency factors as discussed above – whether these represent inherent child characteristics, environmental experiences or both – are important. The risk to a child's mental health is not confined to the specific disorder experienced by their parent; rather, they are at increased risk of a wide range of disorders (Dean et al, 2010).

The most commonly used harmful substance in pregnancy is nicotine, and there is a body of evidence which supports an association between maternal smoking and subsequent child behavioural problems. As noted above, cocaine and opiate use during pregnancy are also associated with childhood disruptive behavioural problems.

Stressful experiences in the later stages of pregnancy have been associated with emotional and behavioural problems in the child (O'Connor et al, 2003). Similarly, high levels of maternal antenatal anxiety are associated with higher rates of behavioural and emotional problems in children beyond the immediate perinatal period, highlighting the potential for long-term adverse effects (O'Connor et al, 2002). Evidence suggests that prenatal anxiety is related to difficult infant temperament postnatally, and that this is independent of any effect of postnatal depression. Both antenatal anxiety and postnatal depression predict child emotional and behavioural problems, but do so independently of each other. There may also be an additive effect (O'Connor et al, 2002). Children whose mothers experienced antenatal depression were more likely to experience depression in adolescence (Pawlby et al, 2009). Further data from the same group observed that depression in pregnancy significantly predicted violence in adolescence, even after controlling for the family environment, the child's later exposure to maternal depression, the mother's smoking and drinking during pregnancy, and the parents' antisocial behaviour (Hay et al, 2010).

This suggests that interventions could usefully be targeted at mothers who have risk factors for anxiety, such as domestic violence and previous abuse (Austin, 2004). Maternal postnatal depression is associated with increased risk of the child developing depression by the age of 16 years (Murray et al, 2011). Children of mothers who develop psychotic illness in the perinatal period are at increased risk of mental health problems later in life (Abbott et al, 2004).

# Child abuse and neglect

In the majority of cases, parents with mental illness do not set out with the intention of harming their children. Instead, their illness interferes with their ability to provide for the needs of their child. This may manifest as physical or emotional neglect. Child sexual abuse may also occur in the context of a parental mental illness. Rarely, a mentally ill parent may murder their child (Stanton & Simpson, 2006).

The exposure of the infant and child to IPV is associated with increased risk of poor mental health and behavioural outcomes. Children who have been exposed to IPV have higher rates of internalising and externalising disorders, including anxiety, depression and post-traumatic stress disorder (Kitzmann et al, 2003). In addition, they may be at increased risk of risk-taking behaviour in adolescence (Bair-Merritt et al, 2006). Whitaker et al (2006) have described the cumulative effect of maternal mental health problems, substance misuse and IPV on child behaviour. Associations between being physically abused as a child, witnessing IPV and becoming a perpetrator of IPV have been described (Gil-Gonzalez et al, 2008).

Children of parents with mental health problems are at increased risk of abuse and neglect (Sidebotham et al, 2006). Indeed, parental mental illness is consistently identified as a risk factor for recurrent maltreatment (Hindley et al, 2006). It is essential that professionals working with parents with mental health problems are alert to the possibilities of child abuse and neglect and are familiar with child protection and safeguarding procedures (Hall & Williams, 2008). An essential component of the management of mental illness during the perinatal period involves considering the capacity of the ill parent to care for their child. In some cases, it is obvious that an ill parent will not cope and that it would be unsafe for a child to remain in their care. Ideally, the other parent or another family member such as a grandparent or aunt/uncle will care for the child until the parent is well enough to resume parental responsibilities. Being 'looked after' or 'accommodated' by Social Services and being fostered by another family are additional risk factors for mental health problems in children and young people (Kerker & Dore, 2006). It is important to remember that having a child accommodated is also a risk factor for a parent.

Flynn *et al* (2007) have examined the characteristics of people who kill infants in the context of the National Confidential Inquiry into Suicide and Homicide by People with Mental Illness. Between 1996 and 2001, in England and Wales, 112 people were convicted of infant homicide. The inquiry found that fathers killed more infants than mothers. Twenty-four per cent had a mental illness at the time of the killing, and 34% had a lifetime history of mental illness. Fifty-three per cent of the men had a history of drug or alcohol misuse. Forty-four per cent of the infants were killed within 3 months of birth and 78% within 6 months. The authors emphasise the need for perinatal assessment and support. In a further review, Spinelli (2005) addressed the historical, cultural and political views of infanticide, and Friedman *et al* (2012) used evolutionary psychology as a theoretical framework to review infanticide laws (see also Chapter 3).

Flynn *et al* (2013) reviewed filicide (the killing of one's own child) in England and Wales between 1997 and 2006. During this period, 297 filicides and 45 filicide–suicides were recorded. Of the parents who killed their children, 66% were fathers. In most cases, the parents were not mentally ill, but mothers were more likely than fathers to be ill, and to have an affective disorder, schizophrenia or another delusional disorder. The authors emphasise the importance of monitoring mentally ill parents caring for children and the need for further research to identify risk factors.

## Paternal mental illness

The bulk of the evidence about the effect of perinatal mental illness describes maternal mental illness. There is, however, increasing evidence of the extent and significance of paternal mental illness during this period. It is unlikely that paternal mental illness is insignificant in terms of child outcome, and our relative lack of information in this area is simply because we have tended to focus research interest on mothers (Phares, 1992; Phares *et al*, 2005). It is a feature of most cultures that mothers are the primary caregivers of small children. Fathers nevertheless have a role, and indeed paternal caregiving is being promoted in Western cultures. It is important that we consider paternal mental health and the impact of mentally ill fathers on children (Currid, 2005). Ten per cent of fathers will have a partner who is affected by mental illness during the perinatal period, and their role in supporting the family system during such illness is important (Condon, 2006).

Kvalevaag *et al* (2013) describe the association between paternal psychological distress during pregnancy and social, emotional and behavioural problems in their children at 36 months of age. Paternal depression in the postnatal period affects children's later emotional, social and behavioural development (Ramchandani *et al*, 2005; Fletcher *et al*, 2011). In a review, Ramchandani & Psychogiou (2009) describe an increased risk of child behavioural and emotional problems associated with most of the psychiatric disorders that affect fathers. The extent of the risk seems to be similar to that associated with maternal mental illness. They also review evidence suggesting that boys may be more vulnerable than girls to paternal psychiatric illness, and that there may be a greater risk to behavioural rather than emotional problems associated with paternal mental illness.

Fathers are not included in therapy with children as often as mothers. However, when they are, although there may not be any immediate benefit to short-term outcome for the child, there are indirect benefits in terms of retention in treatment and improved interparental relationships. Long-term outcome may also be improved (Phares *et al*, 2005).

## Adolescents

There is an increased risk of adverse physical outcomes in adolescent pregnancy (Ganchimeg *et al*, 2014). Studies have shown rates of postnatal depression of around 50% in adolescents, and a similar number report consuming alcohol during their pregnancy. Up to 30% will have used cannabis. Additional risk factors include poor housing, poor nutrition and cognitive and emotional immaturity (Combs-Orme, 1993; McCracken & Loveless, 2014)

Young mothers experience greater levels of risk factors associated with poor outcomes for both mother and child. In comparison to older mothers, young mothers (less than 20 years of age) are exposed to higher levels of socioeconomic deprivation and have more mental health problems, and their partners are more unreliable, antisocial and abusive, and less supportive both economically and emotionally (Moffitt *et al*, 2002; Hodgkinson *et al*, 2014).

The children of teenage mothers have higher levels of emotional and behavioural problems, and poorer educational attainment, and are at increased risk of accidents, injuries and illness. Children of teenage mothers are at increased risk of adverse long-term outcomes, including early school-leaving, unemployment, early parenthood and offending behaviour (Jaffee *et al*, 2001). Social influence and social characteristics both contribute to this risk.

There is less information about adolescent fathers, but they also present with increased vulnerability and also represent a risk for the outcome of the child. They are more likely to have experienced adverse family relationships such as parental separation or domestic violence, and may not have a positive role model of parenting on which to draw (Tan & Quinlivan, 2006).

As with teenage mothers, teenage fathers have increased levels of psychological symptoms, including anxiety and depression (Quinlivan & Condon, 2005). Teenage expectant fathers are stressed about the pending birth. Many are concerned about how they are going to support the baby and the mother, finish school and get a job, as well as about the well-being of the mother and child. Most want to be involved with their children, and their involvement is associated with better behavioural and cognitive outcome for the child (Barret & Robinson, 1990).

Thus, having teenage parents represents an added vulnerability for the child, with potentially adverse consequence for their short- and longer-term outcome. This group is also vulnerable because of the likelihood of suboptimal antenatal and postnatal care. Clinically, this is a group to be vigilant of in antenatal and postnatal monitoring for both maternal and child outcomes.

## Family aspects

When a mother or father has mental health problems, there is an impact on family functioning and dynamics. The roles and responsibilities of the ill parent, both in general and in relation to childcare, may have to be taken over to varying degrees by the other parent, other family members, friends or professionals. This is disruptive for all concerned. There are effects on the child associated with the nature of the parent's illness, and there may also be effects on their attachment to the ill parent.

Other family members and friends will also be affected. The other parent will have to take over all parenting responsibilities, which may compromise their other roles (e.g. work). There may also be effects on their own mental health because of the worry and stress associated with having an ill partner. Grandparents and siblings also often take on childcare responsibilities, and this is associated with negative effects on their own mental health. Grandparents describe the stress of having to look after young children at a time of life when they had not expected this. In addition, they may also take on responsibilities for caring for the ill parent (Gopfert et al, 2004). Similarly, older children who take on the role of carer for the ill parent as well as assuming childcare responsibilities are a vulnerable group (Aldridge & Becker, 2003). The effect of this on the ill parent must also be recognised. Many describe feeling guilty about the burden they feel they represent to their family and struggle with their loss of role. The impact on families of parental mental illness is complex; the response of families is important in the ill parent's recovery and rehabilitation and also in child outcome (Perera et al, 2014).

# Perinatal mental health in gay and lesbian couples

Increasingly, same-sex couples are entering into parenthood. The literature describing the impact of perinatal mental illness in gay and lesbian parents on their children is limited. Ross (2005) discusses the issues facing lesbian women who are pregnant, and highlights that many of the challenges associated with moving into parenthood are equally applicable to same-sex couples, but notes that there may be additional vulnerabilities such as lack of the usual social and familial supports, compounded by the negative impact of discrimination.

Research has considered lesbian mothers and their children from various perspectives. Johnson (2012) describes three waves of research: focusing on lesbian mothers who had their children while in heterosexual relationships; on those who became parents in lesbian relationships; and, finally, on the challenges faced by the families of lesbian parents.

# Intervention

The management of perinatal mental illness is complex and requires the consideration of the needs of the mother, the fetus and infant, and the mother's adjustment to her pregnancy and becoming a mother, together with the needs of the family and particularly other children.

The primary focus for treatment in perinatal mental illness is the ill parent. The natural assumption is that if the parent's mental illness is treated and they recover, then the effects on the child will be minimised – or, at least, that by treating the parent the risk to the child is removed or lessened. The aim must be to restore the parent to normal day-to-day functioning, which will then facilitate their parenting. Increasingly, it is recognised that it is important to consider the outcome of the child in their own right, and that the specific needs of the child must be included in any treatment plan. Some interventions have been developed with the aim of promoting positive child outcomes; however, there continues to be a paucity of evidence about the effects of routine treatment on child outcome. Increasingly, the evidence suggests that it is not enough just to treat the parent's illness, as this will not necessarily ensure a good outcome for the child, and that it is important to intervene specifically to promote parent–child interaction. However, to date, the evidence is for limited effect. There continues to be a paucity of specialist perinatal and infant mental health services across the UK and internationally. The opportunity to intervene to modify child outcome in the case of parental mental illness is therefore limited. Guidance from NICE (2014) reviews the evidence for the treatment of perinatal mental illness and includes impact on child outcome.

## Assessment

Recognition of the potentially detrimental effect on child outcome of parental perinatal mental illness suggests a role for early identification and intervention. This in turn requires mechanisms for screening in the perinatal period. There are well-established mechanisms for parental mental illness, particularly postnatal depression, e.g. the Edinburgh Postnatal Depression Scale (Cox *et al*, 2014). There are less robust mechanisms for screening for other mental health problems, particularly in the antenatal period. Severe mental illness will in most cases be immediately apparent, but children will still be at risk if parents, because of their illness, do not take up available antenatal and postnatal care. It is important that all staff involved in delivering perinatal services are aware of the range of parental mental health problems and the risk/vulnerability factors for children. Infants who are potentially at risk of adverse outcome can then be identified antenatally, and appropriate measures put in place to monitor their well-being.

There are challenges in the definition and measurement of child outcome in the immediate perinatal period. In the longer term, child outcome can be described by examining social, emotional and behavioural adjustment, as well as cognitive function. The measurement of child outcome in the early neonatal period is complicated and is often described in terms of physical parameters such as birth weight and the achievement of milestones, etc. Given the importance of attachment, it is clear that a key outcome is the quality of parent–child interaction. Aspects of the attachment relationship can be measured in a number of ways, including self-report, e.g. the Parenting Stress Index (Abidin, 1986), the Parental Bonding Instrument (Parker, 1989); and observation, e.g. The Parent–Child Early Relational Assessment (Clark, 1985) and the HOME (Home Observation for the Measurement of the Environment) Inventory (Caldwell & Bradley, 1978). The Adult Attachment Interview (Hesse, 2008) explores the adult's experience of attachment (see earlier comments about the importance of the parents' experience of being parented).

Although measures such as these will provide detailed information about parent–child relationships, they are primarily research tools and are difficult to employ in routine day-to-day practice because of the need for training and the time taken to administer and score measures. Self-report measures have limitations in terms of objectivity. The development of clinically appropriate assessment tools which can be used by a range of professionals should be a focus for further work.

In the longer term, a range of outcome measures can be considered, including those which examine child cognitive development, e.g. the Bayley Scales of Infant Development (Bayley, 1993). As children get older, their social, emotional and behavioural adjustment can be assessed by means of parent and nursery teacher self-report scales, e.g. the Strengths and Difficulties Questionnaire (Goodman, 1997). It is recognised that social, emotional and behavioural problems may present early in life and, if untreated, may have significant implications for long-term prognosis. There is an increasing variety of assessment tools to assess mental health problems in infancy and early childhood, which reflects the developing field of infant mental health (DelCarmen-Wiggins & Carter, 2004). These measures include the Child Behaviour Checklist 1.5-5 (Achenbach & Rescorla, 2001) and the Infant Toddler Symptom Checklist (Degangi *et al*, 1995).

## Treatment

The treatment of the range of perinatal mental illnesses is described throughout this book. A basic principle of treatment of parental mental illness, however, is to avoid or minimise any adverse effect on the fetus or infant. The need to treat the mother and the potential risks associated with not doing so must be balanced against any potential risk to the baby. If a mother has taken psychotropic medication during her pregnancy, it is essential that the infant is assessed for evidence of neonatal adaptation syndrome and for other potential adverse effects in the first few weeks of life. In addition, SSRIs (selective serotonin reuptake inhibitors) and SNRIs (serotonin–noradrenaline reuptake inhibitors) may be associated with a serotonergic syndrome in the baby. Babies of mothers who have misused drugs and alcohol during their pregnancy may experience withdrawal symptoms and/or neonatal abstinence syndrome, which must be treated.

The key consideration in the use of pharmacological agents in relation to child outcome is in terms of potential effects on the fetus and the newborn infant. The psychological aspects of pharmacotherapy for the mother must also be considered. Parental concerns about the use of medication in relation to their expected child must be addressed. Parents often raise concerns in the context of a child and adolescent mental health assessment that their child's difficulties may be the result of something they did or a medication they took during pregnancy.

Electroconvulsive therapy (ECT) is rarely used in pregnancy, but it may be considered when a pregnant woman's life is at risk because of mental illness. Halmo *et al* (2014) describe the occurrence of 'bizarre fetal spasms' occurring in the first 2 h following ECT. However, all of the women studied ($n = 3$) were safely delivered of their babies, who were healthy at follow-up. For a review of ECT in pregnancy, see Pompili *et al* (2014).

The evidence presented in this chapter suggests that, in addition to treating the parent, it is important to consider intervening to support parent–child interaction. A range of interventions and opportunities to employ these are described, particularly focusing on mother–infant interaction. However, the evidence base for effectiveness and cost-effectiveness in relation to child outcome and mother–infant interaction is limited (NICE 2014).

Interventions include antenatal programmes such as Mellow Bumps, a targeted intervention for vulnerable women (Birtwell *et al*, 2015), baby massage and parent/mother–child interaction coaching. The use of unqualified staff in delivering such interventions has been explored, with some evidence for effectiveness in some domains of functioning (Cooper *et al*, 2002). Overall, however, the evidence remains limited for any significant and particularly long-term effect on child outcome.

There are a range of models of parent–child psychotherapy, such as psychodynamic and interactional approaches, and attachment-oriented, cognitive–behavioural therapy and family-based interventions, which can be generalised to parents with mental illness (Puura & Kaukonen, 2010). Most of the evidence for effectiveness relates to evaluations of specific programmes, and there is little information available from systematic reviews or randomised controlled trials specifically in relation to the use of such interventions in perinatal mental illness.

Parent management training (PMT) continues to be used extensively in child and adolescent mental health services, and there is evidence for benefit in young children with disruptive behavioural problems (Furlong *et al*, 2012). There is some evidence that such programmes are also beneficial to maternal psychosocial health (anxiety, depression and self-esteem), although more research is needed in this area (Barlow & Coren, 2004). PMT may be useful in supporting parents with mental illness, but the development of such programmes remains limited (Craig, 2004; Van der Zanden *et al*, 2010).

Residential treatment programmes for substance-misusing expectant mothers have been shown to improve the physical outcomes of babies, for example, birth weight and length (Little, 2003). The incorporation of attachment-based parenting interventions into such programmes may improve their effectiveness in terms of parent–child relationships (Suchman *et al*, 2004).

There has been considerable interest in the use of large-scale intensive home-visiting programmes in the promotion of the well-being of children born into adverse circumstances. The majority have included a component of parent training. There is some evidence of benefit in terms of maternal mental health and mother–child interaction (Beeber *et al*, 2004). A number of projects have also explored the use of volunteer home visitors (Taggart *et al*, 2000). In this way, home-based intervention programmes may provide large-scale indirect support of parental (especially maternal) mental health – although, again, the evidence for long-term benefits for mother–child interaction and child outcome is limited (Wan *et al*, 2008).

In addition to the more generic parent training interventions described above, some programmes specifically address parent–infant interaction, e.g. Minding the Baby (Slade *et al*, 2005; Sadler *et al*, 2013) and Watching, Waiting and Wondering (Muir, 1992). Such interventions aim to work with parents to develop their reflective capacities so that they are able to observe and reflect on their infant's emotional life and follow his or her lead.

It is important to consider the potential benefits to the child of being cared for by someone else (Lee *et al*, 2006). In extreme cases, it may not be safe for a child to remain with a parent with severe mental health problems. It is therefore essential that multidisciplinary staff working with parents with mental health problems are aware of their responsibilities in terms of child protection. Parents with mental health problems are often aware of the effect of their illness on their parenting and are concerned about this, often feeling guilty and that they are failing their children. This is particularly so when a child is removed and taken into the care of Social Services or when a parent is admitted to hospital. Evidence suggests that even when the parent and child are separated, parenting remains important and mothers have described their efforts to maintain meaningful relationships with their children (Savvidou *et al*, 2003; Montgomery *et al*, 2006). The aim is always to rehabilitate the parent and child, and, in doing this, close attention must be paid to addressing the parent's feelings of guilt. In extreme cases the child may be rejected.

It is clear that perinatal mental illness is complex and has the potential to adversely affect parents and children across multiple domains of functioning. This suggests the need for a multidisciplinary approach to management. However, there are few specialist multidisciplinary services and little comparative evaluation data describing their effectiveness. In day-to-day clinical practice, it is important that child mental health services develop close working relationships with their colleagues in adult mental health, so that collaborative working can take place where parents are affected by mental health problems. It is estimated that 15–30% of adult mental health patients are parents, and 13% of mothers experience perinatal mental illness. It is remarkable, therefore, that so little joint working takes place routinely. Many adult mental health services do not routinely or reliably collect information about dependent children.

## Conclusions

It is apparent that perinatal mental illness has implications for the immediate and longer-term well-being of the child. A range of factors influence this; however, at this stage in our understanding, it is difficult to predict outcomes for individual children. Why do some children whose parents have mental illness do well and others not? Further work is needed to characterise risk and resilience factors for the child and their parents. Such information will inform the development and refining of interventions, as well as informing us about the most appropriate ways to target preventive interventions.

Much of the evidence available focuses on the immediate impact of perinatal mental illness. Some perinatal mental health problems are short term, but in many cases they represent more enduring psychopathology. The effects of this on the developing child beyond the perinatal period must be considered in terms of the risk to the child's development and general well-being. Equally, a child who is exposed to perinatal mental illness and whose early development is thereby compromised may be exposed to positive experiences later on which may have a self-righting effect.

Children are always part of complex systems, the most immediate of which is their family. Parental mental illness affects everyone who is part of that system (such as grandparents, siblings and partners), and each person's reaction will in turn have an impact on that system and on the child. An awareness of these systemic influences is important in the development and delivery of perinatal mental health interventions and for all practitioners who work with children and families.

Perinatal mental illness is associated with adverse effects on the fetus and infant. Therefore, the outcome for the fetus and infant is an important consideration in the management of parental mental illness. The evidence base for specific interventions is limited. Instead, the focus has been on the effects of treating the parental illness, in terms of both positive and negative effects on the child. There continues to be a paucity of information on how and when to intervene to promote good child outcomes. This remains a priority for future research.

Intervention is complex work, requiring the knowledge and skills of both child and adult mental health practitioners. Despite our increasing awareness of the implications of parental mental health for child outcome, there continues to be relatively little collaborative work between child and adult practitioners in the delivery of perinatal – and indeed all – mental health interventions. Specialist services for families affected by mental illness in the perinatal period are limited. There is a need for closer working between generic child and adult mental health specialists in the day-to-day management of the range of perinatal mental illness, and for there to be further evaluation of the effectiveness of interventions, in both the short and the long term. Work to identify effective models of service delivery incorporating liaison between child and adult mental health services must be a priority for future work.

# References

Abbott R, Dunn VJ, Robling SA, et al (2004) Long term outcome of offspring after maternal severe puerperal disorder. *Acta Psychiatrica Scandinavica*, **110**: 365–373.

Abidin RR (1986) *Parenting Stress Index Manual* (2nd edn). Pediatric Psychology Press.

Abramowitz JA, Moore K, Carmin C, et al (2001) Acute onset of obsessive-compulsive disorder in males following childbirth. *Psychosomatics*, **42**: 429–431.

Achenbach TM, Rescorla LA (2001) *Manual for the ASBEBA School-Age Forms and Profiles*. University of Vermont, Research Centre for Children, Youth and Families.

Ainsworth MDS (1963) The development of infant-mother interaction among the Ganda. In *Determinants of Infant Behaviour* (vol 2) (ed BM Foss): pp. 67–112. Methuen.

Ainsworth MDS, Wittig BA (1969) Attachment and exploratory behaviour of one-year-olds in a strange situation. In *Determinants of Infant Behaviour* (vol 2) (ed BM Foss): pp. 111–136. Methuen.

Alder J, Fink N, Bitzer J, et al (2007) Depression and anxiety during pregnancy: a risk factor for obstetric, fetal and neonatal outcome? A critical review of the literature. *Journal of Maternal-Fetal & Neonatal Medicine*, **20**: 189–209.

Aldridge A, Becker S (2003) *Children Caring for Parents with Mental Illness. Perspectives of Young Carers, Parents and Professionals.* Policy Press.

Alhusen JL (2008) A literature update on maternal fetal attachment. *Journal of Obstetric, Gynaecologic and Neonatal Nursing,* **37**: 315–328.

Alhusen JL, Ray E, Sharps P, *et al* (2015) Intimate partner violence during pregnancy: Maternal and neonatal outcomes. *Journal of Women's Health,* **24**: 100–106.

Allison SJ, Stafford J, Anumba DOC (2011) The effect of stress and anxiety associated with maternal prenatal diagnosis on feto-maternal attachment. *BMC Women's Mental Health,* **11**: 33.

American Psychiatric Association (2013) *Diagnostic and Statistical Manual of Mental Disorders* (5th edn) (DSM-V). APA.

Armstrong DS (2002) Emotional distress and prenatal attachment in pregnancy after perinatal loss. *Journal of Nursing Scholarship,* **34**: 339–345.

Austin MP (2004) Antenatal screening and early intervention for 'perinatal' distress, depression and anxiety: where to from here? *Archives of Women's Mental Health,* **7**: 1–6.

Bair-Merritt MH, Blackstone M, Feudtner C (2006) Physical health outcomes of childhood exposure to intimate partner violence: a systematic review. *Pediatrics,* **117**: e278–e290

Bandstra ES, Morrow CE, Mansoor E, *et al* (2010) Prenatal drug exposure: infant and toddler outcomes. *Journal of Addictive Disorders,* **29**: 245–258.

Barlow J, Coren E (2004) Parent-training programmes for improving maternal psychosocial health. *Cochrane Database Systematic Review,* **1**: CD002020.

Barret RL, Robinson BE (1990) The role of adolescent father in parenting and childrearing. *Advances in Adolescent Mental Health,* **4**: 189–200.

Bauer NS, Gilbert AL, Carroll AE, *et al* (2013) Associations of early exposure to intimate partner violence and parental depression with subsequent mental health outcomes. *JAMA Pediatrics,* **167**: 341–347.

Bayley N (1993) *Bayley Scales of Infant Development* (2nd edn). Psychological Corporation.

Beeber LS, Holditch-Davis D, Belyea MJ, *et al* (2004) In-home intervention for depressive symptoms with low-income mothers of infants and toddlers in the United States. *Health Care Women International,* **25**: 561–580.

Birtwell B, Hammond L, Puckering C (2015) 'Me and my bump': An interpretative phenomenological analysis of the experiences of pregnancy for vulnerable women. *Clinical Child Psychology and Psychiatry,* **20**: 218–238.

Blackmore ER, Cote-Arsenault D, Tang W, *et al* (2011) Previousperinatal loss as a predictor of perinatal depression and anxiety. *British Journal of Psychiatry,* **198**: 373–378.

Bosanac P, Buist A, Burrows G (2003) Motherhood and schizophrenic illnesses: a review of the literature. *Australian and New Zealand Journal of Psychiatry,* **37**: 24–30.

Bowlby J (1958) The nature of the child's tie to his mother. *International Journal of Psychoanalysis,* **39**: 350–373.

Bowlby J (1982) *Attachment* (2nd edn, Vol 1). Basic Books.

Breen D (1975) *The Birth of a First Child.* Tavistock.

Brockington IF (1996) *Motherhood and Mental Health.* Oxford University Press.

Brockington IF (2004) Postpartum psychiatric disorders. *Lancet,* **363**: 303.

Brockington IF, Aucamp HM, Fraser C (2006) Severe disorders of mother-infant relationship: definitions and frequency. *Archives of Women's Mental Health,* **9**: 243–251.

Brown GL, Manglesdorf SC, Neff C (2012) Father involvement, paternal sensitivity and father-child attachment security in the first 3 years. *Journal of Family Psychology,* **26**: 421–430.

Bulik CM, Von Holle A, Siega-Riz AM, *et al* (2009) Birth outcomes in women with eating disorders in the Norwegian Mother and Child cohort study (MoBa). *International Journal of Eating Disorders,* **42**: 9–18.

Caldwell BM, Bradley RH (1978) *Manual for The Home Observation for Measurement of the Environment.* University of Arkansas.

Campion MJ (1995) Mentally handicapped parents. In *Who's Fit to Be a Parent?* Routledge.

Carter AS, Briggs-Gowna MJ, Ornstein Davis N (2004) Assessment of young children's social-emotional development and psychopathology: recent advances and recommendations for practice. *Journal of Child Psychology and Psychiatry*, **45**: 109–134.

Charmandari E, Kino T, Souvatzoglou E, *et al* (2003) Pediatric stress: hormonal mediators and human development. *Hormone Research*, **59**: 161–179.

Chambliss LR (2008) Intimate partner violence and its implications for pregnancy. *Clinical Obstetrics and Gynaecology*, **51**: 385–397.

Clark R (1985) *The Parent-Child Early Relational Assessment. Instrument and manual.* Department of Psychiatry, University of Wisconsin Medical School.

Combs-Orme T (1993) Effects of adolescent pregnancy: implications for social workers. *Family Society*, **74**: 344–354.

Condon J (2006) What about dad? Psychosocial and mental health issues for new fathers. *Australian Family Physician*, **35**: 690–692.

Condon JT (1986) The spectrum of fetal abuse in pregnant women. *Journal of Nervous and Mental Disease*, **174**: 509–516.

Conroy S, Marks MN, Schacht R, *et al* (2010) The impact of maternal depression and personality disorder on early infant care. *Social Psychiatry & Psychiatric Epidemiology*, **45**: 285–289.

Connery HS, Rayburn WF (2014) Substance abuse during pregnancy. *Obstetric Clinics of North America*, **41**: 255–266.

Cooper PJ, Landman M, Tomlinson M, *et al* (2002) Impact of a mother-infant intervention in an indigent peri-urban South African context: pilot study. *British Journal of Psychiatry*, **180**: 76–81.

Cooper PJ, Whelan E, Woolgar M, *et al* (2004) Association between childhood feeding problems and maternal eating disorder: role of the family and environment. *British Journal of Psychiatry*, **184**: 210–215.

Cox J, Holden J, Henshaw C (2014) *Perinatal Mental Health: The Edinburgh Postnatal Depression Scale Manual* (2nd edn). RCPsych Publications.

Craig EA (2004) Parenting programmes for women with mental illness who have young children: a review. *Australian and New Zealand Journal of Psychiatry*, **38**: 923–928.

Culley L, Genders N (1999) Parenting by people with learning disabilities: the educational needs of the community nurse. *Nurse Education Today*, **19**: 502–505.

Currid TJ (2005) Psychological issues surrounding paternal perinatal mental health. *Nursing Times*, **101**: 40–42.

Daniel B (2006) Operationalizing the concept of resilience in child neglect: case study research. *Child Care Health Development*, **32**: 303–309.

Dean K, Stevens H, Mortensen PB, *et al* (2010) Full spectrum of psychiatric outcomes among offspring with parental history of mental disorder. *Archives of General Psychiatry*, **67**: 822–829.

Degangi S, Poisson S, Sickel A, *et al* (1995) *The Infant Toddler Symptom Checklist*. The Psychological Corporation, USA

de Jong-Pleij EA, Ribbert LS, Pistorious LR, *et al* (2013) Three dimensional ultrasound and maternal bonding, a third trimester study and a review. *Prenatal Diagnosis*, **33**: 81–88.

DelCarmen-Wiggins R, Carter A (eds) (2004) *Handbook of Infant, Toddler and Preschool Mental Health Assessment*. Oxford University Press.

Deutsch H (1947) *Psychology of Women. Vol. 2, Motherhood*. Research Books.

Ding XX, Wu YL, Xu SJ, *et al* (2014) Maternal anxiety during pregnancy and adverse birth outcomes: A systematic review and meta-analysis of prospective cohort studies. *Journal of Affective Disorders*, **159**: 103–110.

DiPietro JA (2005) Neurobehavioural assessment before birth. *Mental Retardation Developmental Disability Research Review*, **11**: 4–13.

DiPietro JA (2012) Maternal stress in pregnancy: considerations for fetal development. *Journal of Adolescent Health*, **51** (Suppl 2): S3–S8.

DiPietro JA, Hodgson DM, Costigan KA, *et al* (1996) Fetal antecedents of infant temperament. *Child Development*, **67**: 2568–2583.

DiPietro JA, Hilton SC, Hawkins M, *et al* (2002) Maternal stress and affect influence fetal neurobehavioural development. *Developmental Psychology*, **38**: 659–668.

Eagles JM, Lee AJ, Raja EA, *et al* (2012) Pregnancy outcomes of women with and without a history of anorexia nervosa. *Psychological Medicine*, **42**: 2651–2660.

Elliot RL, Campbell L, Hunter M, *et al* (2014) When I look into my baby's eyes… infant emotion recognition by mothers with borderline personality disorder. *Infant Mental Health*, **35**: 21–32.

Feldman MA (1994) Parenting education for parents with intellectual disabilities: a review of outcome studies. *Research in Developmental Disabilities*, **15**: 299–332.

Fletcher RJ, Freeman E, Garfield C, *et al* (2011) The effects of early paternal depression on children's development. *Medical Journal of Australia*, **195**: 685–689.

Flynn SM, Shaw JJ, Abel KM (2007) Homicide of infants: a cross-sectional study. *Journal of Clinical Psychiatry*, **68**: 1501–1509.

Flynn SM, Shaw JJ, Able KM (2013) Filicide: mental illness in those who kill their children. *PLoS ONE*, **8**: e58981.

Fraiberg S, Adelson E, Shapiro V (1987) Ghosts in the nursery: a psychoanalytic approach to the problems of impaired infant–mother relationships. In *Selected Writings of Selma Fraiberg* (ed L Fraiberg): pp. 100–136. Ohio State University Press.

Friedman SH, Heneghan A, Rosenthal M (2007) Characteristics of women who deny or conceal pregnancy. *Psychosomatics*, **48**: 117–122.

Freidman SH, Heneghan A, Rosenthal M (2009) Disposition and health outcomes among infants born to mothers with no prenatal care. *Child Abuse Neglect*, **33**: 116–122.

Friedman SH, Cavney J, Resnick PJ (2012) Mothers who kill: evolutionary underpinnings and infanticide law. *Behavioural Sciences and the Law*, **30**: 585–597.

Freud A (1963) The concept of developmental lines. *Psychoanalytic Study of the Child*, **18**: 245–265.

Freud A (1970) The concept of the rejecting mother. In *Parenthood: Its Psychology and Psychopathology* (eds EJ Anthony, T Benedek): pp. 376–409. Little, Brown.

Furlong M, McGilloway S, Bywater T, *et al* (2012) Behavioural and cognitive-behavioural group-based parenting programmes for early-onset conduct problems in children aged 3–12 years. *Cochrane Database of Systematic Reviews*, **2**: CD008225.

Ganchimeg T, Ota E, Morisaki N, *et al* (2014) Pregnancy and childbirth outcomes among adolescent mothers: a World Health organization multicountry study. *BJOG*, **121** (Suppl 1): 40–48.

Gilbert AL, Bauer NS, Carroll AE, *et al* (2013) Child exposure to violence and psychological distressassociated withdelayed milestones. *Pediatrics*, **132**: e1577–e1583.

Gil-Gonzalez D, Vives-Cases C, Ruiz MT, *et al* (2008)Childhood experiences of violence in perpetrators as a risk factor for intimate partner violence: a systematic review. *Journal of Public Health*, **30**: 14–22.

Goodman R (1997) The Strengths and Difficulties Questionnaire: a research note. *Journal of Child Psychology and Psychiatry*, **38**: 581–586.

Gopfert MV, Webster M, Seeman MV (eds) (2004) *Parental Psychiatric Disorder: Distressed Parents and Their Families*. Cambridge University Press.

Grote NK, Bridge JA, Gavin AR, *et al* (2010) A metaanalysis of depression during pregnancy and the risk of preterm birth low birth weight and intrauterine growth restriction. *Archives of General Psychiatry*, **67**: 1012–1024.

Halmo M, Spodniakova B, Nosalova P (2014) Fetal spasms after the administration of electroconvulsive therapy in pregnancy: our experience. *Journal of Electroconvulsive Therapy*, **30**: e24–e26.

Hall D, Williams J (2008) Safeguarding, child protection and mental health. *Archives of Diseases in Childhood*, **93**: 11–13.

Hay DF, Pawlby S, Waters CS, et al (2010) Mothers' antenatal depression and their children's antisocial outcomes. Child Development, 18: 149–165.

Hesse E (2008) The Adult Attachment Interview: protocol, method of analysis, and empirical studies. In Handbook of Attachment: Theory, Research, and Clinical Applications (2nd edn) (eds J Cassidy, PR Shaver): pp. 552–598. Guilford.

Hindley N, Rachmandani PG, Jones DPH (2006) Risk factors for recurrence of maltreatment: a systematic review. Archives of Diseases in Childhood, 91: 744–752.

Hobson RP, Patrick M, Crandell L, et al (2005) Personal relatedness and attachment in infants and mothers with borderline personality disorder. Developmental Psychopathology, 17: 329–347.

Hodgkinson S, Beers L, Southammakosane C, et al (2014) Addressing the mental health needs of pregnant and parenting adolescents. Pediatrics, 133: 114–122.

Hogg S (2013) Prevention in Mind. All Babies Count: Spotlight on Perinatal Mental Health. NSPCC.

Howard L, Shah N, Salmon M, et al (2003) Predictors of social services supervision of babies of mothers with mental illness after admission to a psychiatric mother and baby unit. Social Psychiatry and Psychiatric Epidemiology, 38: 450–455.

Howard LM, Thornicroft G, Salmon M et al (2004) Predictors of parenting outcome in women with psychotic disorders discharged from mother and baby units. Acta Psychiatrica Scandinavica, 110: 347–355.

Jablensky AV, Morgan V, Zubrick SR, et al (2005) Pregnancy, delivery, and neonatal complications in a population of women with schizophrenia and major affective disorders. American Journal of Psychiatry, 162: 79–91.

Jaffee S, Caspi A, Moffitt TE, et al (2001) Why are children born to teenage mothers at risk of adverse outcomes in young adulthood? Results from a 20 year longitudinal study. Developmental Psychopathology, 13: 377–397.

Jansson LM, Velez M (2012) Neonatal abstinence syndrome. Current Opinion in Paediatrics, 24: 252–258.

Jenkins A, Millar S, Robbins J (2011) Denial of pregnancy: a literature review and discussion of ethical and legal issues. Journal of the Royal Society of Medicine, 104: 286–291.

Johnson SM (2012) Lesbian mothers and their children: the third wave. Journal of Lesbian Studies, 16: 45–53.

Joseph MA, O'Connor TG, Briskman JA, et al (2014) The formation of secure new attachments by children who were maltreated: an observational study of adolescents in foster care. Developmental Psychopathology, 26: 67–80.

Kapoor A, Dunn E, Kostaki A, et al (2006) Fetal programming of hypothalamo-pituitary-adrenal function: prenatal stress and glucocorticoids. Journal of Physiology, 572: 31–44.

Keegan J, Parva M, Finnegan M, et al (2010) Addiction in pregnancy. Journal of Addictive Diseases, 29: 175–191.

Kent A (2011) Psychiatric disorders in pregnancy. Obstetric, Gynecologic and Reproductive Medicine, 21: 317–322.

Kent L, Laidlaw JD, Brockington IF (1997) Fetal abuse. Child Abuse and Neglect, 21: 181–186.

Kerker BD, Dore MM (2006) Mental health needs and treatment of foster youth: barriers and opportunities. American Journal of Orthopsychiatry, 76: 138–147.

Kim-Cohen J (2007) Resilience and developmental psychopathology. Child and Adolescent Psychiatric Clinics of North America, 16: 271–283.

King-Hele SA, Webb RT, Mortensen PB, et al (2009) Risk of stillbirth and neonatal death linked to maternal mental illness: a national cohort study. Archives of Disease In Childhood. Fetal and Neonatal Edition, 94: F105–F110.

Kitzmann KM, Gaylord NK, Holt AR, et al (2003) Child witness to domestic violence: a meta-analytic review. Journal of Consulting and Clinical Psychology, 71: 339–352.

Knackstedt MK, Hamelmann E, Arck PC (2005) Mothers in stress: consequences for offspring. American Journal of Reproductive Immunology, 54: 63–69.

Knight M, Tuffnell D, Kenyon S, *et al* (eds) (2015) *Saving Lives, Improving Mothers' Care. Surveillance of maternal deaths in the UK 2011–13 and lessons learned to inform maternity care from the UK and Ireland Confidential Enquiries into Maternal Deaths and Morbidity 2009-13*. MBRRACE-UK.

Kochanska G, Kim S (2013) Early attachment organization with both parents and future behavior problems: from infancy to middle childhood. *Child Development*, **84**: 283–296.

Kocherlakota P (2014) Neonatal abstinence syndrome. *Pediatrics*, **134**: e547–e561.

Kopp CB (1982) Antecedents of self-regulation: a developmental perspective. *Developmental Psychology*, **18**: 199–214.

Kopp CB (1989) Regulation of distress and negative emotions: a developmental view. *Developmental Psychology*, **25**: 343–354.

Korenman S, Kaestner R, Joyce T (2002) Consequences of infants of parental disagreement in pregnancy intention. *Perspectives on Sexual and Reproductive Health*, **34**: 198–205.

Kurstjens S, Wolke D (2001) Effects of maternal depression on cognitive development of children over the first seven years of life. *Journal of Child Psychology and Psychiatry*, **42**: 623–636.

Kvalevaag AL, Ramchandani PG, Hove O, *et al* (2013) Paternal mental health and socioemotional and behavioural development. *Pediatrics*, **131**: e462–e469.

Lamb ME (1976) Interactions between eight-month-old children and their fathers and mothers. In *The Role of the Father in Child Development* (ed ME Lamb): pp. 307–327. John Wiley.

Lecanuet J-P, Schaal B (1996) Fetal sensory competencies. *European Journal of Obstetrics & Gynecology and Reproductive Biology*, **68**: 1–23.

Lee L, Halpern CT, Hertz-Picciotto I, *et al* (2006) Child care and social support modify the association between maternal depressive symptoms and early childhood behaviour problems: a US national study. *Journal of Epidemiology and Community Health*, **60**: 305–310.

Lester BM, Lagasse LL (2010) Children of addicted women. *Journal of Addictive Disorders*, **29**: 259–276.

Lindahl V, Pearson JL, Voigt RG, *et al* (2005) Prevalence of suicidality during pregnancy and the postpartum. *Archives of Women's Mental Health*, **8**: 77–87.

Little BB, Snell LM, Van Beveren TT, *et al* (2003) Treatment of substance abuse during pregnancy and infant outcome. *American Journal of Perinatology*, **20**: 255–262.

Macfie J, Swan SA (2009) Representations of the caregiver-child relationship and of the self, and emotion regulation in the narratives of young children whose mothers have borderline personality disorder. *Developmental Psychopathology*, **21**: 993–1011.

Main M (1996) Introduction to the special section on attachment and psychopathology: 2. Overview of the field of attachment. *Journal of Consulting and Clinical Psychology*, **64**: 237–243.

Main M, Solomon J (1986) Discovery of an insecure-disorganized/disoriented attachment pattern. In *Affective Development in Infancy* (eds TB Brazelton, M Yogman). Ablex.

Maldonano-Duran J, Lartigue T, Feintuch M (2000) Perinatal psychiatry: infant mental health interventions during pregnancy. *Bulletin of the Menninger Clinic*, **64**: 317–340.

Mantymaa M, Puura K, Luoma I, *et al* (2003) Infant-mother interaction as a predictor of child's chronic health problems. *Child Care Health and Development*, **29**: 181–191.

McCracken KA, Loveless M (2014) Teen pregnancy: an up-date. *Current Opinion in Obstetrics and Gynaecology*, **26**: 355–359.

Mennella JA, Jagnow CP, Beauchamp GK (2001) Prenatal and postnatal flavour learning by human infants. *Pediatrics*, **107**: E88.

Micali N, Simonoff E, Treasure J (2007) Risk of major adverse perinatal outcomes in women with eating disorders. *British Journal of Psychiatry*, **190**: 255–259.

Minnes S, Lang A, Singer L (2011) Prenatal tobacco, marijuana, stimulant and opiate exposure: outcomes and practice implications. *Addiction Science & Clinical Practice*, **6**: 57–70.

Moffitt TE, E-Risk Study Team (2002) Teen-aged mothers in contemporary Britain. *Journal of Child Psychology and Psychiatry*, **43**: 727–742.

Montgomery P, Tompkins C, Forhuk C, *et al* (2006) Keeping close: mothering with serious mental illness. *Journal of Advanced Nursing*, **54**: 20–28.

Muir M (1992) Watching, waiting and wondering: applying psychoanalytic principles to mother-infant intervention. *Infant Mental Health Journal*, **13**: 319–328.

Murray L, Hipwell A, Hooper R (1996a) The cognitive development of 5-year old children of postnatally depressed mothers. *Journal of Child Psychology and Psychiatry*, **37**: 927–935.

Murray L, Fiori-Cowley A, Hooper R (1996b) The impact of postnatal depression and associated adversity on early mother-infant interactions and later infant outcome. *Child Development*, **67**: 2512–2526.

Murray L, Arteche A, Fearon P, *et al* (2011) Maternal postnatal depression and the development of depression in offspring up to 16 years of age. *Journal of the American Academy of Child and Adolescent Psychiatry*, **50**: 460–470.

NICE (2014) *Antenatal and Postnatal Mental Health: Clinical Management and Service Guidance* [CG192]. National Institute for Health and Care Excellence.

Nirmal D, Thijs I, Bethel J, *et al* (2006) The incidence and outcome of concealed pregnancy among hospital deliveries in an 11 year population-based study in South Glamorgan. *Journal of Obstetrics and Gynaecology*, **26**: 118–121.

O'Connor TG, Rutter M (2000) Attachment disorder behaviour following early severe deprivation: extension and longitudinal follow-up. English and Romanian Adoptees Study Team. *Journal of the American Academy of Child and Adolescent Psychiatry*, **39**: 703–712.

O'Connor TG, Rutter M, Beckett C, *et al* (2000) The effects of global severe privation on cognitive competence: extension and longitudinal follow-up. English and Romanian Adoptees Study Team. *Child Development*, **71**: 376–390.

O'Connor TG, Heron J, Glover V, *et al* (2002) Antenatal anxiety predicts child behavioural/emotional problems independently of postnatal depression. *Journal of the American Academy of Child and Adolescent Psychiatry*, **41**: 1470–1477.

O'Connor TG, Heron J, Golding J, *et al* (2003) Maternal antenatal anxiety and behavioural/emotional problems in children: a test of a programming hypothesis. *Journal of Child Psychology & Psychiatry*, **44**: 1025–1036.

Pajulo M, Savonlathi E, Piha J (1999) Maternal substance abuse: Infant psychiatric interest: a review and hypothetical model of interaction. *American Journal of Drug and Alcohol Abuse*, **25**: 761–769.

Pallitto CC, Garcio-Moreno C, Jansen HA, *et al* (2013) Intimate partner violence, abortion, and unintended pregnancy: results from the WHO Multicountry Study on Women's Health and Domestic Violence. *International Journal of Gynaecology & Obstetrics*, **120**: 3–9.

Park RJ, Senior R, Stein A (2003) The offspring of mothers with eating disorders. *European Journal of Child and Adolescent Psychatry*, **12** (Suppl 1): 110–119.

Parker G (1989) The Parental Bonding Instrument: psychometric properties reviewed. *Psychiatric Dev*, **7**: 317–335.

Pawlby S, Hay DF, Sharp D, *et al* (2009) Antenatal depression predicts depression in adolescent offspring: prospective longitudinal community-based study. *Journal of Affective Disorders*, **113**: 236–243.

Perera DN, Short L, Fernbacher S (2014) 'It's not that straightforward': when family support is challenging for mothers living with mental illness. *Psychiatric Rehabilitation Journal*, **37**: 170–175.

Phares V (1992) Where's poppa? The relative lack of attention to the role of fathers in child and adolescent psychopathology. *American Psychologist*, **47**: 656–674.

Phares V, Fileds S, Kamboukos D, *et al* (2005) Still looking for poppa: the continued lack of attention to the role of fathers in developmental psychopathology. *American Psychologist*, **60**: 735–736.

Pisoni C, Garofoli F, Tzialla C, *et al* (2014) Risk and protective factors in maternal-fetal attachment development. *Early Human Development*, **90** (Suppl): S45–S46.

Pollock PH, Percy A (1999) Maternal antenatal attachment style and potential fetal abuse. *Child Abuse and Neglect*, **23**: 1345–1357.

Pompili M, Dominici G, Giordarno G, *et al* (2014) Electroconvulsive treatment during pregnancy: a systematic review. *Expert Review Neurotherapeutics*, **14**: 1377–1390.

Puura K, Kaukonen P (2010) Parent-infant psychotherapies and indications for inpatient versus outpatient treatments. In *Parenthood and Mental Health: A bridge between infant and adult psychiatry* (eds S Tyano, M Keren, H Herman, *et al*). Wiley-Blackwell.

Quinlivan JA, Condon J (2005) Anxiety and depression in fathers in teenage pregnancy. *Australian and New Zealand Journal of Psychiatry*, **39**: 915–920.

Ramchandani P, Psychogiou L (2009) Paternal psychiatric disorder and children's psychosocial development. *Lancet*, **374**: 646–653.

Ramchandani P, Stein A, Evans J, *et al* (2005) Paternal depression in the postnatal period and child development: a prospective population study. *Lancet*, **365**: 2201–2205.

Raphael-Leff J (1985) Facilitators and regulators; vulnerability to postnatal disturbance. *Journal of Psychosomatic Obstetrics & Gynecology*, **4**: 151–168.

Richards JS, Vasquez AA, Rommelse NN, *et al* (2014) A follow-up study of maternal expressed emotion toward children with attention deficit/hyperactivity disorder (ADHD): relation with severity and persistence of ADHD and comorbidity. *Journal of the American Academy of Child and Adolescent Psychiatry*, **53**: 311–319.

Rilling JK (2013) The neural and hormonal basis of human parental care. *Neuorpsychologia*, **51**: 731–747.

Rokyta R (2008) Fetal pain. *Neuroendocrine Letters*, **29**: 807–814.

Ross LE (2005) Perinatal mental health in lesbian mothers: a review of potential risk and protective factors. *Women & Health*, **41**: 113–128.

Rutter M, O'Connor TG, The English and Romanian Adoptees (ERA) Study Team (2004) Are there biological programming effects for psychological development? Findings from a study of Romanian adoptees. *Developmental Psychology*, **40**: 81–94.

Sable MR, Wilkinson DS (2000) Impact of perceived stress, major life events and pregnancy attitudes on low birth weight. *Family Planning Perspectives*, **32**: 288–294.

Sadler LS, Slade A, Close N, *et al* (2013) Minding the Baby: enhancing reflectiveness to improve early health and relationship outcomes in an interdisciplinary home visiting program. *Infant Mental Health*, **34**: 391–405.

Sands RG, Goldberg-Geln RS, Shin H (2009) The voices of grandchildren and grandparent caregivers: a strengths-resilience perspective. *Child Welfare*, **88**: 25–45.

Sanftner JL, Crowther JH, Crawford PA, *et al* (1996) Maternal influences (or lack thereof) on daughters' eating attitudes and behaviours. *Eating Disorders*, **4**: 147–159.

Savvidou I, Bozikas VP, Hatzigeleki S, *et al* (2003) Narratives about their children by mothers hospitalized on a psychiatric unit. *Family Process*, **42**: 391–402.

Sears RR (1943) *Survey of Objective Studies of Psychoanalytic Concepts*. Social Science Research Council.

Sedgman B, McMahon C, Cairns D, *et al* (2006) The impact of two-dimensional versus three dimensional ultrasound exposure on maternal-fetal attachment and maternal health behaviour. *Ultrasound Obstetrics and Gynecology*, **27**: 245–251.

Shah PS, Balkhair T, Ohlsson A, *et al* (2011) Intention to become pregnant and low birth weight and preterm birth: a systematic review. *Maternal Child Health*, **15**: 205–216.

Sidebotham P, Heron J, ALSPAC Study Team (2006) Child maltreatment in the 'children of the nineties': a cohort study of risk factors. *Child Abuse and Neglect*, **30**: 497–522.

Skala K, Bruckner T (2014) Beating the odds: an approach to the topic of resilience in children and adolescents. *Neuorpsychiatrie*, **28**: 208–217.

Slade A, Sadler L, De Dios-Kenn C, *et al* (2005) Minding the baby: a reflective parenting programme. *Psychoanalytic Study of the Child*, **60**: 74–100.

Sohr-Preston SL, Scaramella LV (2006) Implications of timing of maternal depressive symptoms for early cognitive and language development. *Clinical Child and Family Psychology Review*, **9**: 65–83.

Solmi F, Sallis H, Stahl D, *et al* (2014) Low birth weight in the offspring of women with anorexia nervosa. *Epidemiologic Reviews*, **36**: 49–56.

Sonuga-Barke EJ, Cartwright KL, Thompson MJ, *et al* (2013) Family characteristics, expressed emotion and attention deficit/hyperactivity disorders. *Journal of the American Academy of Child and Adolescent Psychiatry*, **52**: 547–548.

Spinelli MG (2005) Infanticide: contrasting views. *Archives of Women's Mental Health*, **8**: 15–24.

Stanton J, Simpson AL (2006) The aftermath: aspects of recovery described by perpetrators of maternal filicide committed in the context of severe mental illness. *Behavioural Sciences and the Law*, **24**: 103–112.

Stepp DS, Whalen DJ, Pilkonis PA, *et al* (2011) Children of mothers with borderline personality disorder: identifying parenting behaviours as potential targets for intervention. *Personality Disorder*, **3**: 76–91.

Stern NB (1999) Motherhood: the emotional awakening. *Journal of Pediatric Healthcare*, **13**: S8–S12.

Stern D (2002) *The First Relationship: Mother and Infant.* Harvard University Press.

Suchman N, Mayes L, Conti J (2004) Rethinking parenting interventions for drug dependent mothers: from behaviour management to fostering emotional bonds. *Journal of Substance Abuse Treatment*, **29**: 179–185.

Swain JE, Lorberbaum JP, Kose S, *et al* (2007) Brain basis of early parent-infant interactions; psychology, physiology, and in vivo functional neuroimaging studies. *Journal of Child Psychology and Psychiatry*, **48**: 262–87.

Swain JE, Kim P, Spicer J, *et al* (2014) Approaching the biology of human parent attachment behavior: brain imaging, oxytocin and coordinated assessments of mothers and fathers. *Brain Research*, **1580**: 78–101.

Taggart AV, Short SD, Barclay L (2000) 'She has made me feel human again': an evaluation of a volunteer home-based visiting project for mothers. *Health and Social Care in the Community*, **8**: 1–8.

Talge NM, Neal C, Glover V, *et al* (2007) Antenatal maternal stress and long-term effects on child neurodevelopment: how and why? *Journal of Child Psychology and Psychiatry*, **48**: 245–261.

Tan LH, Quinlivan JA (2006) Domestic violence, single parenthood and fathers in the setting of teenage pregnancy. *Journal of Adolescent Health*, **38**: 201–207.

Thomas JM, Chess S, Birch HG (1968) *Temperament and Behaviour Disorders in Children.* New York University Press.

Trad PV (1991) Adaptation to developmental transformation during the various phases of motherhood. *Journal of the American Academy of Psychoanalysis*, **19**: 403–421.

Ullal-Gupta S, Vanden Bosch der Nederlanden CM, Tichko P, *et al* (2013) Linking prenatal experience to the emerging music mind. *Frontiers in Systems Neuroscience*, **7**: 48.

Van der Zanden RA, Speetjens PA, Arntz KS, *et al* (2010) Online group course for parents with mental illness: development and pilot study. *Journal of Medical Internet Research*, **12**: e50.

Vigod SN, Kurdyak PA, Dennis CL, *et al* (2014) Maternal and newborn outcomes among women with schizophrenia: a retrospective population-based cohort study. *BJOG*, **121**: 566–574.

Voegtline KM, Costigan KA, Pater HA, *et al* (2013) Near-term fetal responses to maternal spoken voice. *Infant Behaviour and Development*, **36**: 526–33.

Wan MW, Moulton S, Abel KM (2008) A review of mother–child relational intervention and their usefulness for mothers with schizophrenia. *Archives of Women's Mental Health*, **11**: 171–179.

Waugh E, Bulik CM (1999) Offspring of women with eating disorders. *International Journal of Eating Disorders*, **25**: 123–133.

Whitaker RC, Orzol SM, Khan RS (2006) Maternal mental health, substance use and domestic violence in the year after delivery and subsequent behaviour problems in children at age 3 years. *Archives of General Psychiatry*, **63**: 551–560.

Winnicott DW (1965) *The Maturational Processes and the Facilitating Environment: Studies in the Theory of Emotional Development.* International Universities Press.

Winnicott DW (1970) The mother-infant experience of mutuality. In *Parenthood: Its Psychology and Psychopathology* (eds EJ Anthony, T Benedek): pp. 245–288. Little, Brown.

World Health Organization (1992) *International Classification of Diseases (10th edn).* WHO.

Young Minds (2004) *Mental Health in Infancy.* Young Minds.

# Further reading

Diggins M (ed) (2015) *Parental Mental Health and Child Welfare Work: Volume 1.* Pavilion.

Tyano S, Keren M, Herman H, *et al* (eds) (2010) *Parenthood and Mental Health: A bridge between infant and adult psychiatry.* Wiley-Blackwell.

# CHAPTER 7

# Screening and prevention

Researchers have observed that many pregnant and postpartum women with mental disorder are not identified and adequately treated (Kelly *et al*, 2001; Andersson *et al*, 2003; Coates *et al*, 2004; Smith *et al*, 2004; Thio *et al*, 2006) despite being routinely in contact with health professionals. This chapter aims to address the issues concerning screening and prevention for both current and future disorder during pregnancy and the postpartum period, and to point to best practice.

## Definition of screening

The UK National Screening Committee (NSC) has a very precise definition of screening:

> 'Screening is a process of identifying apparently healthy people who may be at increased risk of a disease or condition. They can then be offered information, further tests and appropriate treatment to reduce their risk and/or any complications arising from the disease or condition' (NSC, 2013).

Another definition of screening is:

> 'The systematic application of a test or inquiry to identify individuals at risk of a specific disorder to benefit from further investigation or direct preventive action among persons who have not sought medical attention on account of that disorder' (Peckham & Dezateux, 1998).

Screening was initially focused on conditions such as cancers, deafness in infants and risk factors for cardiovascular disease. More recently, it has also included psychological disorders. In 2002, the US Preventive Service Task Force (2002) recommended that clinical services screen adults for depression, and several North American colleges and academies now advocate routinely asking patients about depression when taking a medical history. Epidemiologists define 'case finding' as the search for additional disorders in those with medical problems, and this definition fits most closely with the use of screening tools in pregnant and postpartum women.

There was considerable debate and consternation surrounding the NSC's initial recommendation in 2001 that screening for postnatal depression was not justified. They have reviewed their position since then (in 2011) and currently state:

> 'A screening programme for postnatal depression is not recommended. The development of postnatal depression is complex. There is a lack of clarity on the population to be identified by screening and evidence that the use of current screening tools cannot identify risk with sufficient accuracy. There is also insufficient evidence that universal screening and subsequent intervention improve the health outcomes for the mother or the baby. However, as part of a comprehensive clinical assessment, health professionals should be alert to the possibility of postnatal depression and manage it according to current guidance' (NSC, 2011).

The NSC website stated that their position was to be reviewed again in 2014 or 2015, but no update has been issued at the time of writing. Guidance by the National Institute for Health and Care Excellence (NICE, 2007) published in February 2007 advocated asking two questions:

- During the past month, have you often been bothered by feeling down, depressed or hopeless?
- During the past month, have you often been bothered by having little interest or pleasure in doing things?

And, if there is a positive answer to both, asking:

- Is this something you feel you need or want help with?

These questions had been validated in other healthcare settings (e.g. Whooley *et al*, 1997), but not for use in perinatal populations. Since then, a validation study in has been carried out in pregnant and postpartum women, which concluded that a negative response to both questions was accurate at ruling out depression, but that where either response was positive, the third question improved specificity (Mann *et al*, 2012). NICE (2014) continues to recommend their use.

## Screening instruments

Only three instruments have been developed specifically to screen for postnatal depression: the Edinburgh Postnatal Depression Scale (EPDS; Cox *et al*, 1987; Appendix 2), the Postpartum Depression Screening Scale (PDSS; Beck & Gable, 2000) and the Bromley Postnatal Depression Scale (Stein & van den Akker, 1992). Other self-report scales have been used in pregnant and postpartum populations but not all have been validated for this use. Boyd *et al* (2005) reviewed these and five other instruments in detail and critiqued their psychometric properties (reliability, sensitivity, specificity, positive predictive value and concurrent validity). They concluded that the EPDS is the most widely studied and has moderate psychometric soundness, and also discussed some of the implications for clinicians and researchers. Several studies have compared the performance of EPDS with other scales; these are described in Cox *et al* (2014a).

The readability levels of the EPDS and PDSS have been assessed as US third and fourth grade, respectively (Logsdon & Hutti, 2006), and it is stated that 95% of the UK adult population would be able to read the EPDS (Leverton, 2005). However, care should be taken not to assume literacy and those working with non-English-speaking women should consider whether a translation is available (Henshaw & Elliott, 2005; Cox *et al*, 2014b).

### Edinburgh Postnatal Depression Scale

The EPDS was the first instrument developed specifically to screen for postnatal depression (Cox *et al*, 1987). This 10-item paper and pencil self-report questionnaire has since been translated into 57 other languages and validated in many (Cox *et al*, 2014b), and remains the most widely used scale. It takes around 5 min to complete and is simple to score. Response categories are scored 0–3 according to the response, with items 3 and 5–10 being reverse scored, making the total score range 0–30.

The original validation was carried out with Scottish women at 6 weeks postpartum. A cut-off score of 12/13 identified all the women with definite major depression and two of the three women with probable depression, but there were false positives. A French study suggests that the EPDS is better at detecting women with anxious and anhedonic symptoms than those with psychomotor retardation (Guedeney *et al*, 2000). Women from some cultures (e.g. Sylheti or Bengali) 'often prefer' to have the scale read to them than to complete it themselves (Fuggle *et al*, 2002).

The EPDS has been validated for use in pregnancy (Murray & Cox, 1990), some non-childbearing populations (Henshaw & Elliott, 2005; Cox *et al*, 2014a), and adolescent mothers (Venkatesh *et al*, 2014) and fathers (Moran & O'Hara, 2006). However, other instruments have been found to be superior in some non-Western settings, for example, the World Health Organization's Self-Reporting Questionnaire (Pollock *et al*, 2006). It has also been used in mothers with intellectual disability, with a simplified interview reference to an anchor event to emphasise timescales and a pictorial scale to assess severity, (Gaskin & James, 2006). One study of adolescent mothers reported that it may be possible to use three items from the anxiety subscale of the EPDS to make a preliminary diagnosis (Kabir *et al*, 2007), and Venkatesh *et al* (2014) found that three-, seven- and ten-item versions of the EPDS performed equally well in detecting depression in adolescent mothers.

Matthey (2004) has calculated that a four-point change indicates a clinically significant change, and this could be used in research trials. Some researchers and clinicians seem unaware that changing the format or cut-off score used can have a significant impact on the psychometrics of the scale. The variations found and the consequences for research and clinical practice are discussed in Matthey *et al* (2006).

The EPDS copyright is owned by the Royal College of Psychiatrists, and the scale can only be reproduced as published and with the full reference.

## Postpartum Depression Screening Scale

Cheryl Beck and Robert Gable developed the PDSS, a 35-item Likert-type self-report instrument that covers 7 domains (Beck & Gable, 2000). There is also a short form (Beck & Gable, 2002) consisting of the first 7 items of the 35-item version. The PDSS has been validated in Spanish, Chinese, Brazilian Portuguese, Thai and Turkish. It has also been found to be reliable when administered over the telephone, which might be particularly useful in very remote areas (Mitchell *et al*, 2006).

## Bromley Postnatal Depression Scale

This instrument consists of 10 items with open-ended and yes/no questions, and a chart to identify when postnatal depression began. It assesses both current and past episodes of postnatal depression. There is no recommended cut-off score, and only one published study of its psychometric properties has been undertaken (Stein & van den Akker, 1992).

## General Health Questionnaire

Sharp (1988) carried out a validation study of the 30-item General Health Questionnaire (GHQ-30) in early pregnancy and identified the optimum cut-off score as 5/6. However, Martin & Jomeen (2003), assessing the GHQ-12 in late pregnancy, at full term and 28 days after delivery, found that the scoring method had an impact on both the interpretation of data and the prevalence of above-threshold 'cases'. They advised that further research should be undertaken to establish the optimal cut-off before the instrument is used in this population.

The GHQ has been found to have satisfactory sensitivity, specificity and positive predictive values in women who have had a miscarriage (Lok *et al*, 2004) and – although the EPDS performed slightly better – to be a valid measure for screening for postnatal depression, anxiety and adjustment disorders (Navarro *et al*, 2007).

## Hamilton Rating Scale for Depression

Scores on the Hamilton Rating Scale for Depression (HRSD) in women in late pregnancy, and 6 and 16 weeks postpartum were highly correlated with scores on measures that do not include somatic items i.e. the Brief Symptom Inventory and the EPDS (Derogatis & Melisaratos, 1983). Scores on somatic items of the HRSD did not correlate well with the total HRSD score in pregnancy, but did at 6 weeks postpartum. However, scores on HRSD item 1 ('Depression') correlated less well with the total score at 6 weeks postpartum than during pregnancy. Evidence suggests that postpartum women may be less likely to articulate their difficulties as 'depression', and more likely to describe somatic complaints such as low energy or insomnia (Whitton *et al*, 1996).

## Hospital Anxiety and Depression Scale

Factor analysis and internal reliability assessment of the Hospital Anxiety and Depression Scale (HADS) revealed that it does not reliably assess distinct domains of anxiety and depression in early pregnancy (Jomeen & Martin, 2004), or at 12 or 34 weeks (Karimova & Martin, 2003) and is therefore not a suitable screening tool for use in pregnant populations.

## Beck Depression Inventory

Low scores on the Beck Depression Inventory (BDI) are determined mainly by somatic symptoms in pregnant women (Salamero *et al*, 1994), whereas higher scores are determined by depressive symptoms. Caution should therefore be exercised if using the BDI in this population, and low scores should not be interpreted as indicating depressive symptoms. A higher cut-off is advised when used with pregnant women than that usually employed in non-pregnant populations (Holcomb *et al*, 1996).

## Patient Health Questionnaire

The depression-specific version of the Patient Health Questionnaire (PHQ-9) is commonly used in UK primary care, and has been validated for use in pregnant women (Sidebottom *et al*, 2012) and at 1 month postpartum (Gjerdingen *et al*, 2009).

## Other instruments and populations

A research diagnostic criteria-like algorithm based on items from the Self-Rating Depression Scale performed better than the scale itself in pregnant women (Kitamura *et al*, 1999).

Pictorial booklets entitled *How Are You Feeling?* have been developed by the Community Practitioners and Health Visitors Association (Sobowale & Adams, 2005) to assist in the assessment of mental health, and social and physical needs. These are available in Urdu, Bengali, Somali, Chinese, Arabic and English (which may be useful for English-speaking women with intellectual disability or who are non-literate).

Downe *et al* (2007) reviewed the performance of the EPDS, the GHQ, the Punjabi Postnatal Depression Scale and the Doop Chaon© (a visual tool) in screening for depressed mood after delivery in South Asian women living in the UK. They concluded that none of the tools met quality criteria. Qualitative data indicated that the women preferred face-to-face interviews to completing questionnaires.

Somerville and colleagues (2014) have developed and carried out a preliminary validation of the Perinatal Anxiety Screening Scale (PASS) in pregnant and postpartum women, and found that it performed better than the anxiety subscale of the EPDS in detecting anxiety disorders. NICE (2014) recommends asking about anxiety at antenatal booking and postpartum using the 2-item Generalized Anxiety Disorder Scale (Kroenke *et al*, 2007).

There are several studies comparing the performance of different scales in pregnant and postpartum women. Interested readers are directed to Cox *et al* (2014*a*) and Henshaw & Elliott (2005).

Brockington and colleagues (2001) devised and validated the Postpartum Bonding Instrument, a questionnaire to detect mother–infant bonding disorders, which they propose using alongside the EPDS. It has been validated and translated into several languages. The authors suggest the instrument could also be used on a weekly basis to monitor change. Other instruments have been devised to assess mother–infant interaction and bonding (see Chapter 3).

## Internet screening

Participants in one study have described online screening using the EPDS as easy, straightforward and personalised (Drake *et al*, 2014). Other studies, comparing in-person and internet screening using the EPDS and PDSS, found that women from minority ethnic (Hispanic and Asian) communities were more likely to choose internet-based rather than in-person screening, and that the instruments retained their psychometric properties (Le *et al*, 2009).

## Acceptability

Some studies have indicated that screening with the EPDS is acceptable to the majority of postpartum women (Buist *et al*, 2006; Gemmill *et al*, 2006), but not all would agree. In a study undertaken in Oxford, just over half of the women interviewed found screening with the EPDS less than acceptable (irrespective of whether or not they were depressed). Particular issues were problems with how screening was carried out, e.g. the venue, the personal intrusion of it and stigma. Those interviewed had a clear preference for talking about how they felt, rather than filling out a questionnaire (Shakespeare *et al*, 2003). Similar findings are reported by Cubison & Munro (2005) regarding their six-item scale, which they erroneously called the EPDS. The women they interviewed had concerns about how the scale was administered (rushed, without any explanation, with others present and without any discussion about the score). Most were critical of the multiple choice format and some lied when answering it. Others report that some women make a conscious decision not to disclose, and that health professionals may hinder disclosure if they think they do not have the resources to manage women with postnatal depression or there are no services to refer them to (Chew-Graham *et al*, 2009).

# What are we screening for?

This is a crucial question. Is the intention to identify women with current mental disorder, or those at risk of future disorder? This distinction will be borne in mind as we consider screening during pregnancy and in the postpartum period.

## Pregnancy

### Screening for current disorder

Up to one-third of pregnant women are identified as suffering from a current psychiatric disorder (Kelly *et al*, 2001; Andersson *et al*, 2003; Kim *et al*, 2006). Depression is the most common disorder, followed by anxiety. These conditions and others lead to poorer obstetric outcomes during pregnancy and at delivery (Andersson *et al*, 2004).

However, routine antenatal booking assessments do not identify all cases of psychiatric disorder in pregnant women. In a US antenatal care setting, 38% of women had a mental disorder, but only 43% of these had their symptoms recorded, with less than one-fifth having any mention in their records of a formal diagnosis. Just over one-third had evidence of evaluation of their psychiatric problem in their maternity record, but fewer than a quarter had their current treatment outlined (Kelly *et al*, 2001). Similarly, only 26% of pregnant women in public sector obstetric clinics with a mood or anxiety disorder, and 12% experiencing suicidal ideation, had their problem recognised by their healthcare provider (Smith *et al*, 2004). Detection was more likely in this setting if the woman reported domestic violence. Low treatment rates of pregnant women with post-traumatic stress disorder have also been reported (Loveland Cook *et al*, 2004).

Ensuring that screening is universal can be problematic. A US programme, 'Identify, Screen, Intervene, Support', aimed to screen all pregnant women at 32 weeks of gestation with the EPDS. High scorers were to be assessed further (including assessment of suicidal risk) and referred as appropriate: to a brief psychosocial intervention for those with mild to moderate problems, and to the psychiatric team for those with more severe or complex problems (Thoppil *et al*, 2005). They managed to screen 75% of patients.

There are no established biological markers for depression, but Canadian investigators have observed that platelet serotonin levels correlate well with scores on the HRSD and proposed that they might be a useful marker and guide to treatment response (Maurer-Spurej *et al*, 2007). Others have explored the role of corticotropin-releasing hormone (CRH) as a predictor of postnatal depression (see Chapter 2), but studies have produced conflicting results.

### Screening for risk of postnatal depression

Austin & Lumley (2003) reviewed 16 studies which evaluated instruments used to screen women antenatally in order to identify those who are at risk of a postnatal depressive episode. Eleven of the studies used scales devised specifically for this purpose; in seven a study-specific instrument was combined with a standard self-report measure; three used a self-report measure alone; and three used a diagnostic interview. The authors concluded that no instrument met criteria for routine population screening during pregnancy, and postulated that this might have occurred because key risk predictors (personality, past history of abuse or depression, and presence of severe blues after delivery) are not included in many of the instruments in question.

Austin and colleagues then devised the Pregnancy Risk Questionnaire (PRQ), which included identifies risk factors, and carried out a validation study (Austin *et al*, 2005). The PRQ's sensitivity and specificity are better than those of previous scales, although its positive predictive value remains limited.

In Canada, the Antenatal Psychosocial Health Assessment (ALPHA) was developed to screen women for 15 risk factors and identify those most at risk for poorer psychosocial outcomes. When compared against usual care in a randomised controlled trial (RCT), more psychosocial concerns were identified by staff using the ALPHA, particularly those relating to family violence (Carroll *et al*, 2005). However, 65% of clinicians refused to take part in the trial, which raises questions about how easy more routine or widespread use would be.

The Postpartum Depression Predictors Inventory (PDPI), based on 13 risk factors, has been developed and revised (the PDPI-R), and its psychometrics have been tested to some extent (Beck *et al*, 2006). It is designed to be the basis of an interview and is not a self-report scale. It performed well in pregnancy (validated against the EPDS), with a cut-off of 10.5 recommended, although it has not been validated against a standardised interview.

A more recent review and critical analysis (Johnson *et al*, 2012) concluded that the Antenatal Risk Questionnaire fulfilled the reviewers' requirements more comprehensively than the other instruments they assessed.

Systematic enquiry about past psychiatric history, including the nature and severity of the illness and how it was treated, should be used to assess the risk of depression after delivery. Dennis & Ross (2006) observed that mothers with a personal psychiatric history were 4 times more likely to exhibit depressive symptoms at 8 weeks after delivery. A history of previous postnatal depression and depression during the index pregnancy were also predictors, although family psychiatric history was not. Others have found that a family history of postnatal depression is a risk factor (Kimmel *et al*, 2015).

## Screening for substance misuse and social problems

Screening for substance misuse is described in Chapter 5. An assessment should be made of any severe social problems, including domestic violence, following the guidance provided by the Department of Health (2005).

### Screening for risk of severe mental illness

The high risk of recurrence after delivery in women with bipolar disorder, schizoaffective disorder or a history of puerperal psychosis or a severe depressive episode has been outlined in earlier chapters of this book. Failing to identify women at risk and failing to adequately manage that risk is a key factor in maternal suicide and infanticide (Lewis & Drife, 2004).

It is crucial that there is a routine and systematic enquiry at antenatal booking about previous psychiatric illness, including its severity, the clinical presentation and the care received. Almost 10% of women who have a psychiatric admission before pregnancy will develop puerperal psychosis (Harlow *et al*, 2007). The risk increases with the number of hospital admissions, the closer they are in relation to pregnancy, and the length of the most recent admission. Chessick and Dimidjian (2010) advise using brief self-report scales to screen for bipolar disorder and have reviewed the psychometrics of 11 instruments, not all of which have been validated for use in the perinatal period.

General practitioners (GPs) are advised to ensure that details regarding current and past psychiatric history are included in referral to antenatal booking, and to avoid using the term 'postnatal depression' or the acronym 'PND' to describe all types of psychiatric disorder. However, *Maternity Matters* (Department of Health, 2007) encouraged women to refer themselves directly to midwives once they have confirmed they are pregnant, which risks crucial aspects of their medical or psychiatric history not being communicated to those responsible for their maternity care. Hence, the midwife undertaking a booking assessment must seek further details of the history from the woman's GP if she suspects there are or have been problems.

The precise details of previous illness, its severity and the treatment received should be obtained and recorded. When an agreed management plan has been decided upon, it must be communicated to the woman and all health professionals involved, and included in all her records (Royal College of Obstetricians and Gynaecologists (RCOG), 2011).

### Role of midwives and obstetricians

Midwives are the primary providers of antenatal care in the UK, and they are ideally placed to enquire about mental disorder both at the booking appointment and at subsequent visits. In 1999, 94% of maternity units in England and Wales reported that they asked about psychological problems at booking, and 25% undertook formal screening for depression during pregnancy (Tully *et al*, 2002). However, only 16% of units had offered any training to midwives to enable them to carry out this work, and fewer than 25% had policies and guidelines regarding the management of women with depression, let alone any other mental disorder. Results of a survey published in 2006 (Ross-Davie *et al*, 2006) indicate that although midwives have a positive attitude towards women with mental health problems and towards taking on a more developed role in mental health promotion, they also have many gaps in their knowledge, including the signs and symptoms of serious illness and the risk of puerperal psychosis. Midwives feel less confident in managing women with depression or schizophrenia than those with rarer conditions such as HIV, cholestasis and symphysis pubis diastasis. Only 13% have had any post-registration training in mental health.

Like midwives, obstetricians should understand the risk of recurrence of serious mental illness in relation to childbirth, and the timing and likely nature of recurrences. They should be clear about what actions are needed during pregnancy and after delivery (RCOG, 2011).

## Postpartum

Similar to the situation in pregnancy, many women with postpartum depression or anxiety go unrecognised (Thio et al, 2006). Postnatal assessments are usually undertaken between 4 and 6 weeks after delivery, and certainly screening too early in the postpartum period (less than 2 weeks after delivery) is likely to reduce the sensitivity of screening scales, owing to the presence of blues symptoms (Lee et al, 2003).

Around 3–4 months after birth is another opportunity to screen for depression, whether by asking the two questions recommended by NICE (2007) (see above) or by using a self-report questionnaire such as the EPDS to aid the clinical assessment. Using the EPDS in routine screening has been shown to increase the rate of diagnosed depression (Barnett et al, 1993; Hearn et al, 1998; Evins et al, 2000; Georgiopoulos et al, 2001) and treatment (Reay et al, 2010), although more than one-third of those identified as depressed in this study did not access treatment, preferring to use their own resources.

However, the 3–5% of women who suffer from more severe postnatal depressive illnesses and those with psychotic disorders will present much earlier than 6 weeks after delivery. Two-thirds of women with postpartum-onset major depression in a recent study dated the onset of their illness to a mean of 2.2 (±1.7) weeks after delivery (Stowe et al, 2005). Health professionals should not dismiss early symptoms and should assess maternal mental state much earlier than 6 weeks in any woman with a prior history of serious mood disorder or psychosis. A woman with a current or past serious mental illness should be asked about her mental health and symptoms at every postpartum contact.

## Where should we screen?

Screening can take place in a variety of settings, but those most frequently used in UK primary care are women's homes, clinics and children's centres. If others are present at home or the visit is unexpected, it may be inconvenient and lack privacy. Administering a questionnaire in a busy clinic can lead to a woman feeling rushed and, again, privacy may be lacking. In one study, a clear preference was expressed for having the EPDS administered at home (Shakespeare *et al*, 2003). There must be time and privacy to talk to the woman, to explore any issues raised, to ask additional questions to clarify and to answer her questions.

### Child health settings

In the USA, babies are seen 4–6 times per year at 'well baby' clinics, and it has been suggested that this might afford an opportunity for paediatricians to assess maternal depression (Heneghan *et al*, 1998). However, without systematic screening, they did not identify many of the mothers reporting depressive symptoms (Heneghan *et al*, 2000). Barriers appear to be paediatrician's lack of education and training to diagnose and treat maternal depression, and lack of time to take an adequate history (Olson *et al*, 2002; Wiley *et al*, 2004). There is also the question of whether or not they view it as their role. Those who do are more likely to consider changing their practice towards identification of maternal depression. Improving communication skills via video feedback of assessment interviews can improve ability to detect emotional disorders (Wissow *et al*, 1994).

Mothers are concerned about disclosure, owing to fear of judgement and the possibility of being referred to child protection services, and are more likely to disclose if they know their paediatrician well (Heneghan *et al*, 2004).

### Role of health visitors

Health visitors in the UK are qualified nurses or midwives who have undergone further training in health promotion, child health and education. Every family with a child under the age of five has a named health visitor who can advise on everyday concerns such as feeding, sleeping, behaviour problems and parenting in general. Health visitors may also assist with special needs, and may run immunisation programmes, child development checks and parenting classes.

Holden and colleagues (1989) demonstrated in a small RCT that after a short training course, health visitors could deliver an intervention based on Rogerian non-directive counselling which comprised eight 1 h 'listening visits', and that this was an effective intervention for mild to moderate non-psychotic unipolar postnatal depression. Health visitors in most areas have now had some form of training (although the quality and quantity of updates and supervision is very variable), and some form of screening and intervention is available in many parts of the UK.

## *Does screening lead to intervention?*

Screening may not automatically lead to intervention, for a variety of reasons. It is essential that there are clear care pathways so that professionals caring for pregnant or postpartum women know how to access assessment and treatment. The staff undertaking screening should have been trained and have sufficient ongoing supervision, consultation and contact with mental health professionals to enable them to access the pathways. Training will need to be updated and new entrants to the service trained. Workloads, vacancies and high turnover of staff are features of many services; failure in any of these areas can lead to women not receiving the treatment that they need.

Shakespeare (2002) reported on the reasons postpartum women in Oxford were not screened by health visitors (which occurred in one-third to almost half of the total sample). Around a quarter had cultural or language reasons, and others had moved away or were unavailable. Fifteen per cent at 8 weeks and 13% at 8 months refused, and for 26 and 30%, respectively, no reason was given. Recording of EPDS scores was found to be haphazard. Health visitors cited circumstances such as staff shortages and workload issues as the reason for this, but they were also reluctant to label women as depressed, which they felt could have negative consequences.

## What do women think about screening?

Women may be reluctant to disclose their problems or to access mental healthcare. In one study, most women in early pregnancy had not disclosed their emotional distress to their maternity care provider. However, they all expressed willingness to see a mental health professional if they were referred (Birndorf et al, 2001). In an study in an Australian baby health centre, 50% of depressed postpartum mothers identified by screening refused psychiatric referral. The main reason given was the stigma associated with psychiatric treatment; however, women were happy to talk to clinic nursing staff (Robinson & Young, 1982). Even in a setting where screening was routine and had been explained to women, 16% of those with a high EPDS score ignored recommendations for follow-up (Buist et al, 2006). Some mothers fear admission to a psychiatric unit, being locked up or having their baby removed (Hall, 2006). In some cultures, partners and/ or families will actively discourage a woman from disclosing her difficulties.

In 2005, UK parenting website Netmums (http://www.netmums.com) carried out an online survey of members, 63% of whom had been offered screening with the EPDS. Of those, 44% admitted lying to conceal their illness. The most common reason for this was feeling as if admitting being depressed meant admitting you were a failure, followed by not feeling comfortable confiding in the health visitor.

Women may lack knowledge or have misunderstandings about perinatal mental health problems and treatment, as much of the information in the lay press or on websites is inaccurate and misleading (Martinez et al, 2000; Summers & Logsdon, 2005).

There are particular concerns that some of the most vulnerable women – those who are young, less well-educated, poor attenders at appointments, and whose infants have poorer outcomes – are being excluded from health visitor contact (Murray *et al*, 2003). Reasons for this may be mistrust of services and services providers, seeing health visitors as the 'baby police', feeling alienated from healthcare settings, lack of transport, relocation and having multiple demands on their time.

## Prevention

Knowledge of the risk factors for postnatal depression, the risk of recurrence after subsequent deliveries if a woman has had a postpartum episode, and the predictable timing of an episode of depression has led to numerous trials of preventive interventions. Some interventions are delivered during pregnancy, and others are delivered postpartum. Some are targeted at women with any risk factors, others specifically at women who have had a previous episode of depression or psychosis.

## Depression

Several systematic reviews have now addressed the efficacy of various interventions aimed at preventing postnatal depression (Austin, 2003; Bradley *et al*, 2005; Howard *et al*, 2005; Dennis *et al*, 2008; Sado *et al*, 2012; Dennis & Dowswell, 2013; Miller *et al*, 2013; Sockol *et al*, 2013).

### Antidepressants

Nortriptyline is not an effective prophylactic when given to women who have previously had postnatal depression (Wisner *et al*, 2001), but sertraline led to significantly fewer recurrences when given to non-depressed pregnant women with a prior postnatal depression in a RCT (Wisner *et al*, 2004).

### Psychosocial and educational interventions

There is increasing evidence that women who receive a psychosocial or psychological intervention are significantly less likely to develop postpartum depression compared with those receiving standard care (Dennis & Dowswell, 2013; Sockol *et al*, 2013). Promising interventions include the provision of intensive, individualised postpartum home visits provided by public health nurses or midwives, (lay) peer-based telephone support and interpersonal psychotherapy (IPT). Interventions in the postpartum period also significantly reduced the risk of developing depressive symptoms.

### Hormones

Progesterone and progestogens have been suggested as prophylaxis against recurrence of postnatal depression since Katharina Dalton's progesterone trial published in 1985 (Dalton, 1985), in which she claimed that it was an effective prophylactic. However, she used historical controls and the women were not randomised. Four years later she published a controlled trial, reporting similar results, but, again, participants were not randomised (Dalton, 1989). Synthetic progestogens should be used with significant caution in the postpartum period, as they can increase the risk of depressive symptoms. A Cochrane review concluded that 'the role of natural progesterone in the prevention and treatment of postpartum depression has yet to be evaluated in a randomised, placebo-controlled trial' (Dennis *et al*, 2008).

Sichel *et al* (1995) reported a small case series in which four women with a history of puerperal major depression were treated with high-dose oral oestrogen, none of whom experienced a recurrence. However, the risk of venous thromboembolism (VTE) associated with the postpartum period and oestrogen must be considered, and heparinisation may be required. Dennis *et al* (2008) concluded that 'oestrogen therapy may be of modest value for the treatment of severe postpartum depression. Its role in the prevention of recurrent postpartum depression has not been rigorously evaluated'.

Despite the positive association between thyroid antibody status and depression in postpartum women, thyroxine does not prevent the occurrence of postnatal depression (Harris *et al*, 2002).

### Other interventions

Pregnant and recently delivered women often experience sleep disturbance, and this has been proposed as a potential trigger for both postnatal depression and puerperal psychosis. A Canadian centre piloted an intervention for women considered at high risk for recurrence of depression postpartum (those with a personal or family history of depression or with subclinical symptoms during pregnancy). The mothers are offered a hospital stay for 5 nights, during which they sleep in a single room, with their baby spending the night in the nursery. Breastfeeding mothers are encouraged to express milk during the day so that night feeds can be given by staff. Hypnotics are used if required. A case note review of the first 179 patients gave promising results (Steiner *et al*, 2003), but this has yet to be tested in an RCT.

Dietary supplements, including omega-3 fatty acids (Llorente *et al*, 2003; Marangell *et al* 2004; Freeman, 2006; Mozurkewicz *et al*, 2013), calcium carbonate (Harrison-Hohner *et al*, 2001) and selenium (Mokhber *et al*, 2011), have been explored as preventive interventions, with little success to date (Miller *et al* (2013).

Although hypnosis is used to control pain in labour, there are no data from controlled studies supporting its use as a preventive intervention for postnatal depression (Sado *et al*, 2012).

## *Puerperal psychosis*

Two systematic reviews have studied preventive interventions for puerperal psychosis and highlight the paucity of evidence on which to make recommendations (Doucet *et al*, 2011; Essali *et al*, 2013).

Disruption of the sleep–wake cycle, particularly reduced sleep and early waking, is associated with relapse of manic symptoms in non-puerperal populations (Wehr, 1989) and may well be a provoking factor in puerperal psychosis (Sharma, 2003). As far as is possible with a new infant, sleep loss and disruption should be minimised in vulnerable women. This could include support from a partner or family member in helping with night feeds (expressing milk during the day if breastfeeding).

### Drugs

There are studies supporting the efficacy of lithium started in the immediate postpartum or in the last trimester for the prevention of puerperal psychosis (Stewart *et al*, 1991; Austin, 1992; Cohen *et al*, 1995; Bergink *et al*, 2012) but no RCTs. Cohen *et al* (1995) estimated the relative risk of relapse for those not taking mood stabilisers to be 8.6. However, maternal lithium levels must be checked regularly and care taken to avoid toxicity during labour and delivery, when fluid balance may be disrupted, and in the postpartum when renal clearance (increased during pregnancy) returns to pre-pregnancy levels.

A small naturalistic study (part of a larger study of bipolar disorder) examined whether olanzapine alone or in addition to antidepressants and/ or mood stabilisers could prevent a puerperal psychotic episode (Sharma *et al*, 2006). Two (18.2%) of the women who took olanzapine experienced a postpartum episode (depression), compared with eight (57.1%) of those who did not take olanzapine (four depressive episodes, one mixed, one hypomania and two puerperal psychosis). It should be noted that the sample was of women with bipolar I and II disorder, not all of whom had had a previous puerperal psychotic episode, but it is of interest that olanzapine appeared to also prevent depressive episodes. This requires replication under controlled conditions.

### Hormones

Both oestrogen and progesterone have been promoted as prophylactic agents for puerperal psychosis, but with little success. Sichel *et al* (1995) gave seven women with histories of puerperal psychosis high-dose oral oestrogen immediately after delivery. The only woman to relapse postpartum had not been fully adherent to medication. However, transdermal oestradiol administered to 29 women with a diagnosis of bipolar disorder or schizo-affective disorder failed to reduce the rate of relapse (Kumar *et al*, 2003).

To date, there is little evidence to support the use of oestrogen as prophylaxis for puerperal psychosis or recurrence of bipolar disorder postpartum. It should also be remembered that there is an increased risk of VTE in the postpartum period and with the use of oestrogens.

## Conclusion

Mental disorders result in significant morbidity and mortality for pregnant and recently delivered women, and can have lasting effects on their infants and families. As pregnant and postpartum women are in regular contact with health professionals, there are several opportunities for those suffering from or at risk of mental disorder to be detected and treated, or for preventive strategies and monitoring to be put into place.

# References

Andersson L, Sundström-Poromaa I, Bixo M, *et al* (2003) Point prevalence of psychiatric disorders during the second trimester of pregnancy: a population-based study. *American Journal of Obstetrics & Gynecology*, **189**: 148–154.

Andersson L, Sundström-Poromaa I, Wulff M, *et al* (2004) Implications of antenatal depression and anxiety for obstetric outcome. *Obstetrics & Gynecology*, **104**: 467–476.

Austin MP (1992) Puerperal affective psychosis: is there a case for lithium prophylaxis? *British Journal of Psychiatry*, **161**: 692–694.

Austin MP (2003) Targeted group antenatal prevention of postnatal depression: a review. *Acta Psychiatrica Scandinavica*, **107**: 244–250.

Austin MP, Lumley J (2003) Antenatal screening for postnatal depression: a systematic review. *Acta Psychiatrica Scandinavica*, **107**: 10–17.

Austin MP, Hadzi-Pavlovic D, Saint K, *et al* (2005) Antenatal screening for the prediction of postnatal depression: validation of a psychosocial Pregnancy Risk Questionnaire. *Acta Psychiatrica Scandinavica*, **112**: 310–317.

Barnett B, Lockhart K, Bernard D, *et al* (1993) Mood disorders among mothers of infants admitted to a mothercraft hospital. *Journal of Paediatrics and Child Health*, **29**: 270–275.

Beck CT, Gable RK (2000) Postpartum depression screening scale: development and psychometric testing. *Nursing Research*, **49**: 272–282.

Beck CT, Gable RK (2002) *Postpartum Depression Scale Screening Manual*. Western Psychological Services.

Beck CT, Records K, Rice M (2006) Further development of the Postpartum Depression Predictors Inventory-Revised. *Journal of Obstetric, Gynecologic, and Neonatal Nursing*, **35**: 735–745.

Bergink V, Bouvy PF, Vervoort JSP, *et al* (2012) Prevention of postpartum psychosis and mania in women at high risk. *American Journal of Psychiatry*, **169**: 609–615.

Birndorf CA, Madden A, Portera L, *et al* (2001) Psychiatric symptoms, functional impairment, and receptivity toward mental health treatment among obstetrical patients. *International Journal of Psychiatry in Medicine*, **31**: 353–365.

Boyd RC, Le HN, Somberg R (2005) Review of screening instruments for postpartum depression. *Archives of Women's Mental Health*, **8**: 141–153.

Bradley E, Boath E, Henshaw C (2005) The prevention of postpartum depression: a narrative systematic review. *Psychosomatic Obstetrics & Gynecology*, **26**: 185–192.

Brockington I, Oates J, George S, *et al* (2001) A screening questionnaire for mother-infant bonding disorders. *Archives of Women's Mental Health*, **3**: 133–140.

Buist A, Condon J, Brooks J, *et al* (2006) Acceptability of routine screening for perinatal depression. *Journal of Affective Disorders*, **93**: 233–237.

Carroll JC, Reid AJ, Biringer A, *et al* (2005) Effectiveness of the Antenatal Psychosocial Health Assessment (ALPHA) form in detecting psychosocial concerns: a randomized controlled trial. *Canadian Medical Association Journal*, **173**: 253–259.

Chessick CA, Dimidjian S (2010) Screening for bipolar disorder during pregnancy and the postnatal period. *Archives of Women's' Mental Health*, **13**: 233–248.

Chew-Graham CA, Sharp D, Chamberlain E, *et al* (2009) Disclosure of symptoms of postnatal depression, the perspectives of health professionals and women: a qualitative study. *BMC Family Practice*, **10**: 7.

Coates AO, Schaefer CA, Alexander JL (2004) Detection of postpartum depression and anxiety in a large health plan. *Journal of Behavioral Health Services & Research*, **31**: 117–32.

Cohen LS, Sichel DA, Robertson LM, et al (1995) Postpartum prophylaxis for women with bipolar disorder. *American Journal of Psychiatry*, **152**: 1641–1645.

Cox J, Holden J, Henshaw C (2014a) Development of the EPDS. In *Perinatal mental health: the Edinburgh Postnatal Depression Scale Manual* (pp. 22–26). RCPsych Publications.

Cox J, Holden J, Henshaw C (2014b) Appendix 2: Translations of the Edinburgh Postnatal Depression Scale. In *Perinatal mental health: the Edinburgh Postnatal Depression Scale Manual* (pp. 72–191). RCPsych Publications.

Cox JH, Holden JM, Sagovsky R (1987) Detection of postnatal depression: the development of the 10-item Edinburgh Postnatal Depression Scale. *British Journal of Psychiatry*, **150**: 782–786.

Cubison J, Munro J (2005) Acceptability of using the EPDS as a screening tool. In *Screening for Perinatal Depression* (pp. 152–161). Jessica Kingsley.

Dalton K (1985) Progesterone prophylaxis used successfully in postnatal depression. *The Practitioner*, **229**: 507–508.

Dalton K (1989) Successful prophylactic progesterone for idiopathic postnatal depression. *International Journal of Prenatal and Perinatal Studies*, **1**: 323–327.

Dennis CL, Dowswell T (2013) Psychosocial and psychological interventions for preventing postpartum depression. *Cochrane Database of Systematic Reviews*, **2**: CD001134.

Dennis C-L, Ross LE (2006) The clinical utility of maternal self-reported personal and familial psychiatric history in identifying women at risk for postpartum depression. *Acta Obstetricia Gynecologica Scandinavica*, **85**: 1179–1185.

Dennis CL, Ross LE, Herxheimer A (2008) Oestrogens and progestins for preventing and treating postpartum depression. *Cochrane Database of Systematic Reviews*, **4**: CD001690.

Department of Health (2005) *Responding to Domestic Abuse: A Handbook for Health Professionals*. TSO (The Stationery Office).

Department of Health (2007) *Maternity Matters: Choice, Access and Continuity of Care in a Safe Service*. TSO (The Stationery Office).

Derogatis LR, Melisaratos N (1983) The Brief Symptom Inventory: an introductory report. *Psychological Medicine*, **13**: 598–605.

Doucet S, Jones I, Letourneau N, et al (2011) Interventions for the prevention of postpartum psychosis: a systematic review. *Archives of Women's Mental Health*, **14**: 89–98.

Downe SM, Butler E, Hinder S (2007) Screening tools for depressed mood after childbirth in UK-based South Asian women: a systematic review. *Journal of Advanced Nursing*, **57**: 565–583.

Drake H, Howard E, Kinsey E (2014) Online screening and referral for postpartum depression: an exploratory study. *Community Mental Health Journal*, **50**: 305–311.

Essali A, Alabed S, Guul A, et al (2013) Preventive interventions for postnatal psychosis. *Cochrane Database of Systematic Reviews*, **6**:CD009991.

Evins GG, Theofrastous JP, Galvin SL (2000) Postpartum depression: a comparison of screening and routine clinical evaluation. *American Journal of Obstetrics & Gynecology*, **182**: 1080–1082.

Freeman MP (2006) Omega-3 fatty acids and perinatal depression: A review of the literature and recommendations for future research. *Prostaglandins, Leukotrienes and Essential Fatty Acids*, **75**: 291–297.

Fuggle P, Glover L, Khan F, et al (2002) Screening for postnatal depression in Bengali women: preliminary observations from using a translated version of the Edinburgh Postnatal Depression Scale (EPDS). *Journal of Reproductive and Infant Psychology*, **20**: 71–82.

Gaskin K, James H (2006) Using the Edinburgh Postnatal Depression Scale with learning disabled mothers. *Community Practitioner*, **79**: 392–396.

Gemmill AW, Leigh B, Ericksen J, et al (2006) A survey of the clinical acceptability of screening for postnatal depression and non-depressed women. *BMC Public Health*, **6**: 211.

Georgiopoulos AM, Bryan TL, Wollan TL, et al (2001) Routine screening for postpartum depression. *Journal of Family Practice*, **50**: 117–122.

Gjerdingen D, Crow S, McGovern P, et al (2009) Postpartum depression screening at well-child visits: validity of a 2-question screen and the PHQ-9. *Annals of Family Medicine*, **7**: 63–70.

Guedeney N, Fermanian J, Guelfi JD, et al (2000) The Edinburgh Postnatal Depression Scale (EPDS) and the detection of major depressive disorders in early postpartum: some concerns about false negatives. *Journal of Affective Disorders*, **61**: 107–112.

Hall P (2006) Mothers' experiences of postnatal depression: an interpretative phenomenological analysis. *Community Practitioner*, **79**: 256–260.

Harlow BL, Vitonis AF, Sparen P, et al (2007) Incidence of hospitalization for postpartum psychotic and bipolar episodes in women with and without prior prepregnancy or prenatal psychiatric hospitalizations. *Archives of General Psychiatry*, **64**: 42–48.

Harris B, Oretti R, Lazarus J, et al (2002) Randomised trial of thyroxine to prevent postnatal depression in thyroid-antibody-positive women. *British Journal of Psychiatry*, **180**: 327–330.

Harrison-Hohner J, Coste S, Dorato V, et al (2001) Prenatal calcium supplementation and postpartum depression: an ancillary study to a randomized trial of calcium for prevention of preeclampsia. *Archives of Women's Mental Health*, **3**: 141–146.

Hearn G, Iliff A, Jones I, et al (1998) Postnatal depression in the community. *British Journal of General Practice*, **48**: 1064–1066.

Heneghan AM, Silver EJ, Bauman LJ, et al (1998) Depressive symptoms in inner-city mothers of young children: who is at risk? Pediatrics, 102: 1394–1400.

Heneghan AM, Silver EJ, Bauman LJ, et al (2000) Do pediatricians recognize mothers with depressive symptoms? Pediatrics, 106: 1367–1373.

Heneghan AM, Mercer B, DeLeone N (2004) Will mothers discuss parenting stress and depressive symptoms with their child's pediatrician? *Pediatrics*, **113**: 460–467.

Henshaw C, Elliott S (2005) Bibliography of translations and validation studies. In *Screening for Perinatal Depression* (pp. 205–211). Jessica Kingsley.

Holcomb WL, Stone LS, Lustman PJ, et al (1996) Screening for depression in pregnancy: characteristics of the Beck Depression Inventory. *Obstetrics & Gynecology*, **88**: 1021–1025.

Holden JM, Sagovsky R, Cox JL (1989) Counselling in a general practice setting: controlled study of health visitor intervention in treatment of postnatal depression. *BMJ*, **298**: 223–226.

Howard LM, Hoffbrand S, Henshaw C, et al (2005) Antidepressant prevention of postnatal depression. *The Cochrane Database of Systematic Reviews*, **2**: CD004363.

Jomeen J, Martin C (2004) Is the Hospital Anxiety and Depression Scale (HADS) a reliable screening tool in early pregnancy? *Psychology and Health*, **19**: 787–800.

Johnson M, Schmeid V, Lupton SJ, et al (2012) Measuring perinatal mental health risk. *Archives of Women's Mental Health*, **15**: 375–386.

Kabir K, Sheeder J, Kelly L, et al (2007) identifying postpartum depression: 3 questions are as good as 10. *Journal of Pediatric and Adolescent Gynecology*, **20**: S135–S136.

Karimova GK, Martin CR (2003) A psychometric evaluation of the Hospital Anxiety and Depression Scale during pregnancy. *Psychology, Health and Medicine*, **8**: 89.

Kelly RH, Zatick D, Anders TF (2001) The detection and treatment of psychiatric disorders and substance use among pregnant women cared for in obstetrics. *American Journal of Psychiatry*, **158**: 213–219.

Kim HG, Mandell M, Crandall C, et al (2006) Antenatal psychiatric illness and adequacy of prenatal care in an ethnically diverse inner-city obstetric population. *Archives of Women's Mental Health*, **9**: 103–107.

Kimmel M, Hess E, Roy PS, et al (2015) Family history, not lack of medication use, is associated with the development of postpartum depression in a high-risk sample. *Archives of Women's Mental Health*, **18**: 113–21.

Kitamura T, Sugawara M, Shima S, et al (1999) Temporal validity of self-rating questionnaires: improved validity of repeated use of Zung's Self-Rating Depression Scale among women during the perinatal period. *Journal of Psychosomatic Obstetrics & Gynaecology*, **20**: 112–117.

Kroenke K, Spitzer RL, Williams JB, *et al* (2007) Anxiety disorders in primary care: prevalence, impairment, comorbidity, and detection. *Annals of Internal Medicine*, **146**: 317–325.

Kumar C, McIvor RJ, Shima S, *et al* (2003) Estrogen administration does not reduce the recurrence of affective psychosis after childbirth. *Journal of Clinical Psychiatry*, **64**: 112–118.

Le H-N, Perry D, Sheng X (2009) Using the internet to screen for postpartum depression. *Maternal and Child Health Journal*, **13**: 213–221.

Lee DTS, Yip SK, Chui HFK, *et al* (2003) Postdelivery screening for postpartum depression. *Psychosomatic Medicine*, **65**: 357–361.

Leverton T (2005) Advantages and disadvantages of screening in clinical settings. In *Screening for Perinatal Depression* (eds C Henshaw, S Elliott; pp. 34–46). Jessica Kingsley.

Lewis G, Drife J (2004) *Why Mothers Die 2002–2004. The Sixth Report of the Confidential Enquiries into Maternal Death in the United Kingdom*. RCOG Press.

Llorente AM, Jensen CL, Voigt RG, *et al* (2003) Effect of maternal docosahexaenoic acid supplementation on postpartum depression and information processing. *American Journal of Obstetrics & Gynecology*, **188**: 1348–1353.

Logsdon MC, Hutti MH (2006) Readability: an important issue impacting healthcare for women with postpartum depression. *American Journal of Maternal and Child Nursing*, **31**: 351–355.

Lok IH, Lee DTS, Yip S-K, *et al* (2004) Screening for post-miscarriage psychiatric morbidity. *American Journal of Obstetrics & Gynecology*, **191**: 546–550.

Loveland Cook CA, Flick LH, Homan SM, *et al* (2004) Post-traumatic stress disorder in pregnancy: prevalence, risk factors and treatment. *Obstetrics & Gynaecology*, **103**: 710–717.

Mann R, Adamson J, Gilbody S (2012) Diagnostic accuracy of case-finding questions to identify postnatal depression. *Canadian Medical Association Journal*, **184**: e424–e430.

Marangell LB, Martinez JM, Zboyan HA, *et al* (2004) Omega-3 fatty acids for the prevention of postpartum depression: negative data from a preliminary, open-label pilot study. *Depression and Anxiety*, **19**: 20–23.

Martin CR, Jomeen J (2003) Is the 12-item General Health Questionnaire (GHQ-12) confounded by scoring method during pregnancy and following birth? *Journal of Reproductive and Infant Psychology*, **21**: 267–278.

Martinez R, Johnston Robledo I, Ulsh HM, *et al* (2000) Singing 'the baby blues': a content analysis of popular press articles about postpartum affective disturbances. *Women and Health*, **31**: 37–56.

Matthey S (2004) Calculating clinically significant change in postnatal depression studies using the Edinburgh Postnatal Depression Scale. *Journal of Affective Disorders*, **78**: 269–272.

Matthey S, Henshaw C, Elliott SA, *et al* (2006) Variability in use of cut-off scores and formats on the Edinburgh Postnatal Depression Scale-implications for research findings. *Archives of Women's Mental Health*, **9**: 309–315.

Maurer-Spurej E, Pittendreigh C, Misri S (2007) Platelet serotonin levels support depression scores for women with postpartum depression. *Journal of Psychiatry and Neuroscience*, **32**: 23–29.

Miller BJ, Murray L, Beckmann MM, *et al* (2013) Dietary supplements for preventing postnatal depression. *Cochrane Database of Systematic Reviews*, **10**: CD009104.

Mitchell AM, Mittelstaedt ME, Schott-Baer D (2006) Postpartum depression: the reliability of telephone screening. *American Maternal and Child Nurse*, **31**: 382–387.

Mokhber N, Namjoo M, Tara F, *et al* (2011) Effect of supplementation with selenium on postpartum depression: a randomized placebo-controlled trial. *Journal of Maternal-Fetal and Neonatal Medicine*, **24**: 104–108.

Moran TE, O'Hara MW (2006) A partner-rating scale of postpartum depression: The Edinburgh Postnatal Depression Scale - Partner (EPDS-P). *Archives of Women's Mental Health*, **9**: 173–180.

Mozurkewicz E, Chilimigras J, Klemens C, *et al* (2013) The mothers, omega-3 and mental health study. *BMC Pregnancy and Childbirth*, **11**: 46.

Murray D, Cox J (1990) Screening for depression during pregnancy with the Edinburgh Postnatal Depression Scale (EPDS). *Journal of Reproductive and Infant Psychology*, **8**: 99–107.

Murray L, Woolgar M, Murray J, *et al* (2003) Self-exclusion from health care in women at high risk from postpartum depression. *Journal of Public Health Medicine*, **25**: 131–137.

National Institute for Health and Care Excellence (2007) *Antenatal and Postnatal Mental Health. Clinical Management and Service Guidance*. NICE.

National Institute for Health and Care Excellence (2014) *Antenatal and Postnatal Mental Health*. NICE.

National Screening Committee (2011) *The UK NSC Recommendation on Postnatal Depression Screening in Pregnancy*. NSC (https://legacyscreening.phe.org.uk/postnataldepression).

National Screening Committee (2013) *NHS Population Screening Explained*. Public Health England (https://www.gov.uk/guidance/nhs-population-screening-explained).

Navarro P, Ascaso C, Garcia-Esteve L, *et al* (2007) Postnatal psychiatric morbidity: a validation study of the GHQ-12 and the EPDS as screening tools. *General Hospital Psychiatry*, **29**: 1–7.

Olson AL, Kemper KJ, Kelleher KJ, *et al* (2002) Primary care pediatricians' roles and perceived responsibilities in the identification and management of maternal depression. *Pediatrics*, **110**: 1169–1176.

Peckham C, Dezateux C (1998) Issues underlying the evaluation of screening programmes. *British Medical Bulletin*, **54**: 767–778.

Pollock JI, Manaseki-Holland S, Patel V (2006) Detection of depression in women of child-bearing age in non-western cultures: a comparison of the Edinburgh Postnatal Depression Scale and the Self-Reporting Questionnaire-20 in Mongolia. *Journal of Affective Disorders*, **92**: 267–271.

Reay R, Matthey S, Ellwood D, *et al* (2010) Long-term outcomes of participants in a perinatal depression early detection program. *Journal of Affective Disorders*, **129**: 94–103.

Robinson S, Young J (1982) Screening for depression and anxiety in the postnatal period: acceptance or rejection of a treatment offer. *Australian and New Zealand Journal of Psychiatry*, **16**: 47–51.

Ross-Davie M, Elliott SA, Sarkar A, *et al* (2006) A public health role in perinatal mental health: are midwives ready? *British Journal of Midwifery*, **14**: 330–334.

Royal College of Obstetricians and Gynaecologists (2011) *Management of Women with Mental Health Issues during Pregnancy and the Postnatal Period (Good Practice No. 14)*. RCOG.

Sado M, Stickley E, Mori R (2012) Hypnosis during pregnancy, childbirth and the postnatal period for preventing postnatal depression. *Cochrane Database of Systematic Reviews*, **6**: CD009062.

Salamero M, Marcos T, Gutierrez F, *et al* (1994) Factorial study of the BDI in pregnant women. *Psychological Medicine*, **14**: 1031–1035.

Shakespeare J (2002) Health visitor screening for postnatal depression using the EPDS: a process study. *Community Practitioner*, **75**: 381–384.

Shakespeare J, Blake F, Garcia J (2003) A qualitative study of the acceptability of routine screening of postnatal women using the Edinburgh Postnatal Depression Scale. *British Journal of General Practice*, **53**: 614–619.

Sharma V (2003) Role of sleep loss in the causation of puerperal psychosis. *Medical Hypotheses*, **61**: 477–481.

Sharma V, Smith A, Mazmanian D (2006) Olanzapine in the prevention of postpartum psychosis and mood episodes in bipolar disorder. *Bipolar Disorders*, **8**: 400–404.

Sharp DJ (1988) Validation of the 3-item General Health Questionnaire in early pregnancy. *Psychological Medicine*, **18**: 503–507.

Sichel DA, Cohen LS, Robertson LM, *et al* (1995) Prophylactic estrogen in recurrent postpartum affective disorder. *Biological Psychiatry*, **38**: 814–818.

Sidebottom A, Harrison PA, Godecker A, *et al* (2012) Validation of the Patient Health Questionnaire (PHQ)-9 for prenatal depression screening. *Archives of Women's Mental Health*, **15**: 367–374.

Smith MV, Rosenheck RA, Cavaleri MA, et al (2004) Screening for and detection of depression, panic disorder, and PTSD in public-sector obstetric clinics. Psychiatric Services, 55: 407–414.

Sobowale A, Adams C (2005) Screening where there is no screening scale. In Screening for Perinatal Depression (eds C Henshaw, S Elliott): pp. 90–109. Jessica Kingsley.

Sockol LE, Epperson CN, Barber JP (2013) Preventing postpartum depression: a meta-analytic review. Clinical Psychology Review, 33: 1205–1217.

Somerville S, Dedman K, Hagan R, et al (2014) The Perinatal Anxiety Screening Scale: development and preliminary validation. Archives of Women's Mental Health, 17: 443–454.

Stein G, van den Akker O (1992) The retrospective diagnosis of postnatal depression by questionnaire. Journal of Psychosomatic Research, 36: 67–75.

Steiner M, Fairman M, Jansen K (2003) Can postpartum depression be prevented? Archives of Women's Mental Health, 6: S106.

Stewart DE, Klompenhouwer JL, Kendell RE, et al (1991) Prophylactic lithium in puerperal psychosis. The experience of three centres. British Journal of Psychiatry, 158: 393–397.

Stowe ZN, Hostetter AL, Newport DJ (2005) The onset of postpartum depression: Implications for clinical screening in obstetrical and primary care. American Journal of Obstetrics & Gynecology, 192: 522–526.

Summers AL, Logsdon MC (2005) Web sites for postpartum depression: convenient, frustrating, incomplete, and misleading. North American Journal of Maternal Child Nursing, 30: 88–94.

Thio IM, Oakley Browne MA, Coverdale JH, et al (2006) Postnatal depressive symptoms largely go untreated. Social Psychiatry and Psychiatric Epidemiology, 41: 814–818.

Thoppil J, Riutcel TL, Nalesnik SW (2005) Early intervention for perinatal depression. American Journal of Obstetrics & Gynecology, 192: 1446–1448.

Tully L, Garcia J, Davidson L, et al (2002) Role of midwives in depression screening. British Journal of Midwifery, 10: 374–378.

US Preventive Service Task Force (2002) Screening for depression: recommendations and rationale. Annals of Internal Medicine, 136: 760–764.

Venkatesh KK, Zlotnick C, Triche EW, et al (2014) Accuracy of brief screening tools for identifying postpartum depression in adolescent mothers. Pediatrics, 133: e45–e53.

Wehr TA (1989) Sleep loss: a preventable cause of mania and other excited states. Journal of Clinical Psychiatry, 50 (Suppl): 8–16.

Whitton A, Warner R, Appleby L (1996) The pathway to care in post-natal depression: women's attitudes to postnatal depression and its treatment. British Journal of General Practice, 46: 427–428.

Whooley MA, Avins AL, Miranda J, et al (1997) Case-finding instruments for depression. Two questions are as good as many. Journal of General Internal Medicine, 12: 439–445.

Wiley CC, Burke GS, Gill PA, et al (2004) Paediatricians' views of postpartum depression: a self-administered survey. Archives of Women's Mental Health, 7: 231–236.

Wisner KL, Perel JM, Peindl KS, et al (2001) Prevention of recurrent postpartum depression: a randomized clinical trial. Journal of Clinical Psychiatry, 62: 82–86.

Wisner KL, Perel JM, Peindl KS, et al (2004) Prevention of postpartum depression: a pilot randomized clinical trial. American Journal of Psychiatry, 161: 1290–1292.

Wissow LS, Roter DL, Wilson MEH (1994) Pediatrican interview style and mother's disclosure of psychosocial issues. Pediatrics, 93: 289–295.

# Further reading

American College of Obstetricians and Gynecologists Committee on Obstetric Practice Opinion (2010) Screening for Depression During and After Pregnancy. ACOG.

Austin M-P (2014) Marcé International Society position statement on psychosocial assessment and depression screening in perinatal women. Best Practice & Research Clinical Obstetrics & Gynaecology, 28: 179–187.

Beyond Blue: Australian National Guidelines (www.beyondblue.org.au/resources/health-professionals/clinical-practice-guidelines/perinatal-clinical-practice-guidelines).

Dennis C-L, Chung-Lee L (2006) Postpartum depression help-seeking barriers and maternal treatment preferences: a qualitative systematic review. *Birth*, **33**: 323–331.

Morrell CJ, Sutcliffe P, Booth A, *et al* (2016) A systematic review, evidence synthesis and meta-analysis of quantitative and qualitative studies evaluating the clinical effectiveness, the cost-effectiveness, safety and acceptability of interventions to prevent postnatal depression. *Health Technology Assessment*, **20**: 37.

Scottish Intercollegiate Guidelines Network (2012) Management of Perinatal Mood Disorders. *SIGN*.

## Resources

For details of how to obtain the EPDS, the ALPHA scale, the PDSS and 'How are you feeling?' booklets, please see Appendices II and III.

# CHAPTER 8

# Physical treatments during pregnancy

Given the substantial psychiatric morbidity during pregnancy described in Chapters 2 and 4, it is clear that many women will need drug treatment or other physical treatments during pregnancy, either because non-pharmacological interventions have failed or because there is no alternative. However, only about one-third of women who are depressed during pregnancy appear to receive any treatment (Flynn *et al*, 2006). Recent data from publicly insured women in the USA report that 8% use antidepressants during pregnancy (Huybrechts *et al*, 2011), with higher rates in older and Black and minority ethnic women. Another study in the USA observed a rise from 2.5% in 1998 to 8.1% in 2005 in four states (Alwan *et al*, 2011). A large study of privately insured women in the USA ($n = 343\,299$) who delivered between 2006 and 2011 reported that 10.3% were prescribed one or more psychotropic medicines during pregnancy. This rate varied from 6% to 15% between states. The most commonly used psychotropic medicines were selective serotonin reuptake inhibitors (SSRIs; 5.1%) and benzodiazepines (BDZs) or BDZ-like medicines (3.9%). Approximately 1.6% of women used more than one category of psychotropic medicine in pregnancy, most commonly an antidepressant and an anxiolytic (Hanley & Mintzes, 2014). A UK primary study of over 40 000 women between 1989 and 2010 observed rates of 4.69% before pregnancy; 2.81%, 1.31% and 1.34% in the first, second and third trimesters, respectively; and 5.46% 3 months after delivery (Margulis *et al*, 2014). Rates of antidepressant use in pregnancy appeared to be lower in Denmark at 0.2% in 1997, increasing to 3.2% in 2010 (Jimenez-Solem *et al*, 2013). Women with severe mental illness are more likely to be taking more than one drug (mode = 3), with more than a quarter taking 6–10 drugs over the course of their pregnancy (Peindl *et al*, 2007).

There are a number of factors to be taken into consideration in the risk–benefit analysis, not least the impact of untreated psychiatric disorder on the fetus. The risks associated with untreated depression (adverse neonatal outcomes and maternal morbidity, including suicidal ideas and attempts) were reviewed by Bonari *et al* (2004), who concluded:

'When making clinical decisions, clinicians should weigh the growing body of literature suggesting potential adverse effects of untreated depression during pregnancy against the literature that has failed to find risks associated with in utero antidepressant exposure.'

Readers should note that the evidence base in this area is changing rapidly, and specialist drug information services should be contacted for an update before treating a pregnant woman.

# General principles

As no drug is licensed in the UK specifically for women who are pregnant or breastfeeding, the prescriber should follow professional guidance and document informed consent. For more information, see the General Medical Council's guidance on good practice in prescribing (www.gmc-uk. org/guidance/ethical_guidance/14316.asp).

- Each case should have a careful risk–benefit assessment considering all aspects of maternal and fetal well-being, including how a mental health problem and its treatment might affect parenting.
- If the disorder is mild to moderate in severity, use a non-pharmacological intervention.
- Avoid first-trimester exposure if at all possible.
- Use the lowest effective dose for the shortest time.
- We now have more published data on SSRIs than tricyclic antidepressants (TCAs).
- TCAs are toxic in overdose.
- As far as is possible, treat the woman with a drug she has responded to in the past.
- Avoid new depot medication, but it is not usually necessary to discontinue depots if pregnancy occurs during established treatment. The woman should be warned about possible extrapyramidal side-effects in the infant.
- Avoid polypharmacy if at all possible, whether concurrently or sequentially.
- Consider whether medication should be tapered or withdrawn before delivery and when to reinstate afterwards after careful risk assessment.

Cohen and colleagues (2006) demonstrated that 68% of women who discontinued antidepressants during pregnancy relapsed during pregnancy, compared with 26% who maintained their medication, a fivefold increased risk. However, this study was undertaken in a specialist psychiatric clinic population. Yonkers et al (2011), who carried out a community-based study, reported that discontinuing antidepressants made no difference to rates of relapse, unless there had been an episode in the 6 months before conception or there was a history of 4 or more episodes prior to pregnancy.

Some childhood problems, e.g. internalising behaviours in 4- to 5-year-old children (depression, anxiety and withdrawal), are not associated with psychotropic medications being used during pregnancy but are linked to impaired maternal mood (Misri *et al*, 2006).

The potential risks of drugs include maternal and infant toxicity, side-effects or withdrawal symptoms and fetal teratogenicity, both physical and behavioural. These must be balanced against the risk of not treating the mental disorder, which might result in adverse outcomes either as a direct consequence of the disorder or as a result of behaviours associated with the condition in question. For example, smoking or drug use, reduced self-care, poor attendance at antenatal appointments and self-harm are all associated with maternal mental illness. One study has shown that treating depression during pregnancy (with antidepressants, psychotherapy or both) reduces the risk of the infant requiring neonatal intensive care unit (NICU) admission (Li & Ferber, 2012).

In addition, pregnancy physiology may change drug pharmacokinetics (see Table 8.1). The prescriber must be aware of this, as changes to the dose or dosage schedule may be required at various times during pregnancy and after delivery. For example, higher doses might be needed during pregnancy to achieve therapeutic serum levels, as metabolism and volume of distribution increase during pregnancy, but these may need to be reduced rapidly after delivery to avoid toxicity when pharmacokinetics rapidly return to the pre-pregnant state. For further guidance, see National Institute for Health and Care Excellence (NICE), 2014.

# Routes of fetal exposure

## Placental transfer

Psychotropics cross the placenta. Hostetter *et al* (2000a) reported on three pregnant women treated with fluvoxamine, sertraline and venlafaxine, respectively. All three antidepressants, and the metabolites of sertraline and venlafaxine, were found in umbilical cord blood. A larger study examined umbilical cord blood samples taken immediately after delivery, from 38 women who had been taking citalopram, fluoxetine, paroxetine or sertraline. Both antidepressants and metabolites were detectable in 86.8% of umbilical cord samples, with mean ratios of cord to maternal serum levels between 0.29 and 0.89. The lowest ratios were for sertraline and paroxetine. Maternal doses of sertraline and fluoxetine were correlated with umbilical cord blood sample concentrations (Hendrick *et al*, 2003a). Rampono *et al* (2004) found the following cord/maternal concentration ratios:

- fluoxetine 0.67 (norfluoxetine 0.72)
- sertraline 0.63 (desmethylsertraline 0.63)
- paroxetine 0.52
- venlafaxine 1.1 (*O*-desmethylvenlafaxine 1.0).

**Table 8.1 Pregnancy pharmacokinetics**

| Pregnancy-induced change | Outcome |
| --- | --- |
| Increased absorption<br>Reduced absorption | Delayed gastric emptying<br>Longer intestinal transit times<br>Reduced blood flow to legs in late pregnancy may reduce absorption of intramuscular drugs |
| Increased volume of distribution of psychotropics<br>Serum lipids may compete for protein binding sites and alter unbound drug concentrations | Increased plasma volume<br>Increased extracellular fluid<br>Increased body fat |
| Metabolism tissue delivery increased | Up to 50% increase in cardiac output, but less of output goes to liver as it is diverted to uterus<br>Increased activity of CP450 and CYP3A4, but CYP1A2 activity is decreased |
| Excretion can be increased | Increased renal blood flow<br>Increased glomerular filtration rate |
| Side-effects might be worsened | Increased constipation<br>Lowered blood pressure exacerbating orthostatic hypotension |

*Adapted with permission from Jeffries & Bochner (1988).*

The same group later reported median cord/maternal distribution ratios:

- 0.7–0.86 (range) for SSRIs
- 0.72 for venlafaxine
- 1.08 for the O-desmethyl metabolite (Rampono *et al*, 2009).

Heikkinen *et al* (2002) found infant plasma levels of citalopram, desmethylcitalopram and didesmethylcitalopram that were 64%, 66% and 68% of maternal plasma concentrations, respectively. Briggs *et al* (2009) report a case study of a pregnant woman taking duloxetine 60 mg daily. The duloxetine concentration in cord blood at delivery (14 h after a 60 mg extended release dose) was greater than the mother's peak plasma concentration taken 6 h post dose 32 days after delivery. However, a more recent case study of a woman taking duloxetine 60 mg during pregnancy reported a cord/maternal distribution ratio of 0.12 (Boyce *et al*, 2011).

## Amniotic fluid

Amniotic fluid reaches the fetus via several routes: inhalation into the respiratory tract, swallowing and, possibly, transcutaneous absorption. The amount of amniotic fluid swallowed by the fetus increases as pregnancy progresses. Hostetter *et al* (2000a) found fluvoxamine and venlafaxine in amniotic fluid, but sertraline was below the level of detection of the assay.

Metabolites of all three compounds were present. Loughhead *et al* (2006a) examined amniotic fluid in 27 women who were being treated with SSRIs and venlafaxine and undergoing amniocentesis for obstetric reasons. They found antidepressant concentrations were very variable, with the mean concentrations in amniotic fluid 11.6% of those in maternal serum. The highest ratios were for venlafaxine (172%); however, the ratio of amniotic fluid to maternal serum of metabolites was not consistent.

## Risks to the fetus

In addition to routes of exposure, the clinician must consider the different types of risk to the fetus, which include:

- intrauterine death
- teratogenesis and organ malformation
- growth impairment
- neonatal toxicity or withdrawal syndromes after delivery
- long-term neurobehavioural sequelae.

### Intrauterine death

Exposure to a teratogen before 2 weeks of gestation is likely to result in a non-viable 'blighted ovum'. Drugs taken later in pregnancy may cause miscarriage or stillbirth.

### Teratogenesis and organ malformation

A drug is considered to be teratogenic if exposure during pregnancy raises the risk of congenital physical malformations over the baseline level of birth defects, which is 2–4%. The period of maximum vulnerability is 3–12 weeks. The heart and great vessels are formed 5–10 weeks after the last menstrual period (LMP), and the lip and palate between 8 and 24 weeks. The neural tube folds and closes around 5–6 weeks after the LMP. As around half of all conceptions in the UK are unplanned, and most women do not learn of their pregnancy until around 6 weeks of gestation, exposure has often already happened when pregnancy is discovered.

### Withdrawal syndromes and toxicity

Some drugs, having readily crossed the placenta, produce toxicity in the neonate, as their immature metabolism may be unable to process the drug, leading to accumulation. Or, there may be withdrawal symptoms in the infant following delivery as levels of the drug fall rapidly after birth.

## Women's perceptions of drugs

Women taking antidepressants often discontinue them on learning they are pregnant, fearing risk to the fetus. In one study, 87% of women taking antidepressants rated their risk of teratogenicity as greater than 3% (Bonari *et al*,

2004). Fifteen per cent chose to stop taking them despite receiving reassuring information via counselling, saying that the first person they spoke to had advised discontinuation. The women sought information from multiple sources, and there was often some time lapse between diagnosis and starting treatment that was not observed in the control groups on gastrointestinal or antibiotic drugs.

The manner in which the media report issues relating to drug exposure during pregnancy can give rise to great anxiety and lead to discontinuation of medication even when that has not been the core media message (Einarson *et al*, 2005). It is clear that perception of risk, insight into illness and decision-making are complex issues (Misri *et al*, 2013). Wisner *et al* (2000) describe a model which provides a structure for the decision-making process, and give case examples in relation to depression. Walfisch *et al* (2011) reported that maternal teratogenic risk perception and likelihood of terminating the pregnancy were reduced after counselling.

The presence of other potential teratogens that might act in an additive or synergistic way must also be taken into account. These include non-prescribed drugs, herbal and homeopathic remedies, smoking, alcohol and environmental toxins. A study examining the use of complementary therapies by pregnant women found that 87% reported using mega-vitamins, herbs, massage, aromatherapy and yoga, and that they viewed these therapies as safe and effective (Gaffney & Smith, 2004). However, this should not be assumed.

# Drugs

## *Tricyclic antidepressants*

### First-trimester exposure

Early reports suggested an association between TCAs and limb reduction deformities. However, a systematic review of first-trimester exposure studies up to 1995 involving 414 cases failed to indicate an association between exposure to TCAs and increased rates of congenital malformations, concluding that they are relatively safe (Altshuler *et al*, 1996).

McElhatton *et al* (1996) examined outcomes in 689 women, 330 of whom had taken TCAs during pregnancy. The incidence of congenital malformations, spontaneous abortions and late fetal deaths was within the expected range for the general population. Long-term therapy (usually in association with other drugs) was associated with neonatal withdrawal symptoms. There was no increase in the rate of congenital malformations in the prospective study carried out by Ericson *et al* (1999) in which 390 women were taking TCAs (the majority clomipramine). Simon *et al* (2002) also found no association between TCA exposure and congenital malformations or adverse perinatal outcomes in 209 infants.

Subsequently, a Swedish study (Källén & Otterblad Olausson, 2006) examined the rate of congenital cardiac defects in the infants of 6896 women who had taken antidepressants during pregnancy. Nineteen per cent had taken TCAs. They found an increased risk of ventricular or atrial septal defects with clomipramine (odds ratio (OR) = 2.11). The same group (Reis & Källén, 2010) also reported a higher risk of preterm birth, low birth weight (LBW) and neonatal pathology for women taking TCAs compared with antidepressants.

### Obstetric and neonatal outcomes

Källén (2004) found that maternal antidepressant use during pregnancy was associated with an increased risk of preterm birth (OR = 1.96), LBW (OR = 1.98), respiratory distress (OR = 2.21), low Apgar score (OR = 2.33), neonatal convulsions (OR = 1.90) and hypoglycaemia (OR = 1.62). The risk of hypoglycaemia was particularly associated with TCA exposure. Davis *et al* (2007) reported an increase in preterm delivery risk, respiratory distress, endocrine and metabolic disorders and temperature regulation problems.

One study found a higher rate of miscarriage in those taking TCAs when compared with controls (Pastuzak *et al*, 1993), and a meta-analysis of cohort studies from 1966 to 2003 found a miscarriage rate of 12.4% in women taking antidepressants (all classes), a relative risk of 1.45. However, depression itself might have contributed to this increase (Hemels *et al*, 2005). A more recent population study reported an increased risk of miscarriage in women with depression and anxiety, with a further increase if they were taking psychotropic medication (Ban *et al*, 2012). There was weak evidence of an increased risk if taking TCAs. There does not seem to be an increased risk of bleeding in early or mid pregnancy (Lupattelli *et al*, 2014). Others have reported a higher risk of pre-eclampsia with TCAs, compared with SSRIs and SNRIs (Palmsten *et al*, 2013).

Dose requirements increase during the second half of pregnancy to between 1.3 and 2 times the non-pregnant dose (Wisner *et al*, 1993). This increased clearance rapidly returns to normal levels by the end of the second postpartum week. Serum levels of nortriptyline have been shown to rise in the early postpartum weeks, despite stable dosing. This is due to an apparent refractoriness in its processing, which continues until 6–8 weeks after delivery (Wisner *et al*, 1997). In one case, this was attributed to differences in the woman's smoking patterns during pregnancy and after delivery compared with before she was pregnant, and to her being a genetic poor metaboliser (Osborne *et al*, 2014).

Cholestasis has been reported in association with dothiepin (Milkiewicz *et al*, 2003).

Symptoms of poor neonatal adaptation have been observed when TCAs have been used in the third trimester, and a gradual taper and discontinuation before delivery is often suggested. However, women who require TCAs in late pregnancy are likely to be those most at risk of recurrence or worsening of symptoms postpartum, so discontinuation may not be the most appropriate strategy (Altshuler *et al*, 1996). Each individual case requires careful assessment before deciding on tapering. There are also case reports of symptoms (respiratory distress, hypotonia and jitteriness) correlating with serum drug levels, suggesting toxicity (e.g. Schimmel *et al*, 1991).

### Long-term neurodevelopmental outcomes

Follow-up studies of exposed infants at 5 to 86 months of age revealed no effect of TCAs on global IQ, language development or behaviour (Nulman *et al*, 1997, 2002).

## *Selective serotonin reuptake inhibitors*

### Pharmacokinetics

A study tracking fluoxetine and norfluoxetine during pregnancy and after delivery observed low trough samples during pregnancy on doses of 20–40 mg daily and mean norfluoxetine/fluoxetine ratios in late pregnancy 2.4 times higher than at 2 months after delivery. This may be partly due to increased demethylation by CYP2D6 and may mean that the dose has to be increased to achieve therapeutic benefit (Heikkinen *et al*, 2003). Sit *et al* (2008) reported similar findings for citalopram, escitalopram and sertraline. Hostetter *et al* (2000*b*) followed 34 women taking SSRIs throughout pregnancy. Two-thirds required dose increases to maintain euthymia, and the increases tended to occur in the early part of the third trimester. Doses at delivery were around 1.86 times higher than the initial dose. Kim *et al* (2006) observed a high correlation between maternal and fetal (cord blood) fluoxetine and norfluoxetine concentrations at birth, with ratios of 0.91 and 1.04, respectively.

### Miscarriage

A review of 15 studies, most of which were cohort studies published between 1975 and 2009, concluded that only paroxetine and venlafaxine were associated with an increased risk of miscarriage (Broy & Bérard, 2010). Subsequent studies have reported increased risks but could not be certain that the increase was not due to depression itself or to other lifestyle factors not controlled for (e.g. Klieger-Grossman *et al*, 2012; Siegismund Kjaersgaard *et al*, 2013; Andersen, *et al*, 2014). Not all studies control for a past history of miscarriage, which is a risk factor for any subsequent pregnancy. A systematic review of 25 studies published between 1990 and 2012 reported an increased risk (OR = 1.87, 95% CI 1.5–2.33) (Nikfar *et al*, 2012).

### First-trimester exposure

In 2000, a meta-analysis of first-trimester exposure to fluoxetine (Addis & Koren, 2000), covering studies published between 1988 and 1996 and involving 367 women, concluded that there was no evidence that fluoxetine caused an increase in the rate of congenital malformations.

Alwan *et al* (2005) reported an increased rate of craniosynostosis (OR = 1.8) and omphalocele (OR = 3.0) in infants exposed to SSRIs, but a meta-analysis by Einarson & Einarson (2005) again concluded that SSRIs do not increase the rate of congenital malformations. This was also confirmed by a Finnish population study, which concluded that, other than an increased risk of admission to a neonatal unit with third-trimester exposure (OR = 1.6), SSRIs did not increase the risk of malformations, preterm birth, small for gestational age (SGA) or LBW babies (Malm *et al*, 2005). Three studies have reported an increased risk of club foot. The first reported a twofold increase with first-trimester use, highest with paroxetine (Louik *et al*, 2007); the second reported a 50% increase, also highest with paroxetine (Colvin *et al*, 2011). More recently, Yazdy *et al* (2014) reported that after adjustment for maternal smoking and body mass index, the OR for any SSRI use and clubfoot was 1.8 (95% CI 1.1–2.8). When individual SSRIs were examined, ORs were elevated for sertraline (1.6, 95% CI 0.8–3.2), paroxetine (9.2, 95% CI 0.7–484.6), and escitalopram (2.9, 95% CI 1.1–7.2).

Källén & Otterblad Olaussen (2006) found an increased risk of cardiac malformations with paroxetine (OR = 2.22), as did Diav-Citrin *et al* (2005*a*). Alwan *et al* (2005) found that paroxetine accounted for 36% of the SSRI exposures in omphalocele cases (OR = 6.30). Hence, the manufacturer revised the pregnancy subsection of the product information in October 2005 to advise prescribing paroxetine to a pregnant woman only 'if the potential benefit outweighs the potential risk'. Louik *et al* (2007) observed an association between sertraline exposure and omphalocele (OR = 5.7), between sertraline and septal defects (OR = 2.0), and between paroxetine and right ventricular outflow tract obstruction (OR = 3.3).

Five further meta-analyses have now been conducted. The first (Rahimi *et al*, 2006) included studies conducted between 1990 and 2005 and concluded that there was no increase in congenital malformations but that the risk of spontaneous abortion was significantly increased. Bar-Oz *et al* (2007) included studies published between 1985 and 2006, concluding that paroxetine was associated with a significant increase in cardiac congenital malformations (OR = 4.11), but they could not rule out a detection bias. Studies published up to June 2010 were included in a review by Grigoriadis *et al* (2013*a*). They reported no evidence that antidepressants overall were associated with congenital malformations or major congenital malformations, but that there was an increased risk of cardiac malformations. Two drugs were analysed separately (fluoxetine and paroxetine) and were associated with major congenital malformations (fluoxetine) and cardiac malformations (paroxetine). It should be noted that the relative risk (RR) was below 1.5 in all the sub-analyses. Nikfar *et al* (2012) included 25 studies published between 1990 and 2012 and concluded that there was an increased risk of major congenital malformations (OR = 1.272, 95% CI 1.098–1.474) but no increase in the risk of minor congenital malformations or cardiac congenital malformations. Myles and colleagues (2013), who included 26 studies from 1985 to 2011, reported an increased risk of congenital malformations with fluoxetine (OR = 1.14, 95% CI 1.01–1.30) and paroxetine (OR = 1.29, 95% CI 1.11–1.49). Paroxetine was associated with increased risk of cardiac malformations (OR = 1.44, 95% CI 1.12–1.86). Sertraline and citalopram were not significantly associated with congenital malformations.

Subsequently, Huybrechts *et al* (2014a) observed a reduction in risks for cardiac defects with pregnancy use of SSRIs when confounders were adjusted for, and found no association between paroxetine and right ventricular outflow defects or between sertraline and ventricular septal defects. Ban *et al* (2014a) reported no increase in major congenital malformations with exposure to maternal depression or antidepressants, but an increased risk of cardiac congenital malformations with paroxetine (adjusted OR (aOR) = 1.78, 95% CI 1.09–2.88). A large study involving 2.3 million live births and 2288 sibling pairs found no substantial increase in the prevalence of overall cardiac birth defects among infants exposed to SSRIs or venlafaxine *in utero*. Although the prevalence of septal defects and right ventricular outflow tract defects was higher in exposed infants, the lack of an association in the sibling-controlled analyses argues against a teratogenic effect of these drugs (Faru *et al*, 2015).

Some of the conflicting evidence in studies might relate to the apparent dose–response relationship between paroxetine and congenital malformations, with OR = 2.23 for a major malformation and OR = 3.07 for a cardiac malformation if the dose was above 25 mg/day during the first trimester (Bérard *et al*, 2007). ORs also appear to be higher for polytherapy involving paroxetine compared with paroxetine monotherapy (Cole *et al*, 2007a). The methodological issues involved in studies of SSRIs and pregnancy have been reviewed by Grzeskowiak *et al* (2011).

The duration of exposure to antidepressants does not appear to be associated with an increased risk of major congenital malformations (Ramos *et al*, 2008).

## Obstetric and neonatal complications

Cholestasis has been reported in association with both citalopram and paroxetine (Milkiewicz *et al*, 2003). One study found an association between SSRI exposure in late pregnancy and gestational hypertension, but it is not known whether this relationship is causal (Toh *et al*, 2009). A systematic review with only two studies included found no increased risk of weight gain in pregnancy, weight retention postpartum or gestational diabetes (Lopez-Yarto *et al*, 2012). De Vera & Bérard (2012) reported a case–control study in which 45 women (3.7%) had used antidepressants during pregnancy, compared with 300 (2.5%) in the control group. After adjusting for potential confounders, use of antidepressants during pregnancy was significantly associated with increased risk of pregnancy-induced hypertension (OR = 1.53, 95% CI 1.01–2.33). In stratified analyses, use of SSRIs (OR = 1.60, 95% CI 1.00–2.55) – and, more specifically, paroxetine (OR = 1.81, 95% CI 1.02–3.23) – was associated with risk of pregnancy-induced hypertension.

There is a case report of an infant with necrotizing enterocolitis associated with exposure to escitalopram during pregnancy and breastfeeding (Potts et al, 2007). Bodnar et al (2006) describe a case in which poor maternal weight gain was associated with sertraline treatment commencing at 22 weeks gestation and outline the methods used to counteract this. There does not appear to be an increased risk of postpartum haemorrhage (Salkeld et al, 2008; Lupattelli et al, 2014), and Nordeng et al (2012) failed to demonstrate an increased risk of preterm delivery or LBW with adjustment for confounding variables. Jensen et al (2013a) found only a weak association between SSRIs and newer antidepressants and infants born SGA.

Persistent pulmonary hypertension of the newborn is a rare (1.9 per 1000 live births) but serious condition, which has a mortality rate of 10–20%. A meta-analysis carried out by Grigoriadis et al (2013b) reported an increased risk from SSRI exposure in late but not early pregnancy; however, the absolute risk is very low (2.9–3.5 per 1000 infants).

Cohen et al (2000) found no difference in gestational age, Apgar scores, or the timing of hospital to home discharge in infants born to mothers with late rather than early exposure to fluoxetine. Paroxetine use during the third trimester was associated with neonatal distress in a prospective controlled study (Costei et al, 2002). Suri et al (2004) found no adverse obstetric outcomes in 64 women with depression taking fluoxetine. Hendrick et al (2003b) also found no increase in neonatal complications but noted that the three women treated with high doses of fluoxetine (40–80 mg per day) had LBW infants. Zeskind & Stephens (2004) reported more activity and tremulousness, fewer changes in behavioural state and more rapid eye movement sleep in SSRI-exposed infants. Lattimore et al (2005) pooled the above-mentioned studies in a meta-analysis and observed the following ORs:

- prematurity                           1.85
- LBW                                   3.64
- neonatal unit admission               3.30
- poor neonatal adaptation              4.08

A large register study from Denmark reported an association between SSRI use in pregnancy and low Apgar scores, which was independent of maternal depression (Jensen et al, 2013b). Animal studies have shown transient decreases in uterine artery blood flow, fetal $PO_2$, oxygen saturation and fetal pH, plus fetal $PCO_2$ increases with fluoxetine (Morrison et al, 2002). If repeated, this might provide one mechanism for poor outcomes.

Wen et al (2006) carried out a large population cohort study and reported LBW, preterm birth, fetal death, infant death, seizures and use of mechanical ventilation in infants exposed to paroxetine during pregnancy. There are case reports of neonatal subdural, intraventricular and subarachnoid haemorrhage associated with maternal SSRI use. SSRI inhibition of platelet serotonin leading to decreased platelet aggregation is thought to be responsible, although it is not clear that SSRIs increase the rate of intracranial haemorrhage above the expected rate. One meta-analysis of 41 studies of antidepressant use (mostly SSRIs) in pregnancy and preterm birth concluded that there was an increased risk with second- and third-trimester use, which was not eliminated when controlling for maternal depression (Huybrechts *et al*, 2014*b*). Another meta-analysis (Huang *et al*, 2014) reported increased risk of preterm birth and LBW.

Case reports, case series and cohort studies over several years have reported a poor neonatal adaptation syndrome (PNAS) associated with SSRI exposure in late pregnancy. The most common symptoms (in decreasing order of frequency) are: irritability, hypertonia, jitteriness, difficulty feeding, tremor, agitation, seizures, tachypnoea and posturing. More rarely, seizures and electroencephalogram (EEG) abnormalities have been reported. Hayes *et al* (2012) report an increased risk of infant convulsions with third-trimester SSRI use (OR = 1.4, 95% CI 0.7–2.8; OR = 2.8, 95% CI 1.9–5.5; and OR = 4.9 95% CI 2.6–9.5 for one, two and three prescriptions dispensed, respectively). Källén & Reis (2012) reported an OR of 1.82 (CI 1.6–22.05) for any neonatal symptoms after maternal use of SSRIs only, but it was significantly higher (OR = 2.46, 95% CI, 2.06-2.93) when use of SSRIs was combined with one or more other central nervous system (CNS)-active drugs. Use of any of these CNS-active drugs during the second or third trimester was associated with a significantly increased risk for the following: respiratory diagnoses (OR, 1.51, 95% CI 1.41–1.63); hypoglycaemia (OR = 1.49, CI 1.36–1.63) and low Apgar score (OR = 1.33, 95% CI 1.17–1.53).

The syndrome is usually mild and self-limiting, onsets within hours or days of birth, and resolves within 2 weeks. A meta-analysis of studies published up to mid-June 2010 (Grigoriadis *et al*, 2013*c*) reported that exposure to antidepressants in pregnancy was associated with an increased risk of PNAS (OR = 5.07, 95% CI 3.25–7.90), respiratory distress (OR = 2.20, CI 1.81–2.66) and tremors (OR = 7.89, 95% CI 3.33–18.73). Forsberg *et al* (2014) observed severe PNAS in only 3% of infants exposed to antidepressants.

Management is usually supportive care, sometimes in the NICU. More severe cases might need respiratory support, ventilation, fluid replacement or anticonvulsant therapy. Chlorpromazine has been used in three cases of withdrawal from paroxetine and one from fluoxetine (Nordeng *et al*, 2001).

In order to prevent PNAS, it has been suggested that SSRIs should be tapered off (or stopped in the case of fluoxetine) around 2 weeks before the expected date of delivery and resumed afterwards. However, stopping SSRI exposure before the end of pregnancy does not appear to reduce the likelihood of the syndrome occurring. Warburton *et al* (2010) found no difference in the incidence of PNAS in infants born to women who took SSRIs in the last 14 days of pregnancy and those who stopped them before the last 14 days, when maternal illness severity was controlled for. In addition, the timing of delivery is hard to predict and there is the risk of precipitating an antenatal recurrence and/or increasing the risk of a postpartum depressive episode. Sanz *et al* (2005) advise not prescribing paroxetine to pregnant women, or, if this is not possible, using the lowest effective dose. Infants delivered to a woman taking an SSRI must be monitored for adverse events, and any such events must be reported to the Medicines and Healthcare Products Regulatory Agency (see 'Resources' below).

## Long-term neurodevelopmental outcomes

Nulman *et al* (1997, 2002) reported no effect of *in utero* exposure to fluoxetine on global IQ, language development or behaviour. However, lower Apgar scores and lower scores on Bayley psychomotor development indices and the motor quality factor of the Bayley Behavioural Rating Scale than those in non-exposed children have been found in infants exposed to SSRIs (Casper *et al*, 2003). A later study of children exposed to SSRIs, venlafaxine and untreated maternal depression *in utero* found the untreated depression to be a significant risk factor for lower IQ and behavioural problems in children aged between 3 years and 6 years 11 months rather than antidepressant exposure (Nulman *et al*, 2012).

An attenuated response to heel prick pain has also been shown in infants with prenatal SSRI exposure compared with unexposed infants (Oberlander *et al*, 2005). Mulder *et al* (2011) observed increased fetal motor activity in the second trimester and lack of inhibitory control of motor output at times when the fetus was at rest or in non-REM sleep at the end of the third trimester. These effects were dose-related but independent of SSRI drug type. The significance of these findings for later development is not known.

Others have reported alterations in the developing hypothalamic–pituitary–adrenal axis in SSRI-exposed neonates, via changes in corticosteroid-binding globulin levels and infant salivary cortisol levels, even when controlling for maternal depression (Pawluski *et al*, 2012).

More recently, several papers have reported an association between maternal antidepressant (mostly SSRI) use in pregnancy and autism spectrum disorder (ASD) in exposed children. Three of these studies were included in a meta-analysis (Rais & Rais 2014). They found a weak positive association between antidepressant use in pregnancy and ASD (OR = 1.39, 95% CI 1.04–1.85). Two population-based case–control studies published subsequently also reported an increased risk of ASD with *in utero* SSRI exposure (Gidaya *et al*, 2014) and ASD symptoms (Marroun *et al*, 2014), although others have found no association (Hviid *et al*, 2013; Sørensen *et al*, 2013; Clements *et al*, 2015). The last of these did find an association between antidepressant exposure *in utero* and attention-deficit hyperactivity disorder (ADHD). It should be noted that even if there is a causal link with ASD, the absolute risk is likely to be modest at most, and there are several other risk factors, including maternal age, metabolic conditions and low intake of supplemental iron (Schmidt *et al*, 2014).

## Conclusions

There appears to be a small increased risk of congenital malformation with first-trimester exposure to SSRIs, particularly cardiac malformations with paroxetine exposure. There is also evidence of an association between pregnancy exposure to paroxetine and PNAS and, possibly, a small reduction in gestational age. Hence, paroxetine is best avoided if possible, although if a woman becomes pregnant while taking it, a full risk–benefit analysis must be undertaken before switching or stopping medication, particularly if it is the only drug she responds to.

# *Other antidepressants*

## Venlafaxine

Plasma concentrations of venlafaxine reduce from the first to the third trimester, but concentrations of its metabolite *O*-desmethylvenlafaxine do not appear to change (ter Horst *et al*, 2014). Similarly, Klier *et al* (2007) reported reduced bioavailability of venlafaxine across the three trimesters of pregnancy. Hence, the dose may need to be increased to maintain efficacy but reduced again postpartum.

Some studies have reported that venlafaxine does not appear to increase the rate of congenital malformations above the base rate (Einarson *et al*, 2001; Yaris *et al*, 2004; Einarson & Einarson 2005). However, Polen *et al* (2013) found statistically significant associations for anencephaly, atrial septal defect (secundum type or not otherwise specified), coarctation of the aorta, cleft palate, and gastroschisis with periconceptional use of venlafaxine. Sample sizes were very small and confidence intervals were wide. Another case–control study (Lind *et al*, 2013) reported an association with hypospadias (aOR = 2.4, 95% CI 1.0–6.0).

Einarson *et al* (2001) found a non-significant trend towards a higher rate of miscarriage in exposed pregnancies, and an association has also been reported by Broy & Bérard (2010). Ramos *et al* (2010) reported that doses of venlafaxine below 150 mg/day were associated with SGA babies, unlike higher doses or SSRIs. It is possible that better control of the underlying condition with a higher dose is responsible for this finding.

There are reports of a PNAS including restlessness, jitteriness, irritability, tremor, convulsions, hypotonia, hyperreflexia, diarrhoea, hypoglycaemia and poor feeding (e.g. Pakalapati *et al*, 2006). In one case, improvement was achieved by giving the infant 1 mg of venlafaxine. The symptoms had ceased by the 8th day postpartum (de Moor *et al*, 2003). Yaris *et al* (2004) followed up the infants of 10 women who had taken venlafaxine for 12 months until they were 1 year of age and observed no developmental delay. There is also a case report of preterm twins whose mother had taken venlafaxine throughout pregnancy developing necrotising enterocolitis (Treichel *et al*, 2009) and one report of neonatal seizures (Haukland *et al*, 2013).

## Mirtazapine

Mirtazapine is a benzazepine tetracyclic antidepressant. To date, there are only around 300 pregnancy outcomes reported with this drug. An early case study reported a woman who used it only in the first month of pregnancy, with a successful outcome (Simhandl *et al*, 1998). Two cases reported by Kesim & Yaris (2002) resulted in one uneventful delivery of a healthy infant, but the second infant was delivered at 39 weeks by Caesarean section for premature rupture of membranes and experienced neonatal hyperbilirubinaemia but did not require phototherapy. Yaris *et al* (2004) reported on eight women who took mirtazapine during pregnancy. There were no adverse outcomes in seven, but one (who also took alprazolam, diazepam and nefazodone) miscarried.

Forty-one women out of 13 554 in a prescription event monitoring study of mirtazapine became pregnant. Eight experienced miscarriages, 8 had the pregnancy terminated, and there were 24 live births of which 4 were preterm. One of these infants had a patent ductus arteriosus. The outcome of another pregnancy was not known, as the researchers lost contact with this woman (Biswas *et al*, 2003). Four papers report the use of mirtazapine in the treatment of hyperemesis gravidarum in a total of 12 women, one with a twin pregnancy and one who delivered preterm but also had type I diabetes and pre-eclampsia and whose infant had PNAS (Rohde *et al*, 2001; Saks, 2001; Guclu *et al*, 2005; Schwarzer *et al*, 2008). Djulus *et al* (2006) carried out a prospective study with two comparison groups: disease-matched pregnant women diagnosed with depression taking other antidepressants, and pregnant women not exposed to teratogens. There were 77 live births, one stillbirth, 20 miscarriages, 6 therapeutic abortions, and 2 major malformations in the mirtazapine group. The mean ± s.d. birth weight was 3335 g ± 654 and the mean ± s.d. gestational age at delivery was 38.9 weeks ± 2.5 weeks. Most (95%) of the women took mirtazapine in the first trimester, but only 25% of the women took it throughout pregnancy. The rate of miscarriage was higher in both antidepressant groups (19% in the mirtazapine group and 17% in the other antidepressant group) than in the no-teratogen group (11%), but none of the differences were statistically significant. The rate of preterm births was also higher in the mirtazapine group (10%) and in the other antidepressant group (7%) than in the no-teratogen group (2%). The difference was statistically significant between the mirtazapine group and the no-teratogen group ($P = 0.04$). There is also a report of monozygotic twins whose mother was treated with mirtazapine throughout pregnancy and who presented with recurrent hypothermia not attributable to other causes (Sokolover *et al*, 2008). Einarson *et al* (2009) did not find an increased rate of congenital malformations in a prospective cohort study (68 of 928 women took mirtazapine), but 2 infants had congenital malformations (tracheomalacia and vesicourethral reflux). A larger prospective cohort study of over 80 000 pregnancies including 144 exposed to mirtazapine reported the following congenital malformations in the mirtazapine-exposed infants: ventricular septal defect (2 cases), atrial septal defect (1 case), cleft palate (1 case) and hypospadias (1 case). Overall, there was no increase in the rate of congenital malformations. There was an increased rate of preterm delivery, but no separate analysis was performed for mirtazapine exposure (Lennestal & Källen, 2007).

Uguz (2013) described three cases in which low-dose mirtazapine had been added to SSRIs in the second trimester in women suffering from depression and panic disorder. One infant experienced mild tachypnoea for 2 days, but there were no other adverse events. The same author (Uguz, 2014) reported two women suffering from depression and severe nausea, who were treated solely with low doses of mirtazapine from 15 to 28 weeks and from 34 weeks to delivery, with no adverse events.

In a multicentre, observational prospective cohort study by members of the European Network of Teratology Information Services between 1995 and 2011, no statistically significant difference was found between the rates of major birth defects in mirtazapine-exposed and SSRI-exposed pregnancies, although there was a marginally higher rate of birth defects in the mirtazapine and SSRI groups compared with non-exposed controls (357 pregnancies in each group). Overall pregnancy outcome after mirtazapine exposure was similar to that after SSRI exposure (Winterfeld et al, 2015).

## Nefazodone

The limited data available – Einarson et al, 2003 (89 cases); Yaris et al, 2004 (2 cases); Yaris et al, 2005 (2 cases) – have shown no increase in the rates of malformations or complications with nefazodone. This drug has been discontinued in the UK but may still be available elsewhere.

## Bupropion

A controlled study following up 136 women taking bupropion for depression or smoking cessation found no increase in congenital malformations and a miscarriage rate similar to that of other antidepressants (Chan et al, 2005).

A large prospective cohort study compared outcomes of 928 women who had taken an antidepressant during pregnancy with 1243 who had not, and reported no congenital malformations among the bupropion-exposed cohort (n = 113) (Einarson et al, 2009). A retrospective study analysed the prevalence of cardiac and other congenital malformations following first-trimester bupropion exposure (n = 1213) in comparison with bupropion exposure outside the first trimester (n = 1049) and exposure to other antidepressants in the first trimester (n = 4743). No statistically significant difference in rates of congenital malformations was observed between the groups (Cole et al, 2007b).

A retrospective case–control study comparing 6853 infants with major heart defects and 5869 controls (with no major congenital malformations) found that bupropion exposure at any time between 1 month before conception and 3 months after conception was associated with an increased incidence of left outflow tract heart defects (aOR = 2.6, 95% CI 1.2–5.7; $P = 0.01$). Bupropion exposure was observed in 34 (0.5%) of the cases and in 26 (0.4%) of the controls. Recall bias and a limited sample size are possible confounders in this study (Alwan *et al*, 2010). A recent retrospective study reported a slightly elevated aOR (1.6, 95% CI 1.0–2.8) for ventricular septal defects with first-trimester bupropion use, but no increased odds for other defects (Louik *et al*, 2014).

A case report describes the development of fetal cardiac arrhythmia 2 weeks after a woman was treated for depression with bupropion 100 mg daily, initiated at 30 weeks of pregnancy. Bupropion was immediately discontinued and no further problems were reported during pregnancy or at delivery (Leventhal *et al*, 2010). One preliminary report has suggested that *in utero* exposure to bupropion during pregnancy ($P = 0.02$), particularly in the second trimester ($P < 0.001$), was associated with an increased risk of ADHD in the offspring (Figueroa, 2010).

The manufacturer prospectively collected data from 1997 to 2008 involving 1597 pregnancies in which exposure to bupropion had occurred. Outcome data were available for 994 pregnancies. Of 806 first-trimester exposures, there were 651 live-born infants with no congenital malformations, 96 miscarriages, 39 elective terminations, 4 fetal deaths, and 18 live-born infants with congenital malformations. The incidence of congenital malformations following first-trimester exposure in all bupropion-exposed pregnancies was 24/675 (3.6%, 95% CI 2.3–5.3), no greater than the background rate (GlaxoSmithKline, 2008). Retrospective data comprising 28 pregnancies in which congenital malformations were reported were also analysed. There were 25 first-trimester exposures, a second-trimester exposure and 2 third-trimester exposures, with 12 of the exposures reporting cardiac defects.

The UK Teratology Information Service (UKTIS, 2015) has reviewed several large population-based cohort studies and case–control studies and was unable to confirm a suggested association between bupropion exposure during pregnancy and congenital malformations.

## Trazodone

In the 180 cases of trazodone exposure reported by McElhatton *et al* (1996), Rosa (1994), and Einarson *et al* (2003, 2009), there was no increase in the rate of congenital malformations.

UKTIS (2014) state that there is currently no evidence of an association between trazadone exposure and increased risk of congenital malformations, although the number of case reports they have received is too small to assess the likelihood of adverse outcomes following trazadone use in pregnancy.

## Monoamine oxidase inhibitors

There are animal studies reporting an association between monoamine oxidase inhibitors (MAOIs) and fetal growth retardation (Poulson & Robson, 1964), and results from a small case series of women treated with phenelzine and tranylcypromine during pregnancy found a higher rate of abnormalities than would be expected (Heinonen, *et al*, 1977). In addition, a specific diet must be adhered to, and the possibility of hypertensive crisis during pregnancy or labour indicates that MAOIs should be avoided if at all possible, particularly if an operative delivery is likely, as they interact with several anaesthetic agents. Gracious & Wisner (1997) reported the successful treatment of a depressed woman with phenelzine throughout pregnancy and delivery.

## Moclobemide

There is one case report of uneventful pregnancy and delivery of a healthy infant in a woman exposed to moclobemide during pregnancy (Rybakowski, 2001), and seven exposures in the series reported by Yaris *et al* (2005). One of these women took moclobemide in conjunction with amitriptyline and had a preterm delivery.

## Reboxetine

Hackett *et al* (2006*a*) reported outcomes for four women who took reboxetine during pregnancy. One infant out of the four had developmental problems unrelated to reboxetine; the others met normal developmental milestones, and there were no adverse events.

## Duloxetine

UKTIS has followed up 38 cases of duloxetine exposure during pregnancy. There were 34 prospective therapeutic exposures, one overdose and three retrospective cases. Some of these cases were included in the publication by Einarson *et al* (2012). No increased risk of congenital malformations or other adverse events was found, but the numbers were too small to make any firm conclusions. In an analysis of exposures reported to the manufacturer of 400 cases in which the outcome was known, the frequency of adverse events (e.g. miscarriage and preterm delivery) was not higher than that in the general population (Hoog *et al*, 2013).

## St John's wort (hypericum)

A prospective controlled study of 54 women taking St John's wort during pregnancy observed no increase in the rate of congenital malformations over the background rate, and no increase in the rate of preterm birth (Moretti *et al*, 2009). It should be noted that when used concomitantly with other medications metabolised by CYP450, the serum levels of the medications might be reduced (Dougoua, 2006). Einarson *et al* (2000) note that although doctors are very reluctant to recommend hypericum to pregnant patients, 49% of naturopaths surveyed felt comfortable doing so. Pregnant women should therefore be asked routinely whether or not they are taking any herbal remedies.

### Agomelatine

There are currently no published data on the use of agomelatine in human pregnancy.

### Atomoxetine

Atomoxetine is a SNRI used to treat ADHD. There are currently no published data on the use of atomoxetine in human pregnancy.

## Anxiolytics and hypnotics

### Benzodiazepines

Dolovich et al (1998) carried out a meta-analysis of 23 studies examining major malformations (oral clefts in particular) in infants exposed to BDZs during the first trimester. Pooled data from cohort studies revealed no association between fetal exposure to BDZs and major malformations or oral clefts. However, pooled data from case–control studies indicated an increased risk of major malformations or oral cleft. Only pregnancies resulting in live or stillbirths were included in the review, and not those that were terminated – although pregnancies may have been terminated because of first-trimester exposure, in which case this review would underestimate the risk. However, Khan et al (1999) undertook a logistic regression which revealed that the case–control studies exaggerated the odds ratio for the risk of exposure by 55%, and concluded that there is no association.

Subsequently, a large population-based case–control study involving 22 865 cases and 38 151 controls found no excess of congenital malformations (Eros et al, 2002). An analysis of the French Central-East registry of congenital malformations data from 1976 to 1997 found no increased rate of malformations with use of BDZs in general, but when the data were analysed by individual drug, lorazepam was found to be associated with anal atresia (OR = 6.2) (Bonnot et al, 2003). These and other studies carried out between 2001 and 2011 were reviewed by Bellantuono et al (2013), who highlighted many methodological problems and concluded that there appears to be no increased risk of congenital malformations. A large UK population-based cohort study (Ban et al, 2014b) reached the same conclusion.

If a pregnant woman is exposed to BDZ, an ultrasound scan at 20 weeks should be performed to detect any oral or palatal clefts, or other anomalies.

BDZs are thought to be responsible for two major neonatal complications if prescribed in the last trimester of pregnancy. The first of these is neonatal withdrawal, in which hypertonia, hyperreflexia, feeding difficulties, restlessness, irritability, abnormal sleep patterns, poor suckling, bradycardia, apnoea and an increased incidence of low Apgar scores have been reported, particularly where BDZs have been given during labour. Källén & Reis

(2012) found the highest ORs for neonatal symptoms with BDZ compared with other CNS-active drugs.

The second complication is floppy infant syndrome. This includes tremors, hyperactivity, hypothermia, lethargy and feeding problems. Infants do not appear to have long-lasting sequelae of either syndrome and usually recover in a few weeks. A French study of BDZ use in the last month of pregnancy found that 51% of infants developed adverse reactions. Hypotonia was reported in 42% and neonatal withdrawal in 20%, with tremulousness the most common symptom (Swortfiguer et al, 2005).

Advice is therefore to keep to the lowest possible dose, for the shortest possible time. If possible, reduce the dose in late pregnancy and before delivery to reduce the risk of neonatal withdrawal and floppy infant syndrome.

Gopalan et al (2014) discuss the issues in managing BDZ withdrawal in pregnancy using two case examples and provide general guidelines. NICE (2014) advises using BDZs for short-term treatment of severe anxiety or agitation only.

### Benzodiazepine receptor agonists

There are now reports of over 1000 pregnancy exposures to zopiclone and over 2000 to zolpidem, and fewer in relation to zaleplon, with no increase in the rates of congenital malformation above the background rate (Diav-Citrin et al, 1999; Wikner, et al, 2007a; 2007b; Juric et al, 2009, Wikner & Källén, 2011; Ban et al, 2014b). Adverse obstetric and neonatal outcomes have been reported after zolpidem exposure, e.g. increased ORs for preterm delivery, LBW and SGA infants, and delivery by Caesarean section (Juric et al, 2009; Wang et al, 2010). There is a case report of a neural tube defect in an infant exposed to high doses (30–40mg) of zolpidem in the first trimester (Sharma et al, 2011).

The initial management of a pregnant woman with sleep problems should be advice regarding sleep hygiene, such as bedtime routine, avoiding caffeine and reducing activity before sleep. Only if this fails, or the problem is severe and chronic, should medication be considered. Promethazine is a phenothiazine, which is sedative and anxiolytic and has been used for over 50 years for hyperemesis. It has not been associated with any congenital malformations and could be an alternative hypnotic.

### Buspirone

There are no human data in the literature regarding the safety of buspirone in pregnancy.

## Antipsychotics

Typical antipsychotics have been in use for more than 40 years, and the use of atypicals in pregnant women is increasing (Toh et al, 2013; Epstein et al, 2013). In a population-based cohort study (Vigod et al, 2015), women prescribed an antipsychotic medication in pregnancy were not at a higher risk of gestational diabetes (rate ratio 1.10, 95% CI 0.77–1.57) hypertensive disorders of pregnancy (1.12, 95% CI 0.70–1.78), or venous thromboembolism (0.95, 95% CI 0.40–2.27) compared with non-users. The preterm birth rate, although high among antipsychotic users (14.5%) and matched non-users (14.3%), was not relatively different (0.99, 95% CI 0.78–1.26). Birth weight lower than the 3rd centile or higher than the 97th centile was not associated with antipsychotic drug use in pregnancy (rate ratios 1.21, 95% CI 0.81–1.82; and 1.26, 95% CI 0.69–2.29, respectively).

## Typical antipsychotics

There are relatively few data on the use of typical antipsychotics in pregnancy. Barnes *et al* (2011) systematically reviewed prospective cohort and population studies in which first-trimester drug use was examined and concluded that there was no evidence of any increased rate of congenital malformations with any particular drug, but noted that the maximum number of pregnancy exposures in any of the trials was 250 and many had fewer participants. Others have reported lower mean birth weight and a higher rate of SGA in infants exposed to typical antipsychotics, but, again, numbers in the study were small (Newham *et al*, 2008). Lin *et al* (2010) reported higher odds of preterm birth (OR = 2.46, 95% CI 1.50–4.11) in women with schizophrenia who took typical antipsychotics (*n* = 190) compared with those not receiving antipsychotics.

### Phenothiazines

There has been one meta-analysis of the effects of first-trimester low-potency phenothiazines on pregnancy outcomes (Altshuler *et al*, 1996) and a population-wide study in Sweden of a number of antipsychotics, the majority being phenothiazines (Reis & Källen, 2008). There were small increases in the rate of congenital malformations (ORs of 1.2 and 1.55, respectively), but these were of borderline significance (95% CI 1.01–1.45, 0.99–1.41). Gentile (2010) undertook a systematic review and concluded that the data were too few to draw any conclusions regarding teratogenicity.

Other problems reported include:

- cholestatic liver disease and ductopenia associated with pregnancy use of chlorpromazine (e.g. Moradpour *et al*, 1994; Chlumska *et al*, 2001)
- neonatal fever and cyanotic spells (Ben-Amitai & Merlob, 1991)
- extrapyramidal symptoms in exposed infants (e.g. Levy & Wisniewski, 1974).

One infant who was exposed to chlorpromazine and lithium was reported to have 'neurologic depression' for the first 9 days of life (Nielson *et al*, 1983). The use of depot medication may result in more persistent adverse events. One infant exposed to both chlorpromazine and fluphenazine decanoate experienced neurological symptoms for 9 months (O'Connor *et al*, 1981). However, others have reported successful pregnancy outcomes in a woman taking zuclopenthixol decanoate (Janjić et al, 2013), and in a woman taking fluphenazine decanoate (Dadić-Hero et al, 2011).

### Butyrophenones

Haloperidol is reported to have a placental passage ratio (defined as the ratio of umbilical cord to maternal plasma concentrations (ng/ml)) of 65.5% (Newport et al, 2007). Early case reports suggested an association between first trimester exposure to haloperidol and limb deformities. However, controlled studies of antipsychotics used for pregnancy emesis found no increase in abnormalities, and a multicentre prospective controlled study comparing the outcomes in 219 women exposed to haloperidol ($n = 188$) or penfluridol ($n = 27$) found no difference in the rate of congenital malformations between the exposed group and the controls (Diav-Citrin et al, 2005b). There was an increased rate of preterm birth and LBW in the exposed group. There were two cases of limb defects in the haloperidol/penfluridol group, and the authors could neither confirm nor rule out an association because of the sample size.

Other reported adverse events related to maternal haloperidol include severe hypothermia in an infant who was also exposed to benztropine (Mohan et al, 2000) and dyskinetic symptoms (Collins & Comer, 2003). There is a case report of thrombocytosis persisting for 3 months in the infant of a woman treated with haloperidol, biperiden, promethazine hydrochloride, nitrazepam and chlorpromazine (Nako et al, 2001).

A woman who took an overdose of 300 mg haloperidol at 34 weeks gestation (Hansen et al, 1997) became unresponsive and experienced an extrapyramidal reaction but recovered within 48 h. On admission, there was no fetal movement or breathing and the heart rate was non-reactive. The fetal biophysical profile returned to normal 5 days after admission. Pregnancy-induced hypertension and oligohydramnios were detected at 39 weeks, labour was induced and a healthy infant delivered.

One study followed up the children of mothers who took a variety of typical antipsychotics until the children were aged seven (Platt et al, 1988). Children aged seven who had been exposed for more than 2 months in utero were 3 cm taller than controls but shorter at four months of age.

### Diphenylbutylpiperidines

There is a case report of a woman with Gilles de la Tourette syndrome and obsessive–compulsive disorder who took pimozide and fluoxetine during pregnancy until pimozide was withdrawn 2 weeks prior to delivery. A healthy male infant was born (Bjarnason et al, 2006). Five pimozide exposures were reported by Reis & Källén (2008) with no associated problems.

## Atypical antipsychotics

Placental passage rates for atypical antipsychotics appear to be highest for olanzapine, followed by haloperidol, risperidone and quetiapine (Newport *et al*, 2007). One small study observed a significantly higher incidence of large for gestational age (LGA) infants when exposed to atypical antipsychotics ($n = 25$) compared with typical antipsychotics ($n = 45$) and a control group exposed to non-teratogens ($n = 38$) (Newham *et al*, 2008). There has been concern that atypical antipsychotics might increase the risk of gestational diabetes. Two population studies have explored this, and reported an increased risk of gestational diabetes (ORs 1.78, 1.77 and 1.94), with the effect of olanzapine and clozapine no greater than other antipsychotics taken together and the effect disappearing if early pregnancy BMI was controlled for (Reis & Källén, 2008; Bodén *et al*, 2012). There is an increased rate of macrocephaly in olanzapine- and clozapine-exposed pregnancies (OR = 3.02, 95% CI 1.60–5.71), but no increase in SGA or LGA (Bodén *et al*, 2012). A case–control study (133 women taking atypical antipsychotics and healthy controls), in which 96 (72%) of the women taking atypical antipsychotics were also taking other medications, reported more preterm deliveries, more LGA infants, increased NICU admissions and an increased likelihood of PNAS, mainly in those exposed to polytherapy (Sadowski *et al*, 2013). Similar findings are reported from the Australian register of antipsychotic exposures in pregnancy: 136 women took atypical antipsychotics, and higher doses increased the risk of preterm delivery, respiratory distress and admission to NICU (Kulkarni *et al*, 2014). A study from China investigating the developmental effects of atypicals in the offspring of women with schizophrenia assessed 76 exposed infants and 76 control infants whose mothers were healthy and not taking antipsychotics (Peng *et al*, 2013). They reported short-term delayed development at 2 months in cognitive, motor, socio-emotional and adaptive behaviour in the exposed group, but no difference in language, body weight or height. By 12 months the differences had disappeared.

## Olanzapine

Olanzapine is reported to have the highest placental passage ratio (compared with haloperidol, risperidone and quetiapine) at 72.1% (Newport *et al*, 2007). Goldstein *et al* (2000) reported all known cases of exposure to olanzapine up to October 1998. Of the prospectively identified pregnancies ($n = 37$), 14 were aborted (with no fetal anomaly detected), 13% of the remainder ended in miscarriage (the expected rate in controls is 15%) and there were no congenital malformations in the remaining 20. There was one stillbirth at 37 weeks gestation in a case complicated by drug misuse, hepatitis and gestational diabetes. The authors also identified 11 retrospectively reported cases. The two congenital malformations found in this group (Down's syndrome and unilateral renal atresia) were not attributed to olanzapine. A further paper extended the available information on prospectively identified cases to 96 cases of exposure to olanzapine (Ernst & Goldberg, 2002). The rate of major congenital malformations in the olanzapine-exposed group was 8.3%.

McKenna *et al* (2005) reported on 151 pregnancy outcomes in women exposed to atypicals (60 olanzapine; 49 risperidone; 36 quetiapine and 6 clozapine) and pregnant controls. The only outcome that was a statistically significant difference between the two groups was an increased risk of LBW (10% *v.* 2%) in the exposed group. There was no difference in the rates of congenital malformations, miscarriage, gestational age, stillbirth or neonatal distress.

Others have reported increased rates of LBW and NICU admission with olanzapine (Newport *et al*, 2007). Babu *et al* (2010) reported an association with higher birth weight.Other problems reported in single case studies are:

- LGA infant with Erb's palsy (Friedman & Rosenthal (2003)
- developmental dysplasia of the hip (Spyropoulos *et al*, 2006)
- meningocoele and ankyloblepharon (Arora & Prahaj, 2006)
- atrioventricular canal defect and club foot (Yeshayahu, 2007)
- neonatal hypoglycaemia (Rowe *et al*, 2012)
- microcephaly and anopthalmos (Prakash & Chadda, 2014)
- bilateral hip dysplasia (Kulkarni *et al*, 2014).

One case study of a woman who took an overdose of 112.5 mg olanzapine at 16 weeks gestation and continued to take it along with oxazepam reported no adverse events (Dervaux *et al*, 2007). Several other single case reports have reported no adverse outcomes.

In 2008, Reis & Källén reported 79 first-trimester exposures with craniosynostosis and ureteral reflux ($n = 1$), hand/finger reduction ($n = 1$) ventricular septal defect and upper alimentary canal defect ($n = 1$). There were three cases of gestational diabetes. A safety database compiled by the manufacturer reported on 610 pregnancies during which olanzapine was used (Brunner *et al*, 2013). Of these, 73 were terminated (no congenital malformation). There were no adverse events in 82.3% of the pregnancies, 9.8% had preterm deliveries, 8.0% miscarried, 4.4% had perinatal problems and 2.6% had other difficulties (post-partum problems, ectopic pregnancy, post-term birth and stillbirth). These rates were not different from those in the general population.

A recent case report describes a woman being treated for mania with psychotic features while pregnant who developed peripheral oedema during treatment with olanzapine (Vohra, 2013).

## Quetiapine

There are fewer than 300 published pregnancy exposures to quetiapine. Most data come from single case reports or small registry studies, and some are from teratology information services. Newport *et al* (2007) report a placental passage ratio in 21 women taking quetiapine of 24.1%, significantly lower than that for haloperidol and risperidone. Klier *et al* (2007) observed reduced bioavailability of quetiapine across the three trimesters of pregnancy.

McKenna *et al* (2005) reported 36 exposures with no reports of congenital malformations. A post-marketing surveillance study reported six pregnancies, five with first-trimester-only exposure (Twaites *et al*, 2007). There were no congenital malformations in the five live births. A prospective cohort study by Habermann *et al* (2013) reported an increased risk of cardiac defects (mainly septal defects) following first-trimester exposure to atypical antipsychotics as a group (there were 185 quetiapine exposures) compared with non-exposed pregnancies, but this increase was no greater than in pregnancies exposed to typical antipsychotics. There have been no reports of congenital malformations in single case studies, but an Australian registry study (Kulkarni *et al*, 2014) reported atrial septal defect in an infant exposed to quetiapine and zuclopenthixol, and pulmonary atresia and atrial septal defect in an infant exposed only to quetiapine. There are no studies examining the risk of stillbirth, preterm delivery, altered fetal growth or infant development in quetiapine specifically.

### Risperidone

Risperidone has been reported to have a placental passage ratio of 49.2% (Newport *et al*, 2007). Nine pregnancies exposed to risperidone were reported to a post-marketing study of more than 7000 patients (Mackay *et al*, 1998). These resulted in seven live births, two terminations of pregnancy, and no congenital malformations. There is a report of exaggerated hypotension during a spinal anaesthetic for Caesarean section in a woman who was taking risperidone, which has alpha-1 adrenergic antagonistic properties (Williams & Hepner, 2004). A case report described an uncomplicated pregnancy and successful delivery where the mother was taking risperidone long term (Ratnayake & Libretto, 2002). McKenna *et al* (2005) reported 49 exposures with no reported congenital malformations.

A large post-marketing study identified 713 pregnancies exposed to risperidone (Coppola *et al*, 2007). Of 68 prospectively reported exposures with known outcomes, there were congenital malformations in 3.8% and spontaneous abortions in 16.9%, similar to general population rates. Twelve of the retrospectively reported pregnancies involved congenital malformations, and there were 37 infants with perinatal syndromes, including 21 with a possible withdrawal syndrome. Reis & Källén (2008) included 51 infants exposed to risperidone in their study. There were two infants with congenital malformations: Turner's syndrome in one, and anal atresia and lung malformations in the other. Other problems reported include:

- agenesis of the corpus callosum (Ernst & Goldberg, 2002)
- CHARGE syndrome (coloboma, heart defects, choanal atresia, retarded growth, genital anomalies, ear anomalies) (Kulkarni *et al*, 2014)
- abnormal renal collecting tubule and bilateral talipes (Kulkarni *et al*, 2014)

- tardive dyskinesia in a pregnant woman taking low-dose risperidone (Chatterjee & Sharan, 2014).

There are other case reports and registry case series of exposures to risperidone without congenital malformations, and two reports of women who were managed on long-acting injectable risperidone throughout pregnancy with no maternal or infant adverse events (Dabbert & Heinze, 2006; Kim *et al*, 2007).

## Amisulpride

There are no human data in the literature relating to amisulpride and pregnancy.

## Aripiprazole

There are several case reports of pregnancy exposure to aripiprazole. In one, the pregnancy was uneventful but fetal tachycardia necessitated a Caesarean section at full term. The mother experienced failed lactation, but her infant was healthy and developed normally over the 6-month follow-up period (Mendheker *et al*, 2006*a*), as did that of a woman who took 15 mg/day from 29 weeks (Mendheker *et al*, 2006*b*). Another experienced pregnancy-induced hypertension at 39 weeks but delivered a healthy infant (Mervak *et al*, 2008). A woman taking aripiprazole 10 mg/day plus citalopram and acetazolamide (for benign intracranial hypertension) underwent Caesarean section for a breech presentation. Her baby had some mild respiratory distress, which resolved without intervention, and some poor feeding on day 3 (Nguyen *et al*, 2011). Windhager *et al* (2014) reported three cases without any problems and a placental transfer ratio of 56.2%. Lutz *et al* (2010) and Derganc & Savs (2013) also report the deliveries without problems of infants born to women taking 15 mg daily. One infant in a case reported by Watanabe *et al* (2011) had no spontaneous respiration at delivery and poor muscle tone, which resolved within 1 min of respiratory support. These and other cases not easily accessed via the published literature have been reviewed in detail by Gentile (2014).

## Zotepine, ziprasidone, lurasidone and paliperidone

There is one report of an infant born with a cleft palate after fetal exposure to ziprasidone (Peitl *et al*, 2010) and a report of no problems during pregnancy or with the infant following maternal treatment with citalopram and ziprasidone (Werremeyer, 2009). There are no published human data relating to zotepine, lurasidone or paliperidone in pregnancy.

## Clozapine

Dev & Krup (1995) reported on 80 exposures to clozapine. Thirteen pregnancies were terminated and there were eight miscarriages. There were 61 live births to the remaining 59 women, and 5 infants (8.2%) had congenital malformations (95% CI 3.1–18.8). Five infants had neonatal problems.

Other problems included:

- gestational diabetes (Waldman & Safferman, 1993; Dickson & Hogg, 1998)
- floppy infant exposed to clozapine and lorazepam (di Michele *et al*, 1996)
- seizure in an 8-day-old infant (Stoner *et al*, 1997)
- stillbirth (Mendhekar *et al*, 2003)
- reduced fetal heart rate variability (Yogev *et al*, 2002; Coston *et al*, 2012)
- neutropenia (Borisch *et al*, 2012)
- delayed peristalsis (Moreno-Bruna *et al*, 2012)
- craniosynostosis, hypospadias and hypertelorism (Kulkarni *et al*, 2014)
- gastroschisis and horseshoe kidney (Kulkarni *et al*, 2014).

There is a report of fetal serum clozapine levels greater than those in maternal serum, which the authors suggest may be due to the higher concentration of albumin in fetal blood (Barnas *et al*, 1994). A woman attempting suicide when 9 months pregnant took an overdose of clozapine, resulting in the neonatal death of her infant (Klys *et al*, 2007). Nguyen & Lalonde (2003) reviewed 6 cases published in the literature and summarised data from almost 200 cases known to Novartis. They concluded that no specific risk could be attributed to clozapine. There is also a report of four women successfully treated whose infants were followed up for up to 6–10 years (Gáti *et al*, 2001), a single case report of successful pregnancy with no problems with the infant who was followed for 2 years (Sethi, 2006), and a further two uncomplicated cases (Duran *et al*, 2008).

Obstetric anaesthetists have described a case in which they used general anaesthesia for an emergency Caesarean section in an obese woman who had taken clozapine throughout pregnancy (Doherty *et al*, 2006). General anaesthesia was chosen because of the risk of profound hypotension following neuraxial blockade, which can be resistant to vasopressors. They provide a comprehensive account of the issues related to pre-, peri- and postoperative deliveries involving clozapine exposure, including the increased risk of thromboembolism and intestinal paralysis, and the need to monitor temperature in postoperative parturient women. Psychiatrists assessing such women or caring for them in mother and baby units will find this paper a useful resource.

Koren *et al* (2002) identified obesity and a low intake of folate in women with schizophrenia taking atypical antipsychotics. This puts them at higher risk of having infants with neural tube defects.

## Anticholinergics

There are few data relating to anticholinergic drugs and pregnancy. They should only be used for extrapyramidal side-effects in the short term, and only if absolutely necessary. Preferably, the dose of the drug should be reduced during pregnancy.

## Mood stabilisers

### Lithium

Lithium crosses the placenta, and a mean mother–infant lithium ratio of 1.05 has been reported (Newport *et al*, 2005). Early data in the 1970s from case registers based on voluntary submissions suggested that there was an increased incidence of cardiac malformations, particularly Ebstein's anomaly, in infants exposed to lithium in the first trimester. The risk was estimated at 400 times the expected rate in the general population (Nora *et al*, 1974). Cohen *et al* (1994) reviewed the evidence to date, including controlled epidemiological studies, and reported risk ratios of 1.5–3.0 for all congenital malformations and 1.2–7.7 for cardiac malformations. The risk for Ebstein's anomaly rises from 1 in 20000 in the general population to 1 in 1000. A more recent systematic review and meta-analysis identified 62 studies exploring the teratogenic potential of lithium (7 cohort studies, 7 case–control studies and 48 case reports). The odds of Ebstein's anomaly were not significantly different from controls (OR = 0.27, 95% CI 0.004–18.17; $P = 0.54$), but the numbers of events were small. Similarly, although there was no increased risk of congenital malformations, the numbers of infants exposed to lithium were small (McKnight *et al*, 2012). Diav-Citrin *et al* (2014) reported an aOR for cardiac malformations after first trimester exposure of 4.75 (95% CI 1.11–20.36); ORs for other malformations were not significant.

The window of risk for cardiac malformations is between 4 and 9 weeks gestation. If a woman has been exposed during this time, a level II ultrasound and a fetal echocardiogram between 16 and 18 weeks are advised to assess cardiac development. A small study of 15 children exposed to lithium *in utero* found no adverse effects on growth, or on neurological, cognitive or behavioural development at 3–15 years of age (van der Lugt *et al*, 2012).

Assuming the pregnancy is to be continued, a decision has to be made as to whether or not to carry on with lithium. If lithium is continued throughout pregnancy, the lowest dose to achieve therapeutic levels should be used. This might mean a dose increase as pregnancy progresses, owing to increased clearance via the increased glomerular filtration rate (30–50% in the second half of pregnancy). Levels should be checked more frequently: twice weekly in the second trimester, and weekly in the third. Urea, electrolytes and thyroid function should also be checked. Divided doses are said to reduce peak levels, so twice-daily dosage can be considered. In this case, levels should be monitored just before the next dose.

If lithium is to be discontinued, this should be done gradually, as rapid discontinuation can trigger relapse. This same advice applies to women who are contemplating pregnancy and wish to stop treatment before attempting to conceive. Depending on the severity of illness and likelihood of recurrence, lithium may be restarted during the second trimester.

Tapering and discontinuation of lithium 3–4 weeks before delivery is suggested to avoid fetal toxicity and maternal toxicity during labour. There are numerous reports (for reviews, see Pinelli *et al*, 2002; Kozma, 2005) of neonatal problems, including poor respiratory effort and cyanosis, cardiac rhythm disturbances, nephrogenic diabetes insipidus, thyroid dysfunction, goitre, hypoglycaemia, hypotonia and lethargy, hyperbilirubinaemia and LGA infants. Newport *et al* (2005) confirmed in a controlled study that lower Apgar scores, longer hospital stays and higher rates of CNS and neuromuscular complications were observed in infants with higher lithium concentrations at delivery. They demonstrated that withholding lithium for 48 h before delivery reduced maternal concentrations by 0.28 meq/L. This might be a strategy for women in whom it is too risky to discontinue for a longer period. After delivery, the pre-pregnancy dose should be reinstated (renal clearance falls to non-pregnant levels dramatically postpartum). If a woman is taking lithium, she should deliver in hospital and stop lithium during labour. Close monitoring is required by the obstetric team during delivery to maintain fluid balance and avoid toxicity, and a plasma level should be checked 12 h after her last dose.

### Carbamazepine

Carbamazepine is teratogenic. Neural tube defects occur in 0.5–1.0% of infants exposed during pregnancy, which is 5–10 times the rate in the general population; cardiovascular anomalies occur in 1.5–2.0%; cleft lip and palate occur five times more often than in controls; and skeletal and brain malformations have been observed. A meta-analysis of 1255 pregnancies revealed an overall rate of major malformations of 6.7% (OR = 3.0) (Ornoy, 2006). A recent case study highlights the fact that skin eruptions of varying degrees of severity occur in 3% of people taking carbamazepine. Angioedema is a potentially life-threatening complication, which is more common in women and has a peak incidence in the third decade of life (Elias *et al*, 2006). Anticonvulsants taken during pregnancy (of which carbamazepine was the most commonly used) increase the risk of pre-eclampsia, haemorrhage after vaginal delivery and respiratory distress (Pilo *et al*, 2006).

Clearance varies during pregnancy and serum levels may decrease, so monitoring of serum levels during pregnancy is recommended, with dosage adjustment as indicated. Fetal serum levels are 50–80% of maternal serum levels. Carbamazepine is associated with vitamin K deficiency, which can impair clotting. Supplementation with vitamin K is recommended.

### Sodium valproate

Sodium valproate (also known as divalproex semisodium, valproic acid and Depakote) has been used in the treatment of epilepsy for many years. Soon after its introduction, an increase in the rate of neural tube defects was observed, and other congenital malformations have also been noted

– e.g. cranial facial defects and fetal valproate syndrome (brachycephaly, high forehead, shallow orbits, ocular hypertelorism, small nose and mouth, low-set posteriorly rotated ears, long overlapping fingers and toes and hyperconvex fingernails, fingernail hypoplasia, cardiac defects). The use of valproate as a mood stabiliser has increased in recent years (Bowden & Singh, 2005).

Koren *et al* (2006) carried out a meta-analysis of studies published between 1978 and 2005. The RR for any congenital malformation is 2.59 when compared with monotherapy with other anticonvulsants, 3.16 when compared with untreated patients with epilepsy, and 3.77 when compared with the general population. The RR increased if valproate was given with other anticonvulsants and at doses of 600 mg per day. The largest risk appeared to be when doses were >1000 mg/day, a finding replicated by Vajda *et al* (2006) with doses above 1100 mg/day using data from the Australian Pregnancy Register. A study in which valproate was the second most commonly prescribed anticonvulsant reported an increased risk for adverse delivery events (Pilo *et al*, 2006).

The Medicines and Healthcare Products Regulatory Agency, its equivalents in other countries, and NICE (2014) state that valproate is not recommended in women of current or future childbearing potential, and should only be used in pregnancy if absolutely necessary. Folate 5 mg daily is advised, although it is not clear that this reduces the risk. If there is first-trimester exposure, detailed ultrasound at 16–18 weeks and alpha-fetoprotein assay are advised. Clearance during pregnancy is variable.

Other reported problems include a risk of haemorrhage due to impaired vitamin K-dependent clotting factors and the risk of transient neonatal hepatic dysfunction.

There is now clear evidence from the 22 prospective cohort studies and 6 registry studies included in a Cochrane review (Bromley *et al*, 2014) that *in utero* exposure to valproate impairs neurodevelopment. Others have suggested that there may be an increased risk of ASD, but the evidence remains inconclusive at present.

## Lamotrigine

Lamotrigine clearance is increased by up to 300% in the last trimester of pregnancy and can revert quickly after delivery, but it can also rise again. There seems to be considerable individual variation in pharmacokinetic changes during pregnancy, underlining the need to closely monitor serum levels (Petrenaite *et al*, 2005). The mean infant cord level is reported at 66% of maternal serum levels (Clark *et al*, 2013).

Rates of congenital malformation reported range from 0 to 7% (Vajda *et al*, 2003; Cunnington *et al*, 2005; Morrow *et al*, 2006; Mølgaard-Nielsen & Hviid, 2011; Hernández-Diaz *et al*, 2012; Campbell *et al*, 2014). Some studies seem to indicate that doses of lamotrigine of 200 mg daily or below have minimal teratogenic effect. One study has found that doses above this level are associated with a higher risk of malformations (5.4%), higher still if given with valproate (Morrow *et al*, 2006), but Cunnington *et al* (2007) reported no effect of dose on the rate of congenital malformations.

There are also emerging concerns about a possible increased risk of oral clefts (Holmes *et al*, 2006) when lamotrigine monotherapy is used in the first trimester, and of an increased risk of autistic traits and poorer language scores in exposed infants at 36 months (Veiby *et al*, 2013).

If lamotrigine is to be continued after pregnancy, it should be noted that its interaction with combined oral contraceptives could render them less effective.

### Gabapentin

Öhman *et al* (2005) reported six women with epilepsy or pain disorders who took gabapentin throughout pregnancy. One delivered a preterm infant at 32 weeks, and one infant had short-lived hypotonia and cyanosis. A study of 39 women with 48 pregnancy outcomes (97% had first-trimester exposures) found a higher rate of preterm births (22.9%) when all births including 6 twin deliveries were counted, and 9.1% when the twin deliveries were excluded (Montouris, 2003). The malformation rate was 6.8%. One of the women in this study had a bipolar disorder. A more recent prospective comparative study of 223 pregnancy exposures compared to unexposed pregnancies found no difference in the rate of congenital malformations, but found an increased risk of preterm delivery, LBW and admission to NICU. The two exposed infants who had PNAS were also exposed to other psychotropics (Fujii *et al*, 2013).

Clinicians should therefore only prescribe anticonvulsants in women of childbearing age if the benefits outweigh the disadvantages, and must ensure that reliable contraception is in place. Evidence suggests that this practice is far from universal (Wieck *et al*, 2007).

The incidence of teratogenesis increases significantly with all anticonvulsants in polytherapy, particularly if valproate is involved.

### Calcium channel blockers

Calcium channel blockers have been used in obstetrics as antihypertensives, antiarrhythmics and tocolytics for some time. A prospective analysis of 78 women exposed (41% verapamil, 44% nifedipine) found no increase in the rate of congenital malformations or neonatal problems (Magee *et al*, 1996). A meta-analysis (Berkman *et al*, 2003) of 75 tocolytic studies reported that calcium channel blockers are rated as low risk for short-term neonatal harm. They are now beginning to emerge as mood stabilisers, but the safety data are extremely limited in this population.

- Goodnick (1993) reported the treatment of three women with bipolar disorder who became symptomatic during pregnancy.
- The use of verapamil in a sequential series of women with bipolar disorder (some pregnant) is discussed by Wisner *et al* (2002).

- There is a case report of nimodipine use during pregnancy (Yingling *et al*, 2002).

### Stimulants

Infants of mothers taking methylphenidate at doses ranging from 35 to 80 mg daily for ADHD had doses estimated at 0.2% and 0.7% of the maternal weight-adjusted dose (Hackett *et al*, 2005, 2006*b*). Another paper reports a woman 11 months postpartum taking oral immediate-release methylphenidate 5 mg in the morning and 10 mg at noon. The authors estimated that a fully breastfed infant would receive a dose of 0.16% of the maternal weight-adjusted dosage (Spigset *et al*, 2007). Others have found the drug to be undetectable (e.g. Upadhyaya *et al*, 2003). Seven of 8 infants whose mothers were taking either dextroamphetamine or methylphenidate had no methylphenidate-related adverse reactions and development was age-appropriate (Hackett *et al*, 2005). A review of the studies involving 183 first-trimester exposures concluded that there was no substantial increased risk of congenital malformations (Dideriksen *et al*, 2013) and a population-based study of 222 exposures also reported no increased risk of congenital malformations (OR = 0.8, 95% CI 0.3–1.8) (Pottegård *et al*, 2014).

## Rapid tranquillisation of the pregnant woman

If a pregnant woman requires rapid tranquillisation, she should be managed according to NICE (2014) guidance. Particular factors to consider include the following.

- Restraint procedures should take pregnancy into account; any procedures that might compromise the fetus should not be used.
- The woman should not be placed in seclusion after rapid tranquillisation.
- Antipsychotics or BDZs with short half-lives are the preferred medication, and both should be used at the minimum effective dose. If a BDZ is used in late pregnancy, the risks of floppy baby syndrome must be considered.
- Should a woman require rapid tranquillisation close to term, in labour or soon after delivery, paediatric and anaesthetic opinions are advised.

## Non-drug interventions

### *Electroconvulsive therapy*

Anderson & Reti (2009) reviewed the literature on electroconvulsive therapy (ECT) and pregnancy from 1941 to 2007 and included 339 cases. Efficacy data were only available for 68 cases. Thirty-seven of these cases involved women with a diagnosis of depression, and the response rate reported was 84%. Twenty-one were treated for schizophrenia, and the rate of at least partial remission was 61%. The mean number of treatments was 10.7. Fetal or neonatal abnormalities were reported in 25 cases, including:

- death (11 cases)
- transient fetal bradycardia or decelerations (8 cases)
- congenital pulmonary cysts (2 cases)
- great vessel transposition (2 cases).

There were also single reports of peritonitis, club foot, prematurity, congenital blindness, coarctation of the aorta, cortical infarcts, anencephaly, VATER syndrome and intellectual disability. Nine of the deaths were thought to be related to the ECT; other congenital malformations were unlikely to be related to ECT carried out in the second trimester. The most frequent maternal adverse event was induction of preterm labour. A more recent systematic review of the literature (Leiknes *et al*, 2015) reported an overall child mortality rate of 7.1%, fetal bradycardia (43%), preterm labour (28%), uterine contractions (22%) and vaginal bleeding if ECT was used in the first trimester (12%).

ECT may be the treatment of choice if the patient is severely depressed, manic and not responding to lithium, psychotic or catatonic, and the woman's physical health or that of the fetus is at serious risk. The following advice is gleaned from the literature.

- Obstetric assessment including pelvic examination is advised prior to each treatment.
- Assessment of uterine contractions or vaginal bleeding after treatment is recommended.
- Fetal heart monitoring is recommended by most.
- Place the patient in a slightly left lateral position to minimise aortocaval compression.
- As patients beyond the first trimester are at increased risk of regurgitation of gastric contents, anaesthetic assessment is required regarding the use of anticholinergics and whether intubation is advised.
- Pregnancy is accompanied by mild hyperventilation. Respiratory alkalosis caused by excessive hyperventilation, which is sometimes used to reduce the seizure threshold, should be avoided as it can reduce oxygen transfer from maternal to fetal haemoglobin.

## Transcranial magnetic stimulation

There are case reports of pregnant women treated successfully with transcranial magnetic stimulation (TMS) with no adverse events (Nahas *et al*, 1999; Klirova *et al*, 2008). Sayar *et al* (2014) reported on 33 pregnant women suffering from depression who received TMS 6 days per week for 3 weeks. Half achieved full or partial remission, and there were no adverse events.

There is also a case report of a woman who became pregnant while receiving maintenance TMS and delivered without problems (Burton *et al*, 2014).

## Vagus nerve stimulation

Vagus nerve stimulation (VNS) is of interest as a possible intervention for treatment-resistant depression. There is one case report of a woman with unipolar depression who became pregnant during a pilot study of VNS. She continued to receive VNS, along with citalopram and bupropion, throughout her pregnancy and normal delivery. She experienced a short-lived episode of depression lasting 11 days after delivery, which resolved spontaneously. Her daughter was a healthy term infant (Husain *et al*, 2005).

## Bright light therapy

Bright light therapy is also being explored as a possible treatment for depressed pregnant women. Oren *et al* (2002) carried out an open trial of bright light therapy in an A-B-A design for 3–5 weeks in 16 pregnant women with major depression. After 3 weeks of treatment, mean depression ratings improved by 49% and benefits were seen throughout the 5 weeks of treatment, with no evidence of adverse effects of light therapy on pregnancy.

Epperson *et al* (2004) randomly assigned 10 pregnant women with major depressive disorder to a 5-week trial with either a 7000 lux (active) or 500 lux (placebo) light box. At the end of the randomised controlled trial (RCT), the women had the option of continuing in a 5-week extension phase. Results of the RCT were not significant, but after a further 5 weeks, the presence of active *v.* placebo light produced a clear treatment effect with an effect size (0.43) similar to that seen in antidepressant drug trials. This was associated with phase advances of the melatonin rhythm. A more recent RCT included 27 pregnant women with major depression who were treated with 7000 lux or placebo for 1 h/day for 5 weeks. Reductions in depressive symptoms, response and remission rates were significantly greater in the treatment group. No adverse events were reported (Wirz-Justice *et al*, 2011).

## Omega-3 fatty acids

Su *et al* (2001) report on a woman with long-standing schizophrenia who was treated with omega-3 fatty acids during pregnancy. She experienced a reduction in both positive and negative symptoms, with no adverse effects.

## Aromatherapy and massage

Massage and aromatherapy using essential oils has been suggested as an intervention for anxiety in pregnant women and one that might be more acceptable to them than drugs. However, animal studies have shown some essential oils to be responsible for intrauterine growth retardation and congenital anomalies, and there is a lack of both efficacy and safety data in human pregnancy (Bastard & Tiran, 2006).

## Resources

- Pregnancy exposures can be reported via the UKTIS website (www.uktis.org). Health professionals can register for free-to-access information at www.toxbase.org. Bumps (best use of medicines in pregnancy; www.medicinesinpregnancy.org/) has information for professionals and user-friendly fact sheets.
- Mother to Baby (www.mothertobaby.org) is a USA site that has user-friendly fact sheets on drugs and pregnancy.
- Any adverse or suspected adverse event in relation to a drug or herbal medicine must be reported to the Medicines and Healthcare Products Regulatory Agency via the Yellow Card Scheme (https://yellowcard.mhra.gov.uk/).
- Motherisk (www.motherisk.org) is a Canadian website giving advice and providing resources for patients and professionals regarding pregnancy exposures. Helpline numbers can also be found on their website.
- The British Association for Psychopharmacology (www.bap.org.uk/) will publish guidelines on prescribing for pregnant and lactating women in 2015.

## References

Addis A, Koren G (2000) Safety of fluoxetine during the first trimester of pregnancy: a meta-analytical review of epidemiological studies. *Psychological Medicine*, **30**: 89–94.

Altshuler LL, Cohen L, Szuba MP, *et al* (1996) Pharmacologic management of psychiatric illness during pregnancy: dilemmas and guidelines. *American Journal of Psychiatry*, **153**: 592–606.

Alwan S, Reefhuis J, Rasmussen S, *et al* (2005) Maternal use of selective serotonin reuptake inhibitors and risk for birth defects. *Birth Defects Research (Part A): Clinical and Molecular Teratology*, **73**: 291.

Alwan S, Reefhuis J, Botto LD, *et al* (2010) Maternal use of bupropion and risk for congenital heart defects. *American Journal of Obstetrics and Gynecology*, **203**: e51–e56.

Alwan S, Reefhuis J, Rasmussen S, *et al* (2011) Patterns of antidepressant medication use among pregnant women in a United States population. *Journal of Clinical Pharmacology*, **51**: 264–270.

Andersen JT, Andersen NL, Horwitz H, *et al* (2014) Exposure to selective serotonin reuptake inhibitors and the risk of miscarriage. *Obstetrics and Gynecology*, **124**: 655–661.

Anderson EL, Reti IM (2009) ECT in pregnancy: a review of the literature from 1941–2007. *Psychosomatic Medicine*, **71**: 235–242.

Arora M, Prahaj SK (2006) Meningocele and ankyloblepharon following *in utero* exposure to olanzapine. *European Psychiatry*, **21**: 345–346.

Babu GN, Desai G, Tippeswamy H, *et al* (2010) Birth weight and use of olanzapine in pregnancy. *Journal of Clinical Psychopharmacology*, **30**: 331–332.

Ban L, Tata LJ, West J, *et al* (2012) Live and non-live pregnancy outcomes among women with depression and anxiety: a population-based study. *PLoS ONE*, **7**: e43462.

Ban L, Gibson JE, West J, et al (2014a) Maternal depression, antidepressant prescriptions, and congenital anomaly risk in offspring: a population-based cohort study. *BJOG*, **121**: 1471–1481.

Ban L, West J, Gibson J, et al (2014b) First trimester exposure to anxiolytic and hypnotic drugs and the risk of major congenital anomalies: a United Kingdom population-based cohort study. *PLoS ONE*, **9**: e100996.

Barnas C, Bergant A, Hummer M, et al (1994) Clozapine concentrations in maternal and fetal plasma, amniotic fluid, and breast milk. *American Journal of Psychiatry*, **151**: 945.

Barnes TRE, Schizophrenia Consensus Group of the British Association for Psychopharmacology (2011) Evidence-based guidelines for the pharmacological treatment of schizophrenia: recommendations from the British Association for Psychopharmacology. *Journal of Psychopharmacology*, **25**: 567–620.

Bar-Oz B, Einarson A, Boskovic R, et al (2007) Paroxetine and congenital malformations: meta-analysis and consideration of potential confounding factors. *Clinical Therapeutics*, **29**: 918–926.

Bastard J, Tiran D (2006) Aromatherapy and massage for antenatal anxiety: Its effect on the fetus. *Complementary Therapies in Clinical Practice*, **12**: 48–54.

Bellantuono C, Tofani S, Di Sciascio G, et al (2013) Benzodiazepine exposure in pregnancy and risk of major malformations: a critical overview. *General Hospital Psychiatry*, **35**: 3–8.

Ben-Amitai D, Merlob P (1991) Neonatal fever and cyanotic spells from maternal chlorpromazine. *DICP: The Annals of Pharmacotherapy*, **25**: 1009–1010.

Bérard A, Ramos É, Rey É, et al (2007) First trimester exposure to paroxetine and risk of cardiac malformations in infants: the importance of dosage. *Birth Defects Research Part B: Developmental and Reproductive Toxicology*, **80**: 12–17.

Berkman ND, Thorp JM, Lohr KN, et al (2003) Tocolytic treatment for the management of preterm labour: a review of the evidence. *American Journal of Obstetrics & Gynaecology*, **188**: 1648–1659.

Biswas PN, Wilton LV, Shakir SA (2003) The pharmacovigilance of mirtazapine: results of a prescription event monitoring study on 13 554 patients in England. *Journal of Psychopharmacology*, **17**: 121–126.

Bjarnason NH, Rode L, Kim D (2006) Fetal exposure to pimozide: a case report. *Journal of Reproductive Medicine*, **51**: 443–444.

Bodnar LM, Sunder KR, Wisner KL (2006) Treatment with selective serotonin reuptake inhibitors during pregnancy: deceleration of weight gain because of depression or drug? *American Journal of Psychiatry*, **163**: 986–991.

Bodén R, Lundgren M, Brandt L, et al (2012) Antipsychotics during pregnancy; relation to fetal and maternal metabolic effects. *Archives of General Psychiatry*, **69**: 715–721.

Bonari L, Pinto N, Ahn E, et al (2004) Perinatal risks of untreated depression during pregnancy. *Canadian Journal of Psychiatry*, **49**: 726–735.

Bonnot O, Vollset S-E, Godet P-F, et al (2003) Exposition in utero au lorazepam et atresia anale: signal épidémiologique. *Encéphale*, **29**: 553–559.

Borisch C, Kayser A, Weber-Schoendorfer C, et al (2012) Severe neutropenia in a newborn after clozapine therapy during pregnancy. *Reproductive Toxicology*, **34**: 158.

Bowden CL, Singh V (2005) Valproate in bipolar disorder: 2000 onwards. *Acta Psychiatrica Scandinavica*, **111**: 13–20.

Boyce PM, Hackett P, Ilett KF (2011) Duloxetine transfer across the placenta during pregnancy and into milk during lactation. *Archives of Women's Mental Health*, **14**: 169–172.

Briggs GG, Ambrose PJ, Ilett KF, et al (2009) Use of duloxetine in pregnancy and lactation. *Annals of Pharmacotherapy*, **43**: 1898–1902.

Bromley R, Weston J, Adab N, et al (2014) Treatment for epilepsy in pregnancy: neuro-developmental outcomes in the child. *Cochrane Database of Systematic Reviews*, **10**: CD010236.

Broy P, Bérard A (2010) Gestational exposure to antidepressants and the risk of spontaneous abortion: a review. *Current Drug Delivery*, **7**: 76–92.

Brunner E, Falk DM, Jones M, et al (2013) Olanzapine in pregnancy and breastfeeding: a review of data from global safety surveillance. *BMC Pharmacology and Toxicology*, **14**: 38.

Burton C, Gill C, Clarke P, et al (2014) Maintaining remission of depression with repetitive transcranial magnetic stimulation during pregnancy. *Archives of Women's Mental Health,* 17: 247–250.

Campbell E, Kennedy F, Russell A, et al (2014) Malformation risk of antiepileptic drug monotherapies in pregnancy: updated results from the UK and Ireland epilepsy and pregnancy registers. *Journal of Neurology, Neurosurgery and Psychiatry,* 85: 1029–1034.

Casper RC, Fleisher BE, Lee-Ancajas JC, et al (2003) Follow-up of children of depressed mothers exposed or not exposed to antidepressant drugs during pregnancy. *Journal of Pediatrics,* 142: 402–408.

Chan B, Koren G, Fayez I, et al (2005) Pregnancy outcome of women exposed to bupropion during pregnancy: a prospective comparative study. *American Journal of Obstetrics & Gynecology,* 192: 932–936.

Chatterjee B, Sharan P (2014) Tardive dyskinesia in a pregnant woman with low dose, short duration risperidone: possible role of estrogen-induced dopaminergic hypersensitivity. *Journal of Neuropsychiatry and Clinical Neuroscience,* 26: e44–e46.

Chlumska A, Curik R, Boudova L, et al (2001) Chlorpromazine-induced cholestatic liver disease with ductopenia. *Ceskoslovenska Patologie,* 37: 118–122.

Clark CT, Klein AM, Perel JM, et al (2013) Lamotrigine dosing for pregnant patients with bipolar disorder. *American Journal of Psychiatry,* 170: 1240–1247.

Clements CC, Castro VM, Blumenthal SR, et al (2015) Prenatal antidepressant exposure is associated with risk for attention-deficit hyperactivity disorder but not with autistic spectrum disorder in a large health system. *Molecular Psychiatry,* 20: 727–734.

Cohen LF, Jefferson JM, Johnson JW, et al (1994) A reevaluation of risk of *in utero* exposure to lithium. *JAMA,* 271: 146–150.

Cohen LS, Heller VL, Bailey JW, et al (2000) Birth outcomes following prenatal exposure to fluoxetine. *Biological Psychiatry,* 48: 996–1000.

Cohen LS, Altshuler LL, Harlow BL, et al (2006) Relapse of major depression during pregnancy in women who maintain or discontinue antidepressant treatment. *JAMA,* 295: 499–507.

Cole JA, Ephross SA, Cosmatos IS, et al (2007a) Paroxetine in the first trimester and the prevalence of congenital malformations. *Pharmacoepidemiology and Drug Safety,* 16: 1075–1085.

Cole JA, Modell JG, Haight BR, et al (2007b) Bupropion in pregnancy and the prevalence of congenital malformations. *Pharmacoepidemiology and Drug Safety,* 16: 474–484.

Collins K, Comer J (2003) Maternal haloperidol therapy associated with dyskinesia in a newborn. *American Journal of Health-System Pharmacy,* 60: 2253–2255.

Colvin L, Slack-Smith L, Stanley FJ, et al (2011) Dispensing patterns and pregnancy outcomes for women dispensed selective serotonin reuptake inhibitors in pregnancy. *Birth Defects Research A,* 91: 142–152.

Coppola D, Russo L-J, Kwarta Jr FR (2007) Evaluating the postmarketing experience of risperidone use during pregnancy: pregnancy and neonatal exposures. *Drug Safety,* 30: 247–264.

Costei AM, Kozer E, Ho T, et al (2002) Perinatal outcome following third trimester exposure to paroxetine. *Archives of Pediatrics and Adolescent Medicine,* 156: 1129–1132.

Coston A-L, Hoffman P, Equy V, et al (2012) Fetal heart rate variability and clozapine treatment. *Gynecologie, Obstetrique & Fertilité,* 40: 549–552.

Cunnington M, Tennis P, International Lamotrigine Pregnancy Registry Scientific Advisory Committee (2005) Lamotrigine and the risk of malformations in pregnancy. *Neurology,* 64: 955–960.

Cunnington M, Ferber S, Quartey G, et al (2007) Effect of dose on the frequency of major birth defects following fetal exposure to lamotrigine monotherapy in an international observational study. *Epilepsia,* 48: 1207–1210.

Dabbert D, Heinze M (2006) Follow-up of a pregnancy with risperidone microspheres. *Pharmacopsychiatry,* 39: 235.

Dadić-Hero E, Ružić K, Grahovac T (2011) Fluphenazine in the pregnancy. *European Psychiatry*, **26** (Suppl 1): 1092.

Davis RL, Rubanowice D, McPhillips H, *et al* (2007) Risks of congenital malformations and perinatal events among infants exposed to antidepressant medications during pregnancy. *Pharmacoepidemiology and Drug Safety*, **16**: 1086–1094.

Derganc M, Savs AP (2013) The use of aripiprazole in pregnancy: a case report. *European Psychiatry*, **28** (Suppl 1): 1.

Dervaux A, Ichou P, Pierron G, *et al* (2007) Olanzapine exposure during pregnancy. *Australian and New Zealand Journal of Psychiatry*, **41**: 706.

Dev V, Krupp P (1995) The side effects and safety of clozapine. *Reviews in Contemporary Pharmacotherapy*, **6**: 197–208.

Diav-Citrin O, Okotore B, Lucarelli K, *et al* (1999) Pregnancy outcome following first-trimester exposure to zopiclone: a prospective controlled cohort study. *American Journal of Perinatology*, **16**: 157–160.

Diav-Citrin O, Schechtman S, Winbaum D, *et al* (2005a) Paroxetine and fluoxetine in pregnancy: a mulitcenter, prospective controlled study. *Reproductive Toxicology*, **20**: 459.

Diav-Citrin O, Schechtman S, Ornoy S, *et al* (2005b) Safety of haloperidol and penfluridol in pregnancy: a multicentre, prospective, controlled study. *Journal of Clinical Psychiatry*, **66**: 317–322.

Diav-Citrin O, Schechtman S, Tahover E, *et al* (2014) Pregnancy outcome following *in utero* exposure to lithium: a prospective, comparative, observational study. *American Journal of Psychiatry*, **171**: 785–794.

Dickson RA, Hogg L (1998) Pregnancy of a patient treated with clozapine. *Psychiatric Services*, **49**: 1081–1083.

Dideriksen D, Pottegård A, Hallas J, *et al* (2013) First trimester in utero exposure to methylphenidate. *Basic and Clinical Pharmacology and Toxicology*, **112**: 73–76.

Djulus J, Koren G, Einarson TR, *et al* (2006) Exposure to mirtazapine during pregnancy: a prospective, comparative study of birth outcomes. *Journal of Clinical Psychiatry*, **67**: 1280–1284.

Doherty J, Bell PF, King DJ (2006) Implications for anaesthesia in a patient established on clozapine. *International Journal of Obstetric Anesthesia*, **15**: 59–62.

Dolovich LR, Addis A, Vaillancourt JMR, *et al* (1998) Benzodiazepine use in pregnancy and major malformations or oral cleft: meta-analysis of cohort and case-control studies. *BMJ*, **317**: 839–843.

Dougoua JJ, Mills E, Perri D, *et al* (2006) Safety and efficacy of St John's Wort (hypericum) during pregnancy and lactation. *Canadian Journal of Clinical Pharmacology*, **13**: e268–e276.

Duran A, Ugur MM, Turan S, *et al* (2008) Clozapine use in two women with schizophrenia during pregnancy. *Journal of Psychopharmacology*, **22**: 111–113.

Einarson A, Lawrimore T, Brand P, *et al* (2000) Attitudes and practices of physicians and naturopaths toward herbal products, including use during pregnancy and lactation. *Canadian Journal of Clinical Pharmacology*, **7**: 45–49.

Einarson A, Fatoye B, Sarkar M, *et al* (2001) Pregnancy outcome following gestational exposure to venlafaxine: a multicenter prospective controlled study. *American Journal of Psychiatry*, **158**: 1728–1730.

Einarson A, Bonari L, Voyer-Lavigne S, *et al* (2003) A multicentre prospective controlled study to determine the safety of trazodone and nefazodone use during pregnancy. *Canadian Journal of Psychiatry*, **48**: 106–110.

Einarson A, Schachtschneider AK, Halil R, *et al* (2005) SSRIs and other antidepressant use during pregnancy and potential neonatal adverse effects: impact of a public health advisory and subsequent reports in the news media. *BMC Pregnancy and Childbirth*, **5**: 11.

Einarson A, Choi J, Einarson TR, *et al* (2009) Incidence of major malformations in infants following antidepressant exposure in pregnancy: results of a large prospective cohort study. *Canadian Journal of Psychiatry*, **54**: 242–286.

Einarson A, Smart K, Vial T, *et al* (2012) Rates of major malformations in infants following exposure to duloxetine during pregnancy: a preliminary report. *Journal of Clinical Psychiatry*, **73**: 1471.

Einarson TR, Einarson A (2005) Newer antidepressants in pregnancy and rates of major malformations: a meta-analysis of prospective comparative studies. *Pharmacoepidemiology and Drug Safety*, **14**: 823–827.

Elias A, Madhusoodana S, Pudukkadan D, *et al* (2006) Angioedema and maculopular eruptions associated with carbamazepine administration. *CNS Spectrums*, **11**: 352–354.

Epperson CN, Terman M, Terman JS, *et al* (2004) Randomized clinical trial of bright light therapy for antepartum depression: preliminary findings. *Journal of Clinical Psychiatry*, **65**: 421–425.

Epstein RA, Bobo WV, Shelton RC, *et al* (2013) Increasing use of atypical antipsychotics and anticonvulsants during pregnancy. *Pharmacoepidemiology and Drug Safety*, **22**: 794–801.

Ericson A, Källén B, Wilhon B (1999) Delivery outcome after the use of antidepressants in early pregnancy. *European Journal of Clinical Pharmacology*, **55**: 503–508.

Ernst CL, Goldberg JF (2002) The reproductive safety profile of mood stabilizers, atypical antipsychotics and broad-spectrum psychotropics. *Journal of Clinical Psychiatry*, **63** (Suppl 4): 42–55.

Eros E, Czeizel AE, Rockenbauer M, *et al* (2002) A population-based case-control teratologic study of nitrazepam, medazepam, tofisopam, alprazolam and clonazepam treatment during pregnancy. *European Journal of Obstetrics & Gynecology and Reproductive Biology*, **10**: 147–154.

Faru L, Kieler H, Heglund B, *et al* (2015) Selective serotonin reuptake inhibitors and venlafaxine in early pregnancy and risk of birth defects: population based cohort study and sibling design. *BMJ*, **350**: h1798.

Figueroa R (2010) Use of antidepressants during pregnancy and risk of attention-deficit/hyperactivity disorder in the offspring. *Journal of Developmental and Behavioral Pediatrics*, **8**: 641–648.

Flynn HA, Blow FC, Marcus SM (2006) Rates and predictors of depression treatment among pregnant women in hospital-affiliated obstetrics practices. *General Hospital Psychiatry*, **28**: 289–295.

Forsberg L, Navér L, Gustaffson LL, *et al* (2014) Neonatal adaptation in infants prenatally exposed to antidepressants – clinical monitoring using neonatal abstinence score. *PLoS ONE*, **9**: e111327.

Friedman SH, Rosenthal MB (2003) Treatment of perinatal delusional disorder: a case report. *International Journal of Psychiatry in Medicine*, **33**: 391–394.

Fujii H, Goel A, Bernard N, *et al* (2013) Pregnancy outcomes following gabapentin use: results of a prospective comparative study. *Neurology*, **80**: 1565–1570.

Gaffney L, Smith C (2004) The views of pregnant women towards the use of complementary therapies and medicines. *Birth Issues*, **13**: 43–50.

Gáti A, Trixler M, Tényi T (2001) Pregnancy and atypical antipsychotics. *European Neuropsychopharmacology*, **11**: S247.

Gentile S (2010) Antipsychotic therapy during early and late pregnancy. A systematic review. *Schizophrenia Bulletin*, **36**: 518–544.

Gentile S (2014) A safety evaluation of aripiprazole for treating schizophrenia during pregnancy and puerperium. *Expert Opinion on Drug Safety*, **13**: 1733–1742.

Gidaya, NB, Lee BK, Burstyn I, *et al* (2014) In utero exposure to selective serotonin reuptake inhibitors and risk for autism spectrum disorder. *Journal of Autism and Developmental Disorders*, **144**: 255–2567.

GlaxoSmithKline (2008) *The Bupropion Pregnancy Registry. Final Report. 1 September 1997 through 31 March 2008.* GSK.

Goldstein DJ, Corbin LA, Fung MC (2000) Olanzapine-exposed pregnancies and lactation: early experience. *Journal of Clinical Psychopharmacology*, **20**: 399–403.

Goodnick PJ (1993) Verapamil prophylaxis in pregnant women with bipolar disorder. *American Journal of Psychiatry*, **150**: 10.

Gopalan P, Glance JB, Azzam PN (2014) Managing benzodiazepine withdrawal during pregnancy: case-based guidelines. *Archives of Women's Mental Health*, **17**: 167–170.

Gracious BL, Wisner KL (1997) Phenelzine use throughout pregnancy and the puerperium: case report, review of the literature, and management recommendations. *Depression and Anxiety*, **6**: 124–128.

Grigoriadis S, VonderPorten E, Mamisashvili L, *et al* (2013a) Antidepressant exposure during pregnancy and congenital malformations: Is there an association? A systematic review and meta-analysis of the best evidence. *Journal of Clinical Psychiatry*, **74**: e293–e308.

Grigoriadis S, VonderPorten E, Mamisashvili L, *et al* (2013b) Prenatal exposure to antidepressants and persistent pulmonary hypertension of the newborn: systematic review and meta-analysis. *BMJ*, **348**: f6932.

Grigoriadis S, VonderPorten E, Mamisashvili L, *et al* (2013c) The effect of prenatal antidepressant exposure on neonatal adaptation: a systematic review and meta-analysis. *Journal of Clinical Psychiatry*, **74**: e309–e320.

Grzeskowiak LE, Gilbert AL, Morrison JL (2011) Investigating outcomes following the use of selective serotonin reuptake inhibitor for treating depression in pregnancy. *Drug Safety*, **34**: 1027–1048.

Guclu S, Gol M, Dogan E, *et al* (2005) Mirtazapine use in resistant hyperemesis gravidarum: report of three cases and review of the literature. *Archives of Gynecology and Obstetrics*, **272**: 298–300.

Habermann F, Fritzsche J, Fuhlbrück F, *et al* (2013) Atypical antipsychotic drugs and pregnancy outcome: a prospective, cohort study. *Journal of Clinical Psychopharmacology*, **33**: 453–462.

Hackett LP, Ilett KF, Kristensen JH, *et al* (2005) Infant dose and safety of breastfeeding for dexamphetamine and methylphenidate in mothers with attention deficit hyperactivity disorder. *Therapeutic Drug Monitoring*, **27**: 220–221.

Hackett LP, Ilett KF, Rampono J, *et al* (2006a) Transfer of reboxetine into breastmilk, its plasma concentrations and lack of adverse events in the breastfed infant. *European Journal of Clinical Pharmacology*, **62**: 633–638.

Hackett LP, Kristensen JH, Hale TW, *et al* (2006b) Methylphenidate and breast-feeding. *Annals of Pharmacotherapy*, **40**: 1890–1891.

Hanley GE, Mintzes B (2014) Patterns of psychotropic medicine use in pregnancy in the United States from 2006 to 2011 among women with private health insurance. *BMC Pregnancy and Childbirth*, **14**: 242.

Hansen LM, Megerian G, Donnenfeld AE (1997) Haloperidol overdose during pregnancy. *Obstetrics & Gynecology*, **90**: 659–661.

Haukland LR, Kutzsche S, Hovden IAH, *et al* (2013) Neonatal seizures with reversible EEG changes after antenatal venlafaxine exposure. *Acta Paediatrica Scandinavica*, **102**: e524–e526.

Hayes RM, Pingsheng W, Shelton RC, *et al* (2012) Maternal antidepressant use and adverse outcomes: a cohort study of 228,876 pregnancies. *American Journal of Obstetrics & Gynaecology*, **49**: e1–e9.

Heikkinen T, Ekblad U, Kero P, *et al* (2002) Citalopram in pregnancy and lactation. *Clinical Pharmacology and Therapeutics*, **72**: 184–191.

Heikkinen T Ekblad U, Palo P, *et al* (2003) Pharmacokinetics of fluoxetine and norfluoxetine in pregnancy and lactation. *Clinical Pharmacology and Therapeutics*, **73**: 330–336.

Heinonen OP, Slone D, Shapiro S (1977) *Birth Defects and Drugs in Pregnancy*. Publishing Services Group.

Hemels MEH, Einarson A, Koren G, *et al* (2005) Antidepressant use during pregnancy and the rates of spontaneous abortions: a meta-analysis. *Annals of Pharmacotherapy*, **39**: 803–809.

Hendrick V, Stowe ZN, Altshuler LL, et al (2003a) Placental passage of antidepressant medications. American Journal of Psychiatry, 160: 993–996.

Hendrick V, Smith L, Suri R, et al (2003b) Birth outcomes after prenatal exposure to antidepressant medication. American Journal of Obstetrics & Gynecology, 188: 812–815.

Hernández-Diaz S, Smith CR, Shen A, et al (2012) Comparative safety of antiepileptic drugs during pregnancy. Neurology, 78: 1692–1699.

Holmes LB, Wyszynski DF, Baldwin EJ, et al (2006) Increased risk for non-syndromic cleft palate among infants exposed to lamotrigine during pregnancy. Birth Defects Research Part A: Clinical and Molecular Teratology, 76: 96–104.

Hoog SL, Cheng Y, Elpers J, et al (2013) Duloxetine and pregnancy outcomes: safety surveillance findings. International Journal of Medical Sciences, 10: 413–419.

ter Horst PJ, Larmené-Beld KH, Bosman J, et al (2014) Concentrations of venlafaxine and its main metabolite O-desmethylvenlafaxine during pregnancy. Journal of Clinical Pharmacy and Therapeutics, 39: 541–544.

Hostetter A, Ritchie JC, Stowe ZN (2000a) Amniotic fluid and umbilical cord blood concentrations of antidepressants in three women. Biological Psychiatry, 48: 1032–1034.

Hostetter A, Stowe ZN, Strader JR Jr et al (2000b) Dose of selective serotonin uptake inhibitors across pregnancy: clinical implications. Depression and Anxiety, 11: 51–57.

Huang H, Coleman S, Bridge J, et al (2014) A meta-analysis of the relationship between antidepressant use in pregnancy and the risk of preterm birth and low birthweight. General Hospital Psychiatry, 36: 13–18.

Husain MH, Stegman D, Trevino K (2005) Pregnancy and delivery while receiving vagus nerve stimulation for the treatment of major depression: a case report. Annals of General Psychiatry, 4: 16.

Huybrechts KF, Mogun H, Kowal M, et al (2011) National trends in antidepressant medication treatment among publicly insured pregnant women. General Hospital Psychiatry, 35: 265–271.

Huybrechts KF, Palmsten K, Avorn J, et al (2014a) Antidepressant use in pregnancy and the risk of cardiac defects. New England Journal of Medicine, 370: 2397–2407.

Huybrechts KF Sanghani RS, Avorn J, et al (2014b) Preterm birth and antidepressant medication use during pregnancy: a systematic review and meta-analysis. PLoS ONE, 9: e92778.

Hviid A, Melbye M, Pasternak B (2013) Use of selective serotonin reuptake inhibitors during pregnancy and risk of autism. New England Journal of Medicine, 369: 2406–2415.

Janjić V, Milanović DR, Zecević DR, et al (2013) Zuclopenthixol decanoate in pregnancy: successful outcomes in two consecutive offsprings of the same mother. Military-Medical and Pharmaceutical Review, 70: 526–529.

Jeffries WS, Bochner F (1988) The effect of pregnancy on drug pharmacokinetics. The Medical Journal of Australia, 149: 675–677.

Jensen HM, Grøn R, Lidegaard Ø, et al (2013a) The effects of maternal depression and use of antidepressants during pregnancy on risk of a child small for gestational age. Psychopharmacology, 228: 199–205.

Jensen HM, Grøn R, Lidegaard Ø, et al (2013b) Maternal depression, antidepressant use and Apgar scores in infants. British Journal of Psychiatry, 202: 347– 351.

Jimenez-Solem E, Andersen T, Petersen M, et al (2013) Prevalence of antidepressant use during pregnancy in Denmark, a nation-wide cohort study. PLoS ONE, 8: e63034.

Juric S, Newport J, Ritchie JC, et al (2009) Zolpidem (Ambien®) in pregnancy: placental passage and outcome. Archives of Women's Mental Health, 12: 441–446.

Källen B (2004) Neonate characteristics after maternal use of antidepressants in late pregnancy. Archives of Pediatric and Adolescent Medicine, 158: 312–316.

Källen B, Otterblad Olausson P (2006) Antidepressant drugs during pregnancy and infant congenital heart defect. Reproductive Toxicology, 21: 221–222.

Källén B, Reis M (2012) Neonatal complications after maternal concomitant use of SSRI and other central nervous system active drugs during the second or third trimester of pregnancy. Journal of Clinical Psychopharmacology, 32: 608–614.

Kesim M, Yaris F (2002) Mirtazapine use in two pregnant women: is it safe? *Teratology*, **66**: 204.

Khan KS, Wykes C, Gee H (1999) Quality of studies must influence inferences made from meta-analyses. *BMJ*, **319**: 918.

Kim J, Riggs KW, Misri S, *et al* (2006) Stereoselective disposition of fluoxetine and norfluoxetine during pregnancy and breast-feeding. *British Journal of Clinical Pharmacology*, **61**: 155–163.

Kim S-W, Kim K-M, Kim J-M, *et al* (2007) Use of long-acting injectable risperidone before and throughout pregnancy in schizophrenia. *Progress in Neuro-Psychopharmacology and Biological Psychiatry*, **31**: 543–545.

Klieger-Grossman C, Weitzner B, Panchaud A, *et al* (2012) Pregnancy outcomes following use of escitalopram: a prospective comparative cohort study. *Journal of Clinical Pharmacovigilance*, **52**: 766–770.

Klier CM, Mossaheb N, Saria A, *et al* (2007) Pharmacokinetics and elimination of quetiapine, venlafaxine and trazodone during pregnancy and postpartum. *Journal of Clinical Psychopharmacology*, **27**: 720–722.

Klirova M, Novak T, Kopecek M, *et al* (2008) Repetitive transcranial magnetic stimulation (rTMS) in major depressive episode during pregnancy. *Neuroendocrinology Letters*, **29**: 69–70.

Klys M, Rojek S, Rzepecka-Woźniak E (2007) Neonatal death following clozapine self-poisoning in late pregnancy: an unusual case report. *Forensic Science International*, **171**: e5–e10.

Koren G, Cohn T, Chitayat D, *et al* (2002) Use of atypical antipsychotics during pregnancy and the risk of neural tube defects in infants. *American Journal of Psychiatry*, **159**: 136–137.

Koren G, Nava-Ocampo AA, Moretti ME, *et al* (2006) Major malformations with valproic acid. *Canadian Family Physician*, **52**: 441–447.

Kozma C (2005) Neonatal toxicity and transient neurodevelopmental deficits following prenatal exposure to lithium: another clinical reports and review of the literature. *American Journal of Medical Genetics*, **132A**: 441–444.

Kulkarni J, Worsley R, Gilbert H, *et al* (2014) A prospective cohort study of antipsychotic medications in pregnancy: the first 147 pregnancies and 100 one year old babies. *PLoS ONE*, **9**: e94788.

Lattimore KA, Donn SM, Kaciroti N, *et al* (2005) Selective serotonin reuptake inhibitor (SSRI) use during pregnancy and effects on the fetus and newborn: a meta-analysis. *Journal of Perinatology*, **25**: 595–604.

Leiknes KL, Cooke MJ, Jarosch von Schweder L, *et al* (2015) Electroconvulsive therapy during pregnancy: a systematic review of case studies. *Archives of Women's Mental Health*, **18**: 1–39.

Lennestal R, Källen B (2007) Delivery outcome in relation to maternal use of some recently introduced antidepressants. *Journal of Clinical Psychopharmacology*, **27**: 607–613.

Leventhal K, Byatt N, Lundquist R (2010) Fetal cardiac arrhythmia during bupropion use. *Acta Obstetricia et Gynecologica Scandinavica*, **89**: 980–981.

Levy W, Wisniewski K (1974) Chlorpromazine causing extrapyramidal dysfunction in newborn infant of psychotic mother. *New York State Journal of Medicine*, **74**: 684–685.

Li D-K, Ferber J (2012) Treatment of depression during pregnancy and its effect on infant NICU admission. *Pharmacoepidemiology and Drug Safety*, **21** (Suppl 3): 31.

Lin H-C, Chen I-J, Chen Y-H, *et al* (2010) Maternal schizophrenia and pregnancy outcome: does use of antipsychotics make a difference? *Schizophrenia Research*, **116**: 55–60.

Lind JN, Tinker SA, Broussard CS, *et al* (2013) Maternal medication and herbal use and risk for hypospadias: data from the National Birth Defects Prevention Study, 1997–2007. *Pharmacoepidemiology and Drug Safety*, **22**: 783–793.

Lopez-Yarto M, Ruiz-Mirazo E, Holloway A, *et al* (2012) Do psychiatric medications, especially antidepressants, adversely impact on maternal metabolic outcomes? *Journal of Affective Disorders*, **141**: 120–129.

Loughhead AM, Fisher AD, Newport DJ, et al (2006a) Antidepressants in amniotic fluid: another route of fetal exposure. American Journal of Psychiatry, 163: 145.

Loughhead AM, Stowe ZN, Newport J, et al (2006b) Placental passage of tricyclic antidepressants. Biological Psychiatry, 59: 287–290.

Louik C, Lin AE, Werler MM, et al (2007) First-trimester use of selective serotonin-reuptake inhibitors and the risk of birth defects. New England Journal of Medicine, 356: 2675–2683.

Louik C, Kerr S, Mitchell AA (2014) First–trimester exposure to bupropion and risk of cardiac malformations. Pharmacoepidemiology and Drug Safety, 23: 1066–1075.

van der Lugt NM, van de Maat JS, van Kamp IL, et al (2012) Fetal, neonatal and developmental outcomes of lithium-exposed pregnancies. Early Human Development, 88: 375–378.

Lupattelli A, Spigset O, Koren G, et al (2014) Risk of vaginal bleeding and postpartum hemorrhage after use of antidepressants in pregnancy: a study from the Norwegian Mother and Child Cohort Study. Journal of Clinical Psychopharmacology, 34: 143–148.

Lutz UC, Hiemke C, Wiatr G, et al (2010) Aripiprazole in pregnancy and lactation: a case report. Journal of Clinical Psychopharmacology, 30: 204–205.

Mackay FJ, Wilton LV, Pearce GL, et al (1998) The safety of risperidone: a post-marketing study on 7684 patients. Human Psychopharmacology and Clinical Experience Journal, 13: 413–418.

Magee L, Schick B, Donnenfeld A, et al (1996) The safety of calcium channel blockers in human pregnancy: A prospective, multicenter cohort study. American Journal of Obstetrics & Gynecology, 174: 823–828.

Malm H, Klaukka T, Neuvonon PJ (2005) Risks associated with selective serotonin reuptake inhibitors in pregnancy. Obstetrics & Gynecology, 106: 1289–1296.

Margulis AV, Kang EM, Hammad TA, et al (2014) Patterns of prescription of antidepressants and antipsychotics across and within pregnancies in a population-based UK cohort. Maternal and Child Health Journal, 18: 1742–1752.

Marroun HE, White TJH, Noortje JF, et al (2014) Prenatal exposure to selective serotonin reuptake inhibitors and social responsiveness symptoms of autism: population-based study of young children. British Journal of Psychiatry, 205: 95–102.

McElhatton PR, Garbis HM, Elefant E, et al (1996) The outcome of pregnancy in 689 women exposed to therapeutic doses of antidepressants. A collaborative study of the European Network of Teratology Information Services (ENTIS). Reproductive Toxicology, 10: 285–294.

McKenna K, Koren G, Tetelbaum M, et al (2005) Pregnancy outcome of women using atypical antipsychotic drugs: a prospective comparative study. Journal of Clinical Psychiatry, 66: 444–449.

McKnight R, Adida M, Budge K, et al (2012) Lithium toxicity profile: a systematic review and meta-analyis. Lancet, 379: 721–728.

Mendhekar DN, Sharma JB, Srivastava PK, et al (2003) Clozapine and pregnancy. Journal of Clinical Psychiatry, 64: 850.

Mendhekar D, Sunder KR, Andrade C (2006a) Aripiprazole in a pregnant schizoaffective woman. Bipolar Disorders, 8: 299–300.

Mendhekar D, Sharma J, Srilakshmi P (2006b) Use of aripiprazole during late pregnancy in a woman with psychotic illness. Annals Pharmacotherapy, 40: 575.

Mervak B, Collins J, Valenstein M (2008) Case report of aripiprazole usage during pregnancy. Archives of Women's Mental Health, 11: 249–250.

Di Michele V, Ramenghi L, Sabatino G (1996) Clozapine and lorazepam administration in pregnancy. European Psychiatry, 11: 214.

Milkiewicz P, Chilton AP, Hubscher SG, et al (2003) Antidepressant induced cholestasis: hepatocellular redistribution of multidrug resistant protein (MRP2). Gut, 52: 300–303.

Misri S, Corral M, Wardrop AA, et al (2006) Quetiapine augmentation in lactation. A series of case reports. Journal of Clinical Psychopharmacology, 26: 508–511.

Misri S, Eng AB, Abizadeh J, *et al* (2013) Factors impacting decisions to decline or adhere to antidepressant medication in perinatal women with mood and anxiety disorders. *Depression and Anxiety*, **30**: 1129–1136.

Mohan MS, Patole SK, Whitehall JS (2000) Severe hypothermia in a neonate following antenatal exposure to haloperidol. *Journal of Paediatrics and Child Health*, **36**: 412–413.

de Moor RA, Mourad L, ter Haar J, *et al* (2003) Withdrawal symptoms in a neonate following exposure to venlafaxine during pregnancy. *Nederlands Tijdschrift voor Geneeskunde*, **147**: 1370–1372.

Mølgaard-Nielsen D, Hviid A (2011) Newer-generation antiepileptic drugs and the risk of major birth defects. *JAMA*, **305**: 1996–2002.

Montouris G (2003) Gabapentin exposure in human pregnancy: results from the Gabapentin Pregnancy Registry. *Epilepsy and Behavior*, **4**: 310–317.

Moradpour D, Altorfer J, Greminger P, *et al* (1994) Chlorpromazine-induced vanishing bile duct syndrome leading to biliary cirrhosis. *Hepatology*, **20**: 1437–1471.

Moreno-Bruna M-D, de Montgolfier I, Chabaud M, *et al* (2012) Case report: neonatal delayed peristalsis after in-utero exposure to clozapine. *Archives de Pediatrie*, **19**: 913–916.

Moretti ME, Maxson A, Hanna F, *et al* (2009) Evaluating the safety of St. John's Wort in human pregnancy. *Reproductive Toxicology*, **28**: 96–99.

Morrison JL, Chien C, Riggs KW, *et al* (2002) Effect of maternal fluoxetine administration on uterine blood flow, fetal blood gas status, and growth. *Pediatric Research*, **51**: 433–442.

Morrow J, Russell A, Guthrie E, *et al* (2006) Malformation risks of antiepileptic drugs in pregnancy: a prospective study from the UK Epilepsy and Pregnancy Register. *Journal of Neurology, Neurosurgery and Psychiatry*, **77**: 193–198.

Mulder EJH, Ververs FFT, de Heus R, *et al* (2011) Selective serotonin reuptake inhibitors affect neurobehavioral development in the human fetus. *Neuropsychopharmacology*, **36**: 1961–1971.

Myles N, Newall H, Ward H, *et al* (2013) Systematic meta-analysis of individual selective serotonin reuptake inhibitor medications and congenital malformations. *Australian & New Zealand Journal of Psychiatry*, **47**: 1002–1012.

Nahas Z, Bohning DE, Molloy MA, *et al* (1999) Safety and feasibility of repetitive transcranial magnetic stimulation in the treatment of anxious depression in pregnancy: a case report. *Journal of Clinical Psychiatry*, **60**: 50–52.

Nako Y, Tachibana A, Fujiu T, *et al* (2001) Neonatal thrombocytosis resulting from the maternal use of non-narcotic antischizophrenic drugs during pregnancy. *Archives of Disease of in Childhood- Fetal and Neonatal Edition*, **84**: F198–F200.

NICE (2014) *Antenatal and Postnatal Mental Health: Clinical Management and Service Guidance*. National Institute for Health and Care Excellence.

Newham JJ, Thomas SH, MacRitchie K, *et al* (2008) Birth weight of infants after maternal exposure to typical and atypical antipsychotics: prospective comparison study. *British Journal of Psychiatry*, **192**: 333–337.

Newport DJ, Viguera AC, Beach AJ, *et al* (2005) Lithium placental passage and obstetrical outcome: implications for clinical management during late pregnancy. *American Journal of Psychiatry*, **162**: 2162–2170.

Newport DJ, Calamaras MR, DeVane CL, *et al* (2007) Atypical antipsychotic administration during late pregnancy: placental passage and obstetrical outcomes. *American Journal of Psychiatry*, **164**: 1214–1220.

Nguyen H-N, Lalonde P (2003) Clozapine et grossesse. *Encéphale*, **29**: 119–124.

Nguyen T, Teoh S, Hackett P, *et al* (2011) Placental transfer of aripiprazole. *Australian and New Zealand Journal of Psychiatry*, **45**: 500–501.

Nielsen HC, Wiriyathian S, Rosenfeld R, *et al* (1983) Chlorpromazine excretion by the neonate following chronic *in utero* exposure. *Pediatric Pharmacology*, **3**: 1–5.

Nikfar S, Rahimi R, Hendoiee N, *et al* (2012) Increasing the risk of spontaneous abortion and major malformations in newborns following use of serotonin reuptake inhibitors during pregnancy: a systematic review and updated meta–analysis. *Journal of Pharmaceutical Sciences*, **20**: 75.

Nora JJ, Nora AA, Toews WH (1974) Lithium, Ebstein's anomaly and other congenital heart defects. *Lancet*, **i**: 594–595.

Nordeng H, Lindemann R, Perminov KV, *et al* (2001) Neonatal withdrawal syndrome after *in utero* exposure to selective serotonin reuptake inhibitors. *Acta Paediatrica*, **90**: 288–291.

Nordeng H, Van Gelder M, Spigset O, *et al* (2012) Pregnancy outcome after exposure to antidepressants and the role of maternal depression. *Journal of Clinical Psychopharmacology*, **32**: 186–194.

Nulman I, Rovet J, Stewart DE, *et al* (1997) Neurodevelopment of children exposed in utero to antidepressant drugs. *New England Journal of Medicine*, **336**: 258–263.

Nulman I, Rovet J, Stewart DE, *et al* (2002) Child development following exposure to tricyclic antidepressants or fluoxetine throughout fetal life: a prospective, controlled study. *American Journal of Psychiatry*, **159**: 1889–1895.

Nulman I, Koren G, Rovet J, *et al* (2012) Neurodevelopment of children following prenatal exposure to venlafaxine, selective serotonin reuptake inhibitors, or untreated maternal depression. *American Journal of Psychiatry*, **169**: 1165–1174.

Oberlander TF, Grunau RE, Fitzgerald C, *et al* (2005) Pain reactivity in 2-month-old infants after prenatal and postnatal serotonin reuptake inhibitor medication exposure. *Pediatrics*, **115**: 411–425.

O'Connor M, Johnson GH, James DI (1981) Intrauterine effect of phenothiazines. *Medical Journal of Australia*, **1**: 416–417.

Öhman I, Vitols S, Tomson T (2005) Pharmacokinetics of gabapentin during delivery, in the neonatal period, and lactation: does a fetal accumulation occur during pregnancy? *Epilepsia*, **10**: 1621–1624.

Oren DA, Wisner KL, Spinelli M, *et al* (2002) An open trial of morning light therapy for treatment of antepartum depression. *American Journal of Psychiatry*, **159**: 666–669.

Ornoy A (2006) Neuroteratogens in man: An overview with special emphasis on the teratogenicity of antiepileptic drugs in pregnancy. *Reproductive Toxicology*, **22**: 214–226.

Osborne LM, Birndorf CA, Szodkny LE, *et al* (2014) Returning to tricyclic antidepressants for depression during childbearing: clinical and dosing challenges. *Archives of Women's Mental Health*, **17**: 239–246.

Pakalapati RK, Bolisetty S, Austin M-P, *et al* (2006) Neonatal seizures from in utero venlafaxine exposure. *Journal of Pediatrics and Child Health*, **42**: 737–738.

Palmsten K, Huybrechts KF, Michels K, *et al* (2013) Antidepressant use and risk for pre-eclampsia. *Epidemiology*, **24**: 682–691.

Pastuzak A, Schick-Boschetto B, Zuber C, *et al* (1993) Pregnancy outcome following first-trimester exposure to fluoxetine (Prozac). *JAMA*, **269**: 2246–2248.

Pawluski JL, Brain UM, Underhill CM, *et al* (2012) Prenatal SSRI exposure alters neonatal corticosteroid binding globulin, infant cortisol levels, and emerging HPA function. *Psychoneuroendocrinology*, **37**: 1019–1028.

Peindl KS, Masand P, Mannelli P, *et al* (2007) Polypharmacy in pregnant women with major psychiatric illness: a pilot study. *Journal of Psychiatric Practice*, **13**: 385–391.

Peitl MV, Petrić D, Peitl V (2010) Ziprasidone as a possible cause of cleft palate in a newborn. *Psychiatria Danubina*, **22**: 117–119.

Peng M, Gao K, Ding Y, *et al* (2013) Effects of prenatal exposure to atypical antipsychotics on postnatal development and growth of infants: a case-controlled, prospective study. *Psychopharmacology*, **228**: 577–584.

Petrenaite V, Sabers A, Hansen-Schwartz J (2005) Individual changes in lamotrigine plasma concentrations during pregnancy. *Epilepsy Research*, **65**: 185–188.

Pilo C, Wilde K, Winbladh B (2006) Pregnancy, delivery and neonatal complications after treatment with anticonvulsants. *Acta Obstetricia Gynecologica Scandinavica*, **85**: 643–646.

Pinelli JM, Symington AJ, Cunningham KA, *et al* (2002) Case report and review of the perinatal implications of maternal lithium use. *American Journal of Obstetrics & Gynecology*, **187**: 245–249.

Platt JE, Friedhoff AJ, Broman SH, et al (1988) Effects of prenatal exposure to neuroleptic drugs on children's growth. Neuropsychopharmacology, 1: 205–212.

Polen K, Rasmussen S, Riehle-Colarusso T, et al (2013) Association between reported venlafaxine use in early pregnancy and birth defects, National Birth Defects Prevention Study, 1997–2007. Birth Defects Research (Part A), 97: 28–35.

Pottegård A, Hallas J, Anderson JT, et al (2014) First-trimester exposure to methylphenidate: a population-based cohort study. Journal of Clinical Psychiatry, 75: e88–e93.

Potts AL, Young KL, Carter BS, et al (2007) Necrotizing enterocolitis associated with in utero and breast milk exposure to the selective serotonin reuptake inhibitor, escitalopram. Journal of Perinatology, 27: 120–122.

Poulson E, Robson JM (1964) Effects of phenelzine and some related compounds on pregnancy. Journal of Endocrinology, 30: 205–215.

Prakash S, Chadda RK (2014) Teratogenicity with olanzapine. Indian Journal of Psychological Medicine, 36: 91–93.

Rahimi R, Nikfar S, Abdollahi M (2006) Pregnancy outcomes following exposure to serotonin reuptake inhibitors: a meta-analysis of clinical trials. Reproductive Toxicology, 22: 571–575.

Rais TB, Rais A (2014) Association between antidepressant use during pregnancy and autistic spectrum disorders: a meta–analysis. Innovations in Clinical Neuroscience, 11: 18–22.

Ramos E, St-Andre M, Rey E, et al (2008) Duration of antidepressant use during pregnancy and risk of major congenital malformations. British Journal of Psychiatry, 192: 344–350.

Ramos E, St-Andre M, Bérard A (2010) Association between reported venlafaxine use during pregnancy and infants born small for gestational age. Canadian Journal of Psychiatry, 55: 643–652.

Rampono J, Proud S, Hackett PL, et al (2004) A pilot study of newer antidepressant concentrations in cord and maternal serum and possible affects in the neonate. International Journal of Neuropsychopharmacology, 7: 329–334.

Rampono J, Simmer K, Ilett KF, et al (2009) Placental transfer of SSRI and SNRI antidepressants and effects on the neonate. Pharmacopsychiatry, 42: 95–100.

Ratnayake T, Libretto SE (2002) No complications with risperidone treatment before and throughout pregnancy and during the nursing period. Journal of Clinical Psychiatry, 63: 76–77.

Reis M, Källén B (2008) Maternal use of antipsychotics in early pregnancy and delivery outcome. Journal of Clinical Psychopharmacology, 28: 279–288.

Reis M, Källén B (2010) Delivery outcome after maternal use of antidepressant drugs in pregnancy: an update using Swedish data. Psychological Medicine, 40: 1723–1733.

Rohde A, Dembinski J, Dorn C (2003) Mirtazapine (Remergil) for treatment resistant hyperemesis gravidarum: rescue of a twin pregnancy. Archives of Gynecology and Obstetrics, 268: 219–221.

Rosa F (1994) Medicaid antidepressant pregnancy exposure outcomes. Reproductive Toxicology, 8: 444–445.

Rowe M, Gowda BA, Taylor D, et al (2012) Neonatal hypoglycaemia following maternal olanzapine therapy during pregnancy: a case report. Therapeutic Advances in Psychopharmacology, 2: 265–268.

Rybakowski JK (2001) Moclobemide in pregnancy. Pharmacopsychiatry, 34: 82–83.

Sadowski A, Todorow M, Brojeni PY, et al (2013) Pregnancy outcomes following maternal exposure to second-generation antipsychotics given with other psychotropic drugs. BMJ Open, 3: e003062.

Saks BR (2001) Mirtazapine, treatment of depression, anxiety, and hyperemesis gravidarum in the pregnant patient. A report of seven cases. Archives of Women's Mental Health, 3: 165–170.

Salkeld E, Ferris LE, Juurlink DN (2008) The risk of postpartum haemorrhage with selective serotonin reuptake inhibitors and other antidepressants. Journal of Clinical Psychopharmacology, 28: 230–234.

Sanz EJ, De Las Cuevas C, Kiuru A, *et al* (2005) Selective serotonin reuptake inhibitors in pregnant women and neonatal withdrawal syndrome: a database analysis. *Lancet*, **365**: 482–487.

Sayar GH, Ozten E, Tufan E, *et al* (2014) Transcranial magnetic stimulation during pregnancy. *Archives of Women's Mental Health*, **17**: 311–316.

Schimmell MS, Katz EZ, Shaag Y, *et al* (1991) Toxic neonatal effects following maternal clomipramine therapy. *Clinical Toxicology*, **29**: 479–484.

Schmidt RJ Tancredi DJ, Krakowiak P, *et al* (2014) Maternal intake of supplemental iron and risk of autism spectrum disorder. *American Journal of Epidemiology*, **180**: 890–900.

Schwarzer V, Heep A, Gembruch U, *et al* (2008) Treatment resistant hyperemesis gravidarum in a patient with type 1 diabetes mellitus: neonatal withdrawal symptoms after successful antiemetic therapy with mirtazapine. *Archives of Gynecology and Obstetrics*, **277**: 67–69.

Sethi S (2006) Clozapine in pregnancy. *Indian Journal of Psychiatry*, **48**: 196–197.

Sharma A, Sayeed N, Kesh CRJ, *et al* (2011) High dose zolpidem induced fetal neural tube defects. *Current Drug Safety*, **6**: 128–129.

Siegismund Kjaersgaard MI, Parner EK, Vestergaard M, *et al* (2013) Prenatal antidepressant exposure and risk of spontaneous abortion – a population-based study. *PLoS ONE*, **8**: e72095.

Simhandl C, Zhoglami A, Pinder R (1998) Pregnancy during use of mirtazapine. *European Neuropsychopharmacology*, **8**: S146.

Simon GE, Cunningham ML, Davis RL (2002) Outcomes of prenatal antidepressant exposure. *American Journal of Psychiatry*, **159**: 2055–2061.

Sit DK, Perel JM, Helsel JC, *et al* (2008) Changes in antidepressant metabolism and dosing across pregnancy and early postpartum. *Journal of Clinical Psychiatry*, **69**: 652–658.

Sokolover N, Merlob P, Klinger G (2008) Neonatal recurrent prolonged hypothermia associated with maternal mirtazapine treatment during pregnancy. *Canadian Journal of Clinical Pharmacology*, **15**: e188–190.

Sørensen MJ, Grønborg TK, Christensen J, *et al* (2013) Antidepressant exposure in pregnancy and risk of autistic spectrum disorders. *Clinical Epidemiology*, **5**: 449–459.

Spigset O, Brede WR, Zahlsen K (2007) Excretion of methylphenidate in breast milk. *Am J Psychiatry*, **164**: 348.

Spyropoulos AC, Zervas IM, Soldatos CR (2006) Hip dysplasia following a case of olanzapine during pregnancy. *Archives of Women's Mental Health*, **9**: 219–222.

Stoner SC, Sommi RW, Marken P, *et al* (1997) Clozapine use in two full term pregnancies. *Journal of Clinical Psychiatry*, **58**: 364–365.

Su K-P, Shen WW, Huang S-Y (2001) Omega-3 fatty acids as a psychotherapeutic agent for a pregnant schizophrenic patient. *European Neuropsychopharmacology*, **11**: 295–299.

Suri R, Altshuler L, Hendrick V, *et al* (2004) The impact of depression and fluoxetine on obstetrical outcome. *Archives of Women's Mental Health*, **7**: 193–200.

Swortfiguer D, Cissoko H, Giraudeau B, *et al* (2005) Retentissement neonatal de l'exposition aux benzodiazepines en fin de grossesse. *Archives de Pédiatrie*, **12**: 1327–1331.

Toh S, Mitchell AA, Louik C, *et al* (2009) Selective serotonin reuptake inhibitor use and risk of gestational hypertension. *American Journal of Psychiatry*, **166**: 320–328.

Toh S, Qian L, Cheetham CC, *et al* (2013) Prevalence and trends in the use of antipsychotic medications during pregnancy in the U.S., 2001–2007: a population-based study of 585,615 deliveries. *Archives of Women's Mental Health*, **16**: 149–157.

Treichel M, Schwendener Scholl K, Kessler U, *et al* (2009) Is there a correlation between venlafaxine therapy during pregnancy and a higher incidence of necrotizing enterocolitis? *World Journal of Pediatrics*, **5**: 65–67.

Twaites BR, Wilton LV, Shakir SAW (2007) The safety of quetiapine: results of a post-marketing surveillance study on 1728 patients in England. *Journal of Psychopharmacology*, **21**: 392–399.

UKTIS (2014) *Use of Trazodone in Pregnancy*. UK Teratology Information Service.

UKTIS (2015) *Use of Bupriopion in Pregnancy*. UK Teratology Information Service.

Uguz F (2013) Low-dose mirtazapine added to selective serotonin reuptake inhibitors in pregnant women with major depression or panic disorder including symptoms of severe nausea, insomnia and decreased appetite: three cases. *Journal of Maternal, Fetal and Neonatal Medicine,* **26**: 1066–1068.

Uguz F (2014) Low-dose mirtazapine in treatment of major depression developed following severe nausea and vomiting in pregnancy: two cases. *General Hospital Psychiatry,* **36**: e125–e126.

Upadhyaya HP, Brady KT, Liao J, *et al* (2003) Neuroendocrine and behavioral responses to dopaminergic agonists in adolescents with alcohol abuse. *Psychopharmacology,* **166**: 95–101.

Vajda FJ, O'Brien TJ, Hitchcock A, *et al* (2003) The Australian registry of anti-epileptic drugs in pregnancy: experience after 30 months. *Journal of Clinical Neuroscience,* **10**: 543–549.

Vajda FJ, Hitchcock A, Graham J, *et al* (2006) Foetal malformations and seizure control: 52 months data of the Australian Pregnancy Registry. *European Journal of Neurology,* **13**: 645–654.

Veiby G, Daltveit A, Schjølberg S, *et al* (2013) Exposure to antiepileptic drugs in utero and child development: A prospective population-based study. *Epilepsia,* **54**: 1462–1472.

de Vera MA, Bérard A (2012) Antidepressant use during pregnancy and the risk of pregnancy-induced hypertension. *British Journal of Clinical Pharmacology,* **74**: 362–369.

Vigod S, Gomes T, Wilton S, *et al* (2015) Antipsychotic drug use in pregnancy: high dimensional, propensity matched, population based cohort study. *BMJ,* **350**: h2298.

Vohra A (2013) Olanzapine-induced peripheral oedema in a pregnant woman with bipolar affective disorder. *German Journal of Psychiatry,* **16**: 84–86.

Waldman M, Safferman A (1993) Pregnancy and clozapine. *American Journal of Psychiatry,* **150**: 168–169.

Walfisch A, Sermer C, Matok I, *et al* (2011) Perception of teratogenic risk and the rated likelihood of pregnancy termination: association with maternal depression. *Canadian Journal of Psychiatry,* **56**: 761–767.

Wang L-H, Lin C-C, Chen Y-H, *et al* (2010) Increased risk of adverse pregnancy outcomes in women receiving zolpidem during pregnancy. *Clinical Pharmacology and Therapeutics,* **88**: 369–374.

Warburton W, Hertzman C, Oberlander TF (2010) A register study of the impact of stopping third trimester selective serotonin reuptake inhibitor exposure on neonatal health. *Acta Psychiatrica Scandinavica,* **121**: 471–479.

Watanabe N, Kasahara M, Sugibayashi R, *et al* (2011) Perinatal use of aripiprazole: a case report. *Journal of Clinical Psychopharmacology,* **31**: 337–378.

Wen SW, Yang Q, Garner P, *et al* (2006) Selective serotonin reuptake inhibitors and adverse pregnancy outcomes. *American Journal of Obstetrics & Gynecology,* **194**: 961–966.

Werremeyer A (2009) Ziprasidone and citalopram use in pregnancy and lactation in a woman with psychotic depression. *American Journal of Psychiatry,* **166**: 1298.

Wieck A, Rao S, Sein K, *et al* (2007) A survey of antiepileptic prescribing to women of childbearing potential in psychiatry. *Archives of Women's Mental Health,* **10**: 83–85.

Wikner BN, Källén B (2011) Are hypnotic benzodiazepine receptor agonists teratogenic in humans? *Journal of Clinical Psychopharmacology,* **31**: 356–359.

Wikner BN, Stiller CO, Bergman U, *et al* (2007a) Use of benzodiazepines and benzodiazepine receptor agonists during pregnancy: neonatal outcome and congenital malformations. *Pharmacoepidemiology and Drug Safety,* **16**: 1203–1210.

Wikner BN, Stiller CO, Källén B, *et al* (2007b) Use of benzodiazepines and benzodiazepine receptor agonists during pregnancy: maternal characteristics. *Pharmacoepidemiology and Drug Safety,* **16**: 988–994.

Williams JH, Hepner DL (2004) Risperidone and exaggerated hypotension during a spinal anesthetic. *Anesthetics and Analgesia,* **98**: 240–241.

Windhager E, Kim S-W, Saria A, *et al* (2014) Perinatal use of aripiprazole: plasma levels, placental transfer and child outcome in 3 new cases. *Journal of Clinical Psychopharmacology*, **34**: 637–641.

Winterfeld U, Klinger G, Panchaud A, *et al* (2015) Pregnancy outcome following maternal exposure to mirtazapine: a multicenter, prospective study. *Journal of Clinical Psychopharmacology*, **35**: 250–259.

Wirz-Justice A, Bader A, Frisch U, *et al* (2011) A randomized, double-blind, placebo-controlled study of light therapy for antepartum depression. *Journal of Clinical Psychiatry*, **72**: 986–993.

Wisner KL, Perel JM, Wheeler SB (1993) Tricyclic dose requirements across pregnancy. *American Journal of Psychiatry*, **150**: 1541–1542.

Wisner KL, Perel JM, Peindl KS, *et al* (1997) Effects of the postpartum period on nortriptyline pharmacokinetics. *Psychopharmacology Bulletin*, **33**: 243–248.

Wisner KL, Zarin DA, Holmboe ES, *et al* (2000) Risk-benefit decision making for treatment of depression during pregnancy. *American Journal of Psychiatry*, **157**: 1933–1940.

Wisner KL, Peindl KS, Perel JM, *et al* (2002) Verapamil treatment for women with bipolar disorder. *Biological Psychiatry*, **51**: 745–752.

Yaris F, Kadioglu M, Kesim M, *et al* (2004) Newer antidepressants in pregnancy: prospective outcome of a case series. *Reproductive Toxicology*, **19**: 235–238.

Yaris F, Ulku C, Kesim M, *et al* (2005) Psychotropic drugs in pregnancy: a case-control study. *Progress in Neuro-Psychopharmacology and Biological Psychiatry*, **29**: 333–338.

Yazdy MM, Mitchell AA, Louik C, *et al* (2014) Use of selective serotonin-reuptake inhibitors during pregnancy and the risk of clubfoot. *Epidemiology*, **25**: 859–865.

Yeshayahu Y (2007) The use of olanzapine in pregnancy and congenital cardiac and musculoskeletal abnormalities. *American Journal of Psychiatry*, **164**: 1759–1760.

Yingling DR Utter G, Vengalil S, *et al* (2002) Calcium channel blocker, nimodipine, for the treatment of bipolar disorder during pregnancy. *American Journal of Obstetrics & Gynecology*, **187**: 1711–1712.

Yogev Y, Ben-Haroush A, Kaplan B (2002) Maternal clozapine treatment and decreased fetal heart rate variability. *International Journal of Gynecology & Obstetrics*, **79**: 259–260.

Yonkers KA, Gotman N, Smith MV, *et al* (2011) Does antidepressant use attenuate the risk of a major depressive episode in pregnancy? *Epidemiology*, **22**: 848–854.

Zeskind PS, Stephens LE (2004) Maternal selective serotonin reuptake inhibitor use during pregnancy and newborn behaviour. *Pediatrics*, **113**: 368–375.

# Further reading

Galbally M, Snellen M, Lewis A (2014) *Psychopharmacology and Pregnancy: Treatment Efficacy, Risks and Guidelines*. Springer-Verlag.

Yonkers K, Wisner KL, Stewart DE, *et al* (2012) The management of depression during pregnancy: a report from the American Psychiatric Association and American College of Obstetricians and Gynecologists. *Focus*, **10**: 78–89.

# CHAPTER 9

# Physical treatments and breastfeeding

It is without doubt that breastfeeding has enormous health benefits for both infants and their mothers. Bottle-fed infants are more prone to infections, allergies and being overweight at school entry, and are more likely to develop type 1 (insulin-dependent) diabetes and childhood cancers. Mothers who do not breastfeed are at increased risk of obesity, osteoporosis, and ovarian and breast cancer in later life. Breastfeeding can promote mother–infant interaction and increase maternal self-esteem. It is in this context, together with the recommendations from health organisations that breastfeeding must be promoted, that the treatment of mothers with mental illness sits.

There is a rapidly expanding evidence base. Clinicians should ensure that they contact a specialist drug information service before prescribing to ensure that they have the most up-to-date information.

## Factors influencing infant exposure

Most drugs pass into breast milk, and the amount is influenced by several factors (Box 9.1). There are additional factors which influence the amount the infant receives (summarised in Box 9.2).

---

**Box 9.1 Factors affecting drug concentration in breast milk**

- Maternal plasma level: dependent upon dose, timing and route of administration, maternal metabolism and excretion
- Drug half-life
- Lipid solubility: breast milk is fatty and therefore concentrates lipophilic drugs, including psychotropics
- Protein binding: free drugs transfer into breast milk
- Time since delivery: in the early postpartum there are larger gaps between alveolar cells in the breast, increasing the amount of drug that passes from maternal blood. After 4 days this reduces.
- Fat content of milk: lipophilic drugs will show increased transfer in hind milk compared with fore milk.

---

## General guidelines:

- Sick or preterm infants are more vulnerable than healthy term infants, so exercise additional caution.
- If possible use drugs with a short half-life so that there is the possibility of timing feeds when maternal serum levels are lowest, i.e. just before the next dose. Another option is for the mother to express milk when serum levels are highest and discard that sample. However, these should not be hard and fast rules, as they may not be possible with a hungry demand-fed infant and can be one obstacle too many for a depressed mother.
- If maternal sleep deprivation is a problem, advise the mother to express milk if possible (before next dose) and arrange for someone else to undertake night feeds, or consider whether supplementing with formula is a suitable option.
- Monitor the feeding, activity level, sleep and consciousness level of any breastfed infant whose mother is taking psychotropics.
- Be sensitive to the feelings of any mother who has to stop breastfeeding, is unable to or does not want to. It is all too easy to engender guilt and self-blame.
- Use the same drug in pregnancy as in breastfeeding to avoid exposing an infant to two different drugs.

# Antidepressants

Potential risks to an infant from exposure to an antidepressant via breast milk must be balanced against the considerable body of existing knowledge about the adverse effects of untreated maternal depression on infant development (Stein *et al*, 2014). In addition, it is not advisable to change from a drug that the fetus has already been exposed to during pregnancy, as we have no data on exposure to one drug during pregnancy and a different drug during breastfeeding.

---

**Box 9.2 Factors affecting infant plasma drug levels**

- Amount of drug ingested: dependent upon whether the infant is exclusively breastfed or not, whether fore or hind milk is ingested, and timing since last maternal dose. Infants usually require 150 ml/kg/day of milk.
- Infant metabolism: neonates have a reduced capacity to metabolise drugs for at least the first 2 weeks; this could be extended if the infant is preterm or ill.
- Infant excretion: the neonatal kidney is less efficient than that of an adult and the glomerular filtration rate does not become equivalent to that of an adult until 2–5 months.
- Central nervous system exposure: the blood–brain barrier is immature in neonates.

---

## Tricyclic antidepressants

Yoshida & Kumar (1996) reviewed the available literature on tricyclic antidepressants (TCAs) and breastfeeding. Many of these studies were of single cases only; the largest cohort was 15 and the total number of mother–infant pairs was 44. There appeared to be considerable inter-individual variation in the level of TCAs and their metabolites in plasma and milk samples in women taking the same dose.

There are some reports of amitriptyline concentrations being higher in milk than in maternal serum. Levels of TCAs were undetectable in most infants, but there were low levels of 10-hydroxynortriptyline in two babies aged 3 and 8 weeks (Wisner & Perel, 1991). There are two cases of apparent toxicity. One occurred in an infant exposed to doxepin who became pale, sweaty and drowsy with depressed respiration, and recovered on cessation of breastfeeding (Matheson et al, 1985). In the other case, (Frey et al, 1999), the 9-day-old infant became hypotonic with poor feeding and vomiting. His mother had taken doxepin during late pregnancy and while breastfeeding. Otherwise, there were no adverse events associated with TCAs.

The only group to follow up exposed infants was Buist & Janson (1995), who assessed at 3–5 years of age the children of 30 women who had breastfed while taking dothiepin, and the children of 36 non-depressed women. There were no differences in cognitive scores between the two groups. However, marital conflict and child behavioural disturbances were more common in the dothiepin group – a finding which could be explained by the maternal depression.

Following the 1996 review, Yoshida et al (1997a) studied 10 breastfeeding mothers who were taking TCAs, comparing outcomes in them and their infants with 15 mothers and their bottle-fed infants. Maternal plasma levels had a linear relationship with oral dose and closely reflected the concentrations in milk. The daily dose ingested by the infants was around 1% of the maternal dose/kg, and very small amounts of TCAs were detected in infant plasma and urine. There were no acute toxic effects seen in the breastfed infants and no evidence of developmental delay when compared with the bottle-fed babies.

In summary, TCAs have been widely prescribed and, with the exception of doxepin, appear to be relatively safe in breastfeeding. Levels in infant serum are either low or undetectable – although, as Gentile (2014) points out, there are only 107 cases in the literature in which infant outcome is described. TCAs are toxic in overdose, which may be a risk to the mother or to small children in the household who may accidentally ingest them. The main side-effects are sedation, anticholinergic side-effects and postural hypotension, all of which could be problematic for new mothers. The drug with the lowest toxicity in overdose is lofepramine, and those with lowest levels in breast milk are nortriptyline and imipramine.

## Selective serotonin reuptake inhibitors

### Fluoxetine

Fluoxetine is the selective serotonin reuptake inhibitor (SSRI) with the most published data on its use in breastfeeding mothers. Doses of 20–40 mg (Heikkinen *et al*, 2002*a*) and 20 mg or less (Hendrick *et al*, 2001*a*) during pregnancy produce relatively low trough fluoxetine/norfluoxetine concentrations. The first of these studies observed that infants had umbilical vein levels 65% and 72%, respectively, of maternal levels at birth; the estimated infant exposures were 2.4% of maternal dose at 2 weeks of age and 3.8% at 2 months.

There are three single case reports of exposure to fluoxetine via breastfeeding from the early 1990s (Isenberg, 1990; Burch & Wells, 1992; Lester *et al*, 1993). The dose in each case was 20 mg. There were no adverse events in the first two cases, but the infant in the third case developed colic, vomiting and watery stools. Taddio *et al* (1996) reported on 10 women nursing 11 infants. The average daily dose of fluoxetine and its metabolite received by the infant was 6.5%. This was considered safe, as it is less than 10% of the maternal dose. No adverse events were reported during the short period of observation. However, Brent & Wisner (1998) reported a 3-week-old infant breastfed by a mother taking fluoxetine, carbamazepine and buspirone, who had 60–90 second episodes in which her eyes rolled back, her limbs stretched out and she became limp. These did not recur, but at 4 months of age, she began having episodes in which she became limp and unresponsive for a few seconds several times per week. Investigations revealed nothing and she displayed no further symptoms at 1 year of age.

Since then, there has been a report of a term infant whose mother had taken 40 mg fluoxetine throughout pregnancy. During breastfeeding the infant became sleepy, hypotonic, difficult to rouse and pyrexial, fed poorly and began to moan with an expiratory grunt (Hale *et al*, 2001). She had been normal at birth and the symptoms remitted on cessation of breastfeeding. No infectious or metabolic cause was found for her symptoms. It is assumed that having been exposed to fluoxetine *in utero*, and via breast milk in addition, she had high plasma levels of the drug. Exposure to long half-life drugs via breast milk could lead to accumulation and toxicity in neonates, who are unable to metabolise them efficiently. Kristensen *et al* (1999) demonstrated that neonates exposed to fluoxetine during pregnancy and via breast milk had higher concentrations of fluoxetine and norfluoxetine. Stereoselective disposition of fluoxetine and its metabolite in the mother, fetus, breast milk and infant leads to greater exposure of the infant to the biologically active enantiomer S-norfluoxetine (Kim *et al*, 2006).

Epperson *et al* (2003) studied the effect of fluoxetine in breast milk on platelet serotonin and observed that all but one infant experienced little or no decline, suggesting that there were minimal effects on peripheral and central serotonin transporter blockade. In the remaining infant, levels dropped substantially and were associated with a measurable fluoxetine level. Yoshida and colleagues (1998*a*) tracked the development of 4 infants exposed to fluoxetine *in utero* until the age of 12–13 months using the Bayley scales and found no evidence of delay.

Chambers and colleagues (1999) observed an excess of breastfed infants who weighed less than two standard deviations below the mean when their mothers were taking fluoxetine. However, Hendrick *et al* (2003) report that breastfed infants of depressed mothers who were taking antidepressants (citalopram, fluoxetine, fluvoxamine, paroxetine, sertraline or venlafaxine) do not gain any more weight than infants of euthymic mothers or normative values for 6-month-old infants.

Taking all the above in consideration, fluoxetine should be avoided in breastfeeding in very young, preterm or sick infants who may have immature or impaired metabolism. If it is unavoidable, keep to the lowest possible therapeutic dose and monitor the infant's well-being very closely. If high doses, e.g. 60 mg, must be used (such as in the treatment of bulimia nervosa), the mother should be advised not to breastfeed. The advantages and disadvantages of various sampling and analysis methods are discussed by Suri *et al* (2002).

## Paroxetine

The mean estimated dose of paroxetine to infants has been reported at 0.7–0.9% of the maternal dose, with the highest concentrations in breast milk occurring 4–7 h after ingestion (Öhman *et al*, 1999). Others report breast milk concentrations of 1.13% (Begg *et al*, 1999) and 1.1% (Misri *et al*, 2000) of the maternal dose. This last study found infant plasma levels below the assay's ability to detect them, and the second found levels undetectable in all but one infant, whose level was unquantifiable. Paroxetine is certainly present in breast milk (Stowe *et al*, 2000), but again this study found undetectable amounts in infant sera and observed no adverse events.

Merlob *et al* (2004) did not find any effect of paroxetine on infant weight at 6 and 12 months and observed no adverse events other than one infant being reported as irritable. Developmental milestones in those infants exposed were normal. The low levels of paroxetine found in infant plasma, the lack of adverse events and the fact that it has no active metabolites make paroxetine a potential choice for breastfeeding mothers.

## Sertraline

Sertraline has a weak metabolite and has been detected in breast milk, but only low or undetectable levels have been observed in infant plasma (Altshuler *et al*, 1995; Mammen *et al*, 1997; Stowe *et al*, 1997; Kristensen *et al*, 1998; Epperson *et al*, 2001; Perel *et al*, 2003; Stowe *et al*, 2003). Breast milk levels peak between 1 and 9 h post-ingestion, with the lowest levels occurring 1 h before the next dose.

Mean estimates of infant exposure range from 0.54 to 0.90% of the maternal dose for sertraline, and from 0.49 to 1.32% for *N*-desmethylsertraline.

Epperson *et al* (2001) demonstrated unaltered platelet serotonin uptake in the infants of nursing mothers, suggesting that peripheral or central serotonin transport is unaffected by exposure to sertraline via breast milk. No adverse events have been reported, other than withdrawal symptoms in an infant breastfed after the mother had taken 200 mg sertraline daily throughout pregnancy (Kent & Laidlaw, 1995). Hendrick *et al* (2001*b*) compared concentration of sertraline, paroxetine and fluvoxamine in breastfeeding women. Sertraline was detected in the serum of 24% of exposed infants, but the levels were low and there were no adverse events reported. The likelihood of a detectable infant serum level was increased if the mother's dose was 100 mg or above. Overall, there have now been more than 100 cases reported, with no adverse events identified.

### Citalopram

Spigset *et al* (1997) demonstrated in two cases a relative dose for the infant of 1.8% of maternal dose, which is less than that reported for fluoxetine, but higher than for paroxetine and sertraline. Rampono and colleagues (2000) studied seven women and found infant doses of 3.7% for citalopram and 1.4% for desmethylcitalopram. There were no adverse events. Lepola *et al* (2000) reported on seven women and found an infant dose of 0.03%. Two case reports later that year reported infant doses of 5.4% (Schmidt *et al*, 2000) and 4.8% (Jensen *et al*, 1997). The latter study found levels in milk higher than in maternal serum, and the mother in the study by Schmidt *et al* reported that her infant slept uneasily after 2–3 nights of citalopram treatment.

Heikkinen *et al* (2002*b*) monitored 11 women taking citalopram and 10 matched controls. They found infant doses of 0.3% at 2 weeks and 0.2% at 2 months. All infants were followed up for 1 year, and there were no differences in weight or development between the exposed infants and the controls. In a prospective cohort study, Lee *et al* (2004*a*) assessed 31 breastfeeding women taking citalopram, 12 non-breastfeeding women with depression taking citalopram and 31 healthy women matched by age and parity. They found no differences between the groups in the rate of adverse events and no events related to citalopram, but seven women in the depressed control groups were taking other SSRIs.

### Escitalopram

Ilett *et al* (2005) reported on five lactating mothers taking escitalopram and their infants. Relative infant doses in milk were 4.5 ±1.8% for escitalopram and 1.7 ±0.7% for desmethylescitalopram. Both were undetectable in infant plasma in the two infants sampled. Castberg & Spigset (2006) published a case report of a breastfeeding woman treated with escitalopram, initially alone and then in combination with valproate. The relative doses of escitalopram to the infant were 5.1% when used alone and 7.7% when valproate was added. Rampono *et al* (2006) studied eight breastfeeding women and reported a mean relative infant dose of escitalopram and its major metabolite of 5.3%. No adverse effects were reported.

### Duloxetine

An open-label study observed the pharmacokinetics of 40 mg duloxetine in 6 nursing mothers (Lobo *et al*, 2008). The mean milk:plasma ratio was 0.25, and the infant dose was estimated at 0.14% of the maternal dose. Two single case reports have been published: one reported an absolute infant dose of 7.6 µg/L and a relative infant dose of 0.81% (Boyce *et al*, 2011), while the other reported a relative infant dose of 0.82% of the mother's weight-adjusted dose (Briggs *et al*, 2009).

### Fluvoxamine

Early single case reports estimated the milk:plasma ratio for fluvoxamine as 0.29 (Wright *et al*, 1991; Yoshida *et al*, 1997b). A later case study found a higher milk:plasma ratio (1.32) and a mean infant dose of 1.58% of the maternal dose (Hägg & Spigset, 2000). Piontek and colleagues (2001) studied two mother–infant pairs and found infant serum levels too low to quantify, as did Hendrick *et al* (2001b) (mean infant dose 1.38%) and Kristensen *et al* (2002) (0.8%). Fluvoxamine has no active metabolites. The only adverse event potentially related to fluvoxamine was jaundice that resolved spontaneously despite continuation of the drug and breastfeeding.

## Venlafaxine and desvenlafaxine

A small case series of three mothers and their infants found that the mean dose of venlafaxine received by the infants was 7.6% of the maternal weight-adjusted dose (Ilett *et al*, 1998). There were no adverse effects. Hendrick and colleagues (2001c) studied two mother–infant pairs. No venlafaxine was detectable in infant serum; low levels of the metabolite O-desmethylvenlafaxine (O-DV) were detected, but there were no adverse effects. Ilett *et al* (2002) reported on six women and their infants. Mean maternal plasma values for venlafaxine and O-DV were 2.5 and 2.74, respectively, which led to mean relative infant doses of 3.2% for venlafaxine and 3.2% for O-DV. There were no adverse events observed in the infants.

An infant whose mother had been taking venlafaxine 375 mg daily during pregnancy presented with symptoms of lethargy, poor sucking ability, and dehydration at 2 days of age. The symptoms subsided over 1 week of breastfeeding, and the authors concluded that they were probably withdrawal symptoms that were reduced by the venlafaxine in breast milk (Koren *et al*, 2006). A prospective study of 13 women and their nursing infants reported a mean milk:plasma ratio of 275.3% (CI 1.448–4.057). There were statistically significant time courses of excretion for venlafaxine ($R = 0.36$, $F = 6.82$, $P < 0.02$), O-DV ($R = 0.48$, $F = 4.41$, $P < 0.009$), and combined venlafaxine/O-DV ($R = 0.51$, $F = 5.16$, $P < 0.004$), with the highest venlafaxine and O-DV concentrations in the breast milk occurring

8 h after maternal ingestion. Infant plasma concentrations for combined venlafaxine/O-DV were 37.1% of maternal plasma concentrations. The relative infant venlafaxine/O-DV dose was 8.1%. The theoretical and relative infant doses for O-DV were 197% and 224% higher, respectively, than those for venlafaxine. No adverse events were observed or reported in the nursing infants (Newport *et al*, 2009). Rampono *et al* (2011) studied 10 breastfeeding pairs where the mother was being treated with desvenlafaxine. They reported an infant exposure estimate of 4.8% (3.5–6.2%), and the relative infant dose was 6.8% (5.5–8.1%) of the weight-adjusted maternal dose.

## Monoamine oxidase inhibitors

Pons *et al* (1990) studied the pharmacokinetics of moclobemide and its metabolites in six lactating women. Concentrations in milk were highest 3 h after the dose and absent after 12 h. On average, the concentration in milk was 72% of the maternal serum concentration. An infant would receive an estimated 1% of the maternal dose. There are no published safety data relating to phenelzine, tranylcypromine, moclobemide or isocarboxazid; these drugs should be avoided in breastfeeding mothers.

## Mirtazapine

Maternal levels of mirtazapine in breast milk remain low if the dose remains below 120 mg daily, and exclusively breastfed infants receive an average of 1.5% (range 0.6–2.8%) of the maternal dose of mirtazapine and 0.4% (range 0.1–0.7%) of its metabolite desmethylmirtazapine (Aichhorn *et al*, 2004; Klier *et al*, 2007; Kristensen *et al*, 2007). Tonn *et al* (2009) reported on the overweight infant of a mother breastfeeding while taking mirtazapine 15 mg daily. The mother was concerned about possible over-sedation. The infant's serum level was 10 ng/ml, higher than in the previous reports.

## Trazodone

Peak trazodone levels in breast milk occur around 2 h after the dose, and it has been estimated that an exclusively breastfed infant would receive 0.65% of the maternal weight-adjusted dosage (Verbeeck *et al*, 1986), although the active metabolite was not measured. The infant of a mother who took trazodone 200 mg daily for 12 weeks, starting at 4 weeks postpartum, was followed up at 12 months of age; no adverse effects on growth and development were found (Misri *et al*, 1991). Another woman took trazodone 75 mg in addition to venlafaxine 75 mg and quetiapine 75 mg daily before conception, during pregnancy and during breastfeeding. Her breastfed infant's development was tested at 12 months and was within normal limits (Misri *et al*, 2006).

## Nefazodone (withdrawn in the UK)

Infant intake of nefazodone and its active metabolite hydroxynefazodone are estimated at 6.2% and 2.0%, respectively (Dodd *et al*, 1999). There is one report of a premature (36 weeks adjusted gestational age) infant becoming drowsy and lethargic, not feeding well and being unable to maintain normal body temperature when her mother was taking 300 mg nefazodone daily (Yapp *et al*, 2000). Symptoms resolved on cessation of breastfeeding, and no other cause was found on investigation. This case highlights the fact that preterm infants have immature metabolic systems.

Dodd and colleagues (2000) report on two mothers who breastfed while taking nefazodone. There was inter-individual variation in the amount of drug in milk, unrelated to dose. Milk:plasma ratios were 3.17 and 0.14; infant doses were 2.2% and 0.4%. There were no developmental difficulties in the infants.

## Bupropion

There is one case report of a mother breastfeeding her 14-month-old son while taking bupropion (Briggs *et al*, 1993). Neither the drug nor its metabolites were detectable in the single plasma sample taken from the infant. Similarly, assays in two mother–infant pairs found no detectable levels of bupropion or hydroxybupropion (its most active metabolite) in infant serum, and no problems were reported (Baab *et al*, 2002).

Haas and colleagues (2004) assessed the concentration of bupropion and all its active metabolites (hydroxybupropion, erythrobupropion and threohydrobupropion) in the milk of ten postpartum volunteers in an attempt to determine the average infant exposure. The calculated dose in breast milk was 6.75 mg/kg/day. Taking into account the metabolites, the total exposure to the infant would be 2% of the weight-adjusted maternal dose. There were no adverse events in the women. There is a report of a 6-month-old infant experiencing a seizure, but no milk or plasma level of bupropion was taken at the time, so a causal relationship cannot be confirmed (Ginsberg, 2004). However, there are reports of seizures in adults taking bupropion.

## Others

Hackett *et al* (2006) sampled four women taking reboxetine during pregnancy and their infants. The mean milk:plasma ratio was 0.06, and the relative infant dose was 2.0%. As noted in Chapter 8, one infant out of the four had developmental problems unrelated to reboxetine; the others met normal developmental milestones, and no adverse events were reported. There are no published data on agomelatine and atomoxetine.

## St John's wort (hypericum) and other herbal medicines

Klier and colleagues (2002) observed that hyperforin rather than hypericin was excreted into breast milk, albeit in very small amounts (milk:plasma ratio < 1), and that it was undetectable in infant plasma. No side-effects were seen in either mother or infant. Lee *et al* (2003) reported a prospective cohort study of 33 women who were breastfeeding while taking hypericum. Outcomes were compared with disease-matched controls not taking any medication, and with well women of a similar age and parity. There were more reports of colicky or drowsy infants in the hypericum group, but these did not require medical attention. There were no differences in reports of decreased milk production and infant weight gain over the first year among the groups.

Five women and two infants had breast milk and maternal and infant plasma sampled over an 18 h period (Schäfer *et al*, 2005). Their hyperforin milk:plasma ratios ranged from 0.04 to 0.13, and infant plasma levels were 0.17% and 0.15% of maternal levels. The relative mean dose per kg received by the infant was 0.9–2.5% of the maternal dose, and there were no maternal or infant adverse events. A systematic review (Dugoua *et al*, 2006) concluded that use of hypericum during lactation 'appeared to be of minimal risk' but may cause side-effects. They also drew attention to the fact that taking it concomitantly with other psychotropics might lower their serum levels by hypericum induction of CYP450 enzymes. Budzynska *et al* (2012) undertook a systematic review of breastfeeding and herbal medicines covering 1970–2010. The most commonly studied herbs were St John's wort, garlic and senna. The methodology of many studies was poor, many did not report safety data, and the review only included studies in English.

## Benzodiazepines and hypnotics

Benzodiazepines (BDZs) and their metabolites are excreted in breast milk. Some studies in breastfeeding mother–infant dyads have observed infant serum levels one-third to one-sixth of maternal levels when mothers were taking high doses (Erkkola & Kanto, 1972). However, other studies have observed lower levels of BDZs, including clonazepam (Birnbaum *et al*, 1999) and lormetazepam (Humpel *et al*, 1982). The mean infant dose of alprazolam was reported as 3% in a study of eight women (Oo, *et al*, 1995). Where higher concentrations do occur, there has usually also been *in utero* exposure. If BDZs are required while breastfeeding, using a short half-life drug intermittently will reduce the risk of higher infant serum levels. However, there are reports of infants appearing restless and irritable (Anderson & McGuire, 1989) and drowsy (Ito *et al*, 1993) with alprazolam. Infants should be monitored for signs of central nervous system (CNS) depression and apnoea. Iqbal *et al* (2002) comprehensively reviewed the literature relating to diazepam, chlordiazepoxide, clonazepam, lorazepam and alprazolam and breastfeeding.

Lebedevs and colleagues (1992) studied temazepam in ten breastfeeding mothers and their infants. The dose was 10–20 mg at night, and several of the mothers were taking other drugs in addition. The milk:plasma ratio ranged from <0.09 to <0.63 and the milk concentration was below the limit of detection for the assay in several samples. Zolpidem is excreted in breast milk in very small amounts (0.004–0.019% of the administered dose), and most of this takes place in the 3 h after the dose (Pons *et al*, 1989). The milk:plasma ratio at 3 h was 0.13. No infant samples were taken. Kelly *et al* (2012) reported data from 124 women contacting the Canadian Motherisk programme for advice about the safety of BDZs. The most commonly used BDZs were lorazepam (52%), clonazepam (18%) and midazolam (15%). There were only two reports of infant sedation, and adverse outcomes were not related to BDZ dose, number of hours breastfed or any demographic trait. The mothers who reported adverse effects in themselves were more likely to be taking other CNS depressants.

## Mood stabilisers

### Lithium

Single case studies of lithium exposure via breastfeeding have given rise to estimates of concentrations in infant serum of between 30 and 200% of maternal levels (Tunnessen & Hertz, 1972; Schou & Amdisen, 1973; Sykes *et al*, 1976; Skausig & Schou, 1977). One infant is reported to have become cyanotic, floppy, lethargic and hypotonic, but recovered. Another experienced an upper respiratory tract infection and developed a lithium level twice that of the maternal level. The infant recovered after breastfeeding was discontinued. Moretti *et al* (2003) reported on 11 bipolar mothers taking between 600 and 1500 mg lithium daily. There was wide variation in the dose the infant received via breast milk (0–30%), but no adverse events were reported. There are also risks of thyroid dysfunction, tremor, poor muscle tone and electrocardiogram (ECG) changes. A further series of 10 mother–infant pairs was reported by Viguera *et al* (2007). They also observed a wide range in the dose received by the infant (25–92% of maternal serum level) with a mean of 24%. Although no development delays were reported by the sample, four infants had abnormalities of thyroid-stimulating hormone (TSH), blood urea nitrogen or serum creatinine levels. More recently, Bogen *et al* (2012) reported on three women, all of whom took lithium during pregnancy and while breastfeeding, and their four infants. One infant was exposed to lithium only; the others were also exposed to other psychotropics. Infant serum lithium levels ranged from 10 to 17%. Two infants had feeding problems and one had hypotonia. The National Institute for Health and Care Excellence (NICE, 2014) advises that lithium should not be routinely offered to a woman who is breastfeeding because of the risk of toxicity in infants, whose renal excretion will be immature.

## Anticonvulsants

Bar-Oz et al (2000) reviewed the use of anticonvulsants during breastfeeding, concluding that 'phenytoin, carbamazepine and valproic acid [...] are generally considered safe for use during breast feeding'. Hägg & Spigset (2000) similarly concluded that these drugs are compatible with breastfeeding. In this chapter we will focus on those anticonvulsants used as mood stabilisers.

### Carbamazepine

Carbamazepine and its active metabolite, the 10,11-epoxide, have been studied in more than 25 breastfeeding mothers. The vast majority of these involved women with epilepsy who were also taking other drugs and were taking carbamazepine during pregnancy. Concentrations in breast milk ranged from 7 to 95% of the maternal serum level, but most were between 25 and 65%. Adverse events included cholestatic hepatitis, hyperbilirubinaemia and increased gamma-glutamyltransferase (GGT) levels (Frey et al, 1990; Merlob et al, 1992), a seizure (Brent & Wisner, 1998) and poor suckling (Froescher et al, 1984). NICE (2014) therefore recommends that carbamazepine should not be routinely offered to a woman who is breastfeeding.

### Valproate

There are over 90 reports of valproate in breast milk, and only one has reported any adverse outcome so far. Hence, the American Academy of Pediatrics considers it safe to breastfeed while taking it. The infant of a mother taking 600 mg sodium valproate daily (and who had done so throughout pregnancy) developed thrombocytopenic purpura and anaemia (Stahl et al, 1997). The majority of reports have involved mothers with epilepsy, some of whom were also taking other anticonvulsants. However, there are two studies on mothers with bipolar disorders.

Wisner & Perel (1998) reported on two mothers who breastfed while taking valproate. When steady state had been achieved, the infant serum levels were 1.5 and 6% of maternal values. Piontek et al (2000) assessed serum valproate levels in six mother–infant pairs. The mothers were taking doses of 750–1000 mg daily, and all but one had serum levels within the therapeutic range of 56.2–79 mg/ml. The infant serum levels were 0.9–2.3% of maternal levels, and none of the infants experienced any adverse events.

### Lamotrigine

Case reports suggest extensive passage of lamotrigine through the placenta and into breast milk (Rambeck et al, 1997; Tomson et al, 1997). Öhman and colleagues (2000) monitored lamotrigine levels in nine pregnant women and their ten infants through delivery and lactation. They confirmed extensive passage over the placenta and into breast milk, but also noted a slow elimination in the neonate and a profound increase in maternal serum concentrations following delivery. Lamotrigine serum concentrations in the infant were 23–50% of maternal serum concentrations. Lamotrigine is metabolised by glucuronidation, a process that is immature in neonates – this could lead to accumulation, although no adverse events were noted in this cohort. A further study adds to these concerns. Four women taking lamotrigine and their infants were studied; lamotrigine levels in the infants ranged from 20 to 43% of the maternal drug level. This had not declined by 2 months of age, but no short-term adverse effects were reported (Liporace *et al*, 2004). Gentile (2005) published a case report of a successful outcome in a mother and infant where lamotrigine had been taken throughout pregnancy and breastfeeding. More recently, Clark *et al* (2013) found mean infant serum levels to be 32.5% of maternal serum levels, assessed in 8 mother–infant pairs.

### Gabapentin

Öhman *et al* (2005) reported five breastfeeding mother–infant pairs in which the mother had taken gabapentin during pregnancy and while breastfeeding. The milk:plasma ratio was 1.0 before nursing, and the estimated dose to the infant was 1.3–1.8% of the maternal dose. When sampled 2–3 weeks after delivery, two of the infants had detectable concentrations of gabapentin, although these were below the levels of the normal range of the assay, and one had undetectable levels. No adverse events were reported. Kristensen *et al* (2006) report a further case in which the milk:plasma ratio was 0.86 and the estimated infant dose was 2.34%. There were no adverse events.

### Verapamil

The literature contains two reports of mothers breastfeeding while taking verapamil (Andersen, 1983). In the first, the infant was exposed *in utero* and during lactation to 240 mg. The infant's verapamil level was 2.1 ng/mL at 4 days postpartum. In the second case, the mother received 240 mg verapamil after delivery, and no verapamil (or its metabolite norverapamil) could be detected in the infant's serum at 3 months postpartum. At typical doses, the neonatal intake of verapamil is estimated to be about one-hundredth of the maternal dose.

# Antipsychotics

Gentile (2008) systematically reviewed the literature published between 1950 and 2008 and stated that 'no conclusions can be drawn about the risk/benefit profile of the majority of antipsychotic medications', with two exceptions.

- Clozapine should be contraindicated because of the possibility of inducing life-threatening events in the infant.

- Olanzapine is associated with an increased risk of extrapyramidal symptoms in breastfed babies.

## Typical antipsychotics

Haloperidol is 90% protein-bound, so limited amounts are available for absorption into breast milk. Whalley *et al* (1981) observed a milk:plasma ratio of around 0.6 and a low concentration of haloperidol in the infant's urine. No adverse events were reported, and the child appeared to be developing normally at 6 months and 1 year. Yoshida and colleagues (1998*b*) reported on 12 breastfeeding mothers who were taking haloperidol, chlorpromazine or trifluoperazine. Nine of the women took haloperidol (five of these also took chlorpromazine and one imipramine), and the mean ratio of foremilk to plasma was 2.8 and of foremilk to hind milk 3.6, i.e. there was a higher concentration in milk than in plasma. One mother had particularly high plasma and milk concentrations, but no sample was taken from the baby (who had some developmental delay). Seven women took chlorpromazine and two trifluoperazine. Overall the estimated infant dose for the drugs was 3% of maternal dose/kg. There were some concerns about the infants of women who were prescribed both haloperidol and chlorpromazine, but it is acknowledged that illness and other factors may have been involved.

In another report of two cases, one of the women took flupentixol and nortriptyline while breastfeeding; the other took zuclopentixol. Estimated daily infant doses were 0.5 and 0.3%, respectively, for the antipsychotics, and 2.3% for nortriptyline (Matheson & Skjaeraasen, 1988).

## Atypical antipsychotics

### Olanzapine

Ernst & Goldberg (2002) and Patton *et al* (2002) reported a total of 21 infants exposed to olanzapine via breastfeeding. Five experienced adverse events, including sedation, jaundice, cardiomegaly, cardiac murmur, shaking, poor feeding, lethargy, and an inability to roll from back to front at 7 months (development was normal by 11 months). A case report (Kircheiner *et al*, 2000) gave an account of an infant whose plasma levels of olanzapine were one-third of maternal levels but who appeared to experience no adverse events. Gentile (2004) summarised the milk:plasma ratios and infant doses in two studies of 12 infants and reported milk:plasma ratios between 0.10 and 0.84, with relative infant doses from 0.22 to 2.5%. Gilad *et al* (2011) followed up 37 mother–infant pairs in a prospective controlled study. The rate of adverse events in the infants (respiratory distress, hypotonia and feeding difficulties) was no greater in those exposed to olanzapine than in the controls. Brunner *et al* (2013) reported adverse events in 15.6% of infants (*n* = 102) exposed to olanzapine. The most common events were somnolence, irritability, tremor and insomnia.

## Risperidone

Hill *et al* (2000) reported milk:plasma ratios of 0.42 for risperidone and 0.24 for 9-hydroxyrisperidone. The likely infant doses of the drug and metabolite were 0.84% and 3.46%, respectively. A similar study of two breastfeeding women (Ilett *et al*, 2004) revealed milk:plasma ratios of < 0.5%, and relative infant doses were 2.3% and 2.8%. There were no adverse events reported. Aichhorn and colleagues (2005) reported a case in which milk levels were tenfold lower than maternal plasma levels, and the infant dose was well below 10%. Again, there were no adverse events.

## Quetiapine

Lee *et al* (2004*b*) reported a case in which a woman who had taken quetiapine during pregnancy also breastfed her infant while taking it. Levels of quetiapine in milk fell to almost the pre-dose levels by 2 h, and the estimated infant dose was 0.09–0.43% of the maternal dose. The infant was followed up until 4.5 months of age, and no problems were observed. In another case, a woman breastfed for 12 weeks without any adverse events in the infant (Ritz, 2005), and Gentile (2006) reported a woman who took quetiapine and fluvoxamine with 5 mg folic acid daily throughout pregnancy. A Caesarean section was performed, owing to pre-existing uterine myoma, and she supplemented breastfeeding with formula. Her infant experienced no problems. Rampono *et al* (2007) observed a milk:plasma ratio of 0.29 and a relative infant dose of 0.09% in a 3-month-old infant, and also observed no adverse events.

Misri and colleagues (2006) investigated the effects of adding quetiapine to antidepressant therapy in six postpartum women who had panic disorder or obsessive–compulsive disorder. Medication was detected in breast milk in half the sample, but there was only one case in which this medication was quetiapine, and the participant in question had taken a dose of 400 mg daily. Two infants showed evidence of mild developmental delays.

## Clozapine

There are reports of clozapine concentrations in breast milk being higher than in maternal serum (e.g. Barnas *et al*, 1994). The authors state that this is most likely due to the lipophilic nature of the drug. There are also reports of sedation, agranulocytosis (Trixler & Tényi, 1997) and cardiovascular instability (Dev & Krup, 1995), so breastfeeding while taking clozapine is not advised by NICE (2014). It has been noted that some clinicians might allow women with schizophrenia already on clozapine to continue while breastfeeding; however, if this is the case, it is essential that regular full blood counts be taken from the infant as well as the mother (Goodwin & Young, 2005).

### Aripiprazole

There are two case reports of infants exposed to aripiprazole via breastfeeding (Schlotterbeck *et al*, 2007; Lutz *et al*, 2010). Neither aripiprazole nor its metabolite were detectable in the three milk samples taken, and the estimated relative infant dose was less than 0.7% in the case reported by Lutz *et al* (2010). In the case reported by Schlotterbeck *et al* (2007), the concentration of aripiprazole in milk was 20% of the maternal serum level, and the milk:plasma ratio was 0.18:0.20.

### Others

There is one case of ziprasidone exposure during breastfeeding, in which ziprasidone was undetectable in milk for the first 10 days of treatment and the relative infant dose was 1.2% (Schlotterbeck *et al*, 2009). There are no published human data on zotepine, lurasidone or paliperidone in relation to breastfeeding.

## Non-drug interventions

There are no published data on electroconvulsive therapy (ECT), transcranial magnetic stimulation or light therapy and breastfeeding, but provided short-acting anaesthetic agents are used for ECT and any existing drugs the patient might be taking are not contraindicated, breastfeeding should be possible soon after treatment. If a mother needs to sleep for some time after each treatment, then expressing milk beforehand can enable someone else to feed the infant should this be needed before she wakes.

## References

Aichhorn W, Whitworth AB, Weiss U, *et al* (2004) Mirtazapine and breast-feeding. *American Journal of Psychiatry*, **161**: 2325.

Aichhorn W, Stuppaeck C, Whitworth AB (2005) Risperidone and breast-feeding. *Journal of Psychopharmacology*, **19**: 211–213.

Altshuler LL, Burt VK, McMullen M, *et al* (1995) Breastfeeding and sertraline: a 24-hour analysis. *Journal of Clinical Psychiatry*, **56**: 243–245.

Andersen HJ (1983) Excretion of verapamil in human milk. *European Journal of Clinical Pharmacology*, **25**: 279–280.

Anderson PO, McGuire GC (1989) Neonatal alprazolam withdrawal; possible effects of breast feeding. *Annals of Pharmacotherapy*, **23**: 614.

Baab SW, Peindl KS, Piontek CM, *et al* (2002) Serum bupropion levels in 2 breastfeeding mother-infant pairs. *Journal of Clinical Psychiatry*, **63**: 910–911.

Barnas C, Bergant A, Hummer M, *et al* (1994) Clozapine concentrations in maternal and fetal plasma, amniotic fluid, and breast milk. *American Journal of Psychiatry*, **151**: 945.

Bar-Oz B, Nulman I, Koren G, *et al* (2000) Anticonvulsants and breast feeding: a critical review. *Paediatric Drugs*, **2**: 113–126.

Begg EJ, Duffull SB, Saunders DA, *et al* (1999) Paroxetine in human milk. *British Journal of Clinical Pharmacology*, **48**: 142–147.

Birnbaum CS, Cohen LS, Bailey JW, *et al* (1999) Serum concentrations of antidepressants and benzodiazepines in nursing infants: a case series. *Pediatrics*, **104**: e11.

Bogen L, Sit D, Genovese A, *et al* (2012) Three cases of lithium exposure and exclusive breastfeeding. *Archives of Women's Mental Health*, **15**: 19–72.

Boyce P, Hackett LP, Ilett KF (2011) Duloxetine transfer across the placenta during pregnancy and into milk during lactation. *Archives of Women's Mental Health*, **14**: 169–172.

Brent NB, Wisner KL (1998) Fluoxetine and carbamazepine concentrations in a nursing mother/infant pair. *Clinical Pediatrics*, **37**: 41–44.

Briggs G, Samson J, Ambrose P, *et al* (1993) Excretion of bupropion in breast milk. *Annals of Pharmacotherapy*, **27**: 431–433.

Briggs GG, Ambrose PJ, Ilett KF, *et al* (2009) Use of duloxetine in pregnancy and lactation. *Annals of Pharmacotherapy*, **43**: 1898–1902.

Brunner E, Falk DM, Jones M, *et al* (2013) Olanzapine in pregnancy and breastfeeding: a review of data from global safety surveillance. *BMC Pharmacology and Toxicology*, **14**: 38.

Budzynska K, Gardner ZE, Dugoa J-J, *et al* (2012) Systematic review of breastfeeding and herbs. *Breastfeeding Medicine*, **7**: 489–503.

Buist A, Janson H (1995) Effect of exposure to dothiepin and nordothiepin in breast milk on child development. *British Journal of Psychiatry*, **167**: 370–373.

Burch KJ, Wells BG (1992) Fluoxetine/norfluoxetine concentrations in human milk. *Pediatrics*, **89**: 676–677.

Castberg I, Spigset O (2006) Excretion of escitalopram in breast milk. *Journal of Clinical Psychopharmacology*, **26**: 536–537.

Chambers CD, Anderson PO, Thomas RG, *et al* (1999) Weight gain in infants breastfed by mothers who take fluoxetine. *Pediatrics*, **104**: e61–e65.

Clark CT, Klein AM, Perel JM, *et al* (2013) Lamotrigine dosing for pregnant patients with bipolar disorder. *American Journal of Psychiatry*, **170**: 1240–1247.

Dev V, Krup P (1995) The side-effects and safety of clozapine. *Reviews in Contemporary Pharmacotherapy*, **6**: 197–208.

Dodd S, Buist A, Burrows GD, *et al* (1999) Determination of nefazodone and its pharmacologically active metabolites in human blood and breast milk by high-performance liquid chromatography. *Journal of Chromatography B: Biomedical Sciences and Applications*, **730**: 249–255.

Dodd S, Maguire KP, Burrows GD, *et al* (2000) Nefazodone in the breast milk of nursing mothers: a report of two patients. *Journal of Clinical Psychopharmacology*, **20**: 717–718.

Dugoua JJ, Mills E, Perri D, *et al* (2006) Safety and efficacy of St John's Wort (hypericum) during pregnancy and lactation. *Canadian Journal of Clinical Pharmacology*, **13**: e268–e276.

Epperson N, Czarkowski KA, Ward-O'Brien D, *et al* (2001) Maternal sertraline treatment and serotonin transport in breast-feeding mother-infant pairs. *American Journal of Psychiatry*, **158**: 1631–1637.

Epperson CN, Jatlow PJ, Czarkowski K, *et al* (2003) Maternal fluoxetine treatment in the postpartum period: effects on platelet serotonin and plasma drug levels in breastfeeding mother-infant pairs. *Pediatrics*, **112**: e425–e429.

Erkkola R, Kanto J (1972) Diazepam and breast-feeding. *Lancet*, **i**: 1235–1236.

Ernst CL, Goldberg JF (2002) The reproductive safety profile of mood stabilizers, atypical antipsychotics, and broad-spectrum psychotropics. *Journal of Clinical Psychiatry*, **63**: 42–55.

Frey B, Schubiger G, Musy JP (1990) Transient cholestatic hepatitis in a neonate associated with carbamazepine exposure during pregnancy and breast-feeding. *European Journal of Pediatrics*, **150**: 136–138.

Frey OR, Scheidt P, von Brennendorff AI (1999) Adverse effects in a newborn infant breast-fed by a mother treated with doxepin. *Annals of Pharmacotherapy*, **33**: 690–692.

Froescher W, Eichelbaum M, Niesen M, *et al* (1984) Carbamazepine levels in breast milk. *Therapeutic Drug Monitoring*, **6**: 266–271.

Gentile S (2004) Clinical utilization of atypical antipsychotics in pregnancy and lactation. *Annals of Pharmacotherapy*, **38**: 1265–1271.

Gentile S (2005) Lamotrigine in pregnancy and lactation. *Archives of Women's Mental Health*, **8**: 57–58.

Gentile S (2006) Quetiapine-fluvoxamine combination during pregnancy and while breastfeeding. *Archives of Women's Mental Health*, **9**: 158–159.

Gentile S (2008) Infant safety with antipsychotic therapy in breast–feeding: a systematic review. *Journal of Clinical Psychiatry*, **69**: 666–673.

Gentile S (2014) Tricyclic antidepressants in pregnancy and puerperium. *Expert Opinion on Drug Safety*, **13**: 207–225.

Gilad O, Merlob P, Stahl B, *et al* (2011) Outcome of infants exposed to olanzapine during breastfeeding. *Breastfeeding Medicine*, **6**: 55–58.

Ginsberg DL (2004) Bupropion-associated seizure in a breastfeeding infant. *Primary Psychiatry*, **11**: 26–27.

Goodwin G, Young A (2005) Using guidelines in real clinical situations: clozapine and breast feeding in bipolar disorder. *Journal of Psychopharmacology*, **19**: 317–318.

Haas JS, Kaplan CP, Barenboim D, *et al* (2004) Bupropion in breast milk: an exposure assessment for potential treatment to prevent post-partum tobacco use. *Tobacco Control*, **13**: 52–56.

Hackett LP, Ilett KF, Rampono J, *et al* (2006) Transfer of reboxetine into breastmilk, its plasma concentrations and lack of adverse events in the breastfed infant. *European Journal of Clinical Pharmacology*, **62**: 633–638.

Hägg S, Spigset O (2000) Anticonvulsant use during lactation. *Drug Safety*, **22**: 425–440.

Hale TW, Shum S, Grossberg M (2001) Fluoxetine toxicity in a breastfed infant. *Clinical Pediatrics*, **40**: 681–684.

Heikkinen T, Ekblad U, Palo *et al* (2002a) Pharmacokinetics of fluoxetine and norfluoxetine in pregnancy and lactation. *Clinical Pharmacology and Therapeutics*, **73**: 330–337.

Heikkinen T, Ekblad U, Kero P, *et al* (2002b) Citalopram in pregnancy and lactation. *Clinical Pharmacology and Therapeutics*, **72**: 184–191.

Hendrick V, Stowe ZN, Altshuler LL, *et al* (2001a) Fluoxetine and norfluoxetine concentrations in nursing infants and breast milk. *Biological Psychiatry*, **50**: 775–782.

Hendrick V, Fukuchi A, Altshuler L, *et al* (2001b) Use of sertraline, paroxetine and fluvoxamine by nursing women. *British Journal of Psychiatry*, **179**: 163–166.

Hendrick V, Altshuler L, Wertheimer A, *et al* (2001c) Venlafaxine and breast-feeding. *American Journal of Psychiatry*, **158**: 2089–2090.

Hendrick V, Smith LM, Hwang S, *et al* (2003) Weight gain in breastfed infants of mothers taking antidepressants. *Journal of Clinical Psychiatry*, **64**: 410–412.

Hill RC, McIvor RJ, Wojnar-Horton RE, *et al* (2000) Risperidone distribution and excretion into human milk: case report and estimated infant exposure during breast-feeding. *Journal of Clinical Psychopharmacology*, **20**: 285–286.

Humpel M, Stoppelli I, Milia S, *et al* (1982) Pharmacokinetics and biotransformation of the new benzodiazepine, lormetazepam, in man. III. Repeated administration and transfer to neonates via breast milk. *European Journal of Clinical Pharmacology*, **21**: 421–425.

Ilett KF, Hackett LP, Dusci LJ, *et al* (1998) Distribution and excretion of venlafaxine and O-desmethylvenlafaxine in human milk. *British Journal of Clinical Pharmacology*, **45**: 459–462.

Ilett KF, Kristensen JH, Hackett LP, *et al* (2002) Distribution of venlafaxine and its O-desmethyl metabolite in human milk and their effects in breastfed infants. *British Journal of Clinical Pharmacology*, **53**: 17–22.

Ilett KF, Hackett LP, Kristensen JH, *et al* (2004) Transfer of risperidone and 9-hydroxyrisperidone into human milk. *Annals of Pharmacotherapy*, **38**: 273–276.

Ilett KF, Hackett LP, Kristensen JH, *et al* (2005) Estimation of infant dose and assessment of breastfeeding safety for escitalopram use in postnatal depression. *Therapeutic Drug Monitoring*, **27**: 144.

Iqbal MM, Sobhan T, Ryals T (2002) Effects of commonly used benzodiazepines on the neonate, and the nursing infant. *Psychiatric Services*, **53**: 39–49.

Isenberg KE (1990) Excretion of fluoxetine in human breast milk. *Journal of Clinical Psychiatry*, **51**: 169.

Ito S, Blajchman A, Stephenson M, *et al* (1993) Prospective follow-up of adverse reactions in breastfed infants exposed to maternal medication. *American Journal of Obstetrics & Gynecology*, **168**: 1393–1399.

Jensen PN, Olesen OV, Bertelsen A, *et al* (1997) Citalopram and desmethylcitalopram concentrations in breast milk and in serum of mother and infant. *Therapeutic Drug Monitoring*, **19**: 236–239.

Kelly LE, Poon S, Madadi P, *et al* (2012) Neonatal benzodiazepines exposure during breastfeeding. *Journal of Pediatrics*, **161**: 448–451.

Kent LS, Laidlaw JD (1995) Suspected congenital sertraline dependence. *British Journal of Psychiatry*, **167**: 412–413.

Kim J, Riggs KW, Misri S, *et al* (2006) Stereoselective disposition of fluoxetine and norfluoxetine during pregnancy and breast-feeding. *British Journal of Clinical Pharmacology*, **61**: 155–163.

Kircheiner J, Berghofer A, Bolk-Weischedel D (2000) Healthy outcome under olanzapine treatment in a pregnant woman. *Pharmacopsychiatry*, **33**: 78–80.

Klier CM, Schäfer MR, Schmid-Siegel B, *et al* (2002) St. John's wort (*Hypericum perforatum*): is it safe during breastfeeding? *Pharmacopsychiatry*, **35**: 29–30.

Klier CM, Schmid-Siegel B, Schäfer MR, *et al* (2006) St. John's wort (*Hypericum perforatum*) and breastfeeding: plasma and breast milk concentrations of hyperforin for 5 mothers and 2 infants. *Journal of Clinical Psychiatry*, **67**: 305–309.

Klier CM, Mossaheb N, Lee A, *et al* (2007) Mirtazapine and breastfeeding: maternal and infant plasma levels. *American Journal of Psychiatry*, **164**: 348–349.

Koren G, Moretti M, Kapur B (2006) Can venlafaxine in breast milk attenuate the norepinephrine and serotonin reuptake neonatal withdrawal syndrome. *Journal of Obstetrics and Gynecology Canada*, **28**: 299–302.

Kristensen JH, Ilett KF, Dusci LJ, *et al* (1998) Distribution and excretion of sertraline and N-desmethylsertraline in human milk. *British Journal of Clinical Pharmacology*, **45**: 453–457.

Kristensen JH, Ilett LP, Yapp P, *et al* (1999) Distribution and excretion of fluoxetine and norfluoxetine in human milk. *British Journal of Clinical Pharmacology*, **48**: 521–527.

Kristensen JH, Hackett LP, Kohan R, *et al* (2002) The amount of fluvoxamine in milk is unlikely to be a cause of adverse effects in breastfed infants. *Journal of Human Lactation*, **18**: 139–143.

Kristensen JH, Ilett KF, Hackett LP, *et al* (2006) Gabapentin and breastfeeding: a case report. *Journal of Human Lactation*, **22**: 426–428.

Kristensen JH, Ilett KF, Rampono J, *et al* (2007) Transfer of the antidepressant mirtazapine into breast milk. *British Journal of Clinical Pharmacology*, **63**: 322–327.

Lebedevs TH, Wojnar-Horton RE, Yapp P, *et al* (1992) Excretion of temazepam in breast milk. *British Journal of Clinical Pharmacology*, **33**: 204–206.

Lee A, Minhas R, Matsuda N, *et al* (2003) The safety of St. John's wort (*Hypericum perforatum*) during breastfeeding. *Journal of Clinical Psychiatry*, **64**: 966–968.

Lee A, Woo J, Ito S (2004a) Frequency of infant adverse events that are associated with citalopram use during breast-feeding. *American Journal of Obstetrics & Gynecology*, **190**: 218–221.

Lee A, Giesbrecht G, Dunn E, *et al* (2004b) Excretion of quetiapine in breast milk. *American Journal of Psychiatry*, **161**: 1715–1716.

Lepola U, Penttinen J, Koponen H, *et al* (2000) Citalopram treatment and breast-feeding. *Biological Psychiatry*, **47**: S149.

Lester BM, Cucca J, Andreozzi L, *et al* (1993) Possible association between fluoxetine hydrochloride and colic in an infant. *Journal of the American Academy of Child and Adolescent Psychiatry*, **32**: 1253–1255.

Liporace J, Kao A, D'Abreu (2004) Concerns regarding lamotrigine and breast-feeding. *Epilepsy and Behavior*, **5**: 102–105.

Lobo ED, Loghin C, Knadler MP, *et al* (2008) Pharmacokinetics of duloxetine in breast milk and plasma of healthy postpartum women. *Clinical Pharmacokinetics*, **47**: 103–109.

Lutz UC, Hiemke C, Wiatr G, *et al* (2010) Aripiprazole in pregnancy and lactation: a case report. *Journal of Clinical Psychopharmacology*, **30**: 204–205.

Mammen OK, Perel JM, Rudolph G, *et al* (1997) Sertraline and norsertraline levels in three breastfed infants. *Journal of Clinical Psychiatry*, **58**: 100–103.

Matheson I, Skjaeraasen J (1988) Milk concentrations of flupenthixol, nortriptyline and zuclopenthixol and between-breast differences in two patients. *European Journal of Clinical Pharmacology*, **35**: 217–220.

Matheson I, Pande H, Alertsen AP (1985) Respiratory depression caused by N-desmethyl doxepin in breast milk. *Lancet*, **16**: 1124.

Merlob P, Mor N, Litwin A (1992) Transient hepatic dysfunction in an infant of an epileptic mother treated with carbamazepine during pregnancy and breastfeeding. *Annals of Pharmacotherapy*, **26**: 1563–1565.

Merlob P, Stahl B, Sulkes J (2004) Paroxetine during breast-feeding: infant weight gain and maternal adherence to counsel. *European Journal of Pediatrics*, **163**: 135–139.

Misri S, Sivertz K (1991) Tricyclic drugs in pregnancy and lactation: a preliminary report. *International Journal of Psychiatry in Medicine*, **21**: 157–171.

Misri S, Kim J, Riggs W, *et al* (2000) Paroxetine levels in postpartum depressed women, breast milk and infant serum. *Journal of Clinical Psychiatry*, **61**: 828–832.

Misri S, Corral M, Wardrop AA, *et al* (2006) Quetiapine augmentation in lactation: a series of case reports. *Journal of Clinical Psychopharmacology*, **26**: 508–511.

Moretti ME, Koren G, Verjee Z, *et al* (2003) Monitoring lithium in breast milk: an individualized approach for breastfeeding mothers. *Clinical Pharmacology and Therapeutics*, **25**: 364–366.

Newport DJ, Ritchie JC, Knight BT, *et al* (2009) Venlafaxine in human breast milk and nursing infant plasma: determination of exposure. *Journal of Clinical Psychiatry*, **70**: 1304–1310.

NICE (2014) *Antenatal and Postnatal Mental Health: Clinical Management and Service Guidance*. National Institute for Health and Care Excellence.

Öhman R, Hagg S, Carleborg L, *et al* (1999) Excretion of paroxetine into breast milk. *Journal of Clinical Psychiatry*, **60**: 519–523.

Öhman I, Vitols S, Tomson T (2000) Lamotrigine in pregnancy: pharmacokinetics during delivery, in the neonate and during lactation. *Epilepsia*, **41**: 709–713.

Öhman I, Vitols S, Tomson T (2005) Pharmacokinetics of gabapentin during delivery, in the neonatal period, and lactation: does a fetal accumulation occur during pregnancy? *Epilepsia*, **46**: 1621–1624.

Oo CY, Kuhn RJ, Desai N, *et al* (1995) Pharmacokinetics in lactating women; prediction of alprazolam transfer into milk. *British Journal of Clinical Pharmacology*, **40**: 231–236.

Patton SW, Misri S, Corral MR, *et al* (2002) Antipsychotic medication during pregnancy and lactation in women with schizophrenia: evaluating the risk. *Canadian Journal of Psychiatry*, **47**: 959–965.

Perel JM, Wisner KL, Reiter C, *et al* (2003) Sertraline therapy of postpartum depression, maternal therapeutic drug monitoring and infant exposure during breastfeeding. *Therapeutic Drug Monitoring*, **25**: 518.

Piontek CM, Baab S, Peindl KS (2000) Serum valproate levels in 6 breast-feeding mother-infant pairs. *Journal of Clinical Psychiatry*, **61**: 170–172.

Piontek CM, Wisner KL, Perel JM, *et al* (2001) Serum fluvoxamine levels in breastfed infants. *Journal of Clinical Psychiatry*, **62**: 111–113.

Pons G, Francoual C, Guillet P, *et al.* (1989) Zolpidem excretion in breast milk. *European Journal of Clinical Pharmacology*, **37**: 245.

Pons G, Schoerlin P, Tam YK, *et al* (1990) Moclobemide excretion in human breast milk. *British Journal of Clinical Pharmacology*, **29**: 27–31.

Rambek B, Cullman G, Stories SRG, *et al* (1997) Concentrations of lamotrigine in a mother on lamotrigine treatment and her newborn child. *European Journal of Clinical Pharmacology*, **52**: 481–484.

Rampono J, Kristensen JH, Hackett LP, et al (2000) Citalopram and desmethylcitalopram in human milk; distribution, excretion and effects in breast fed infants. British Journal of Clinical Pharmacology, 50: 263–268.

Rampono J, Hackett LP, Kristensen JH, et al (2006) Transfer of escitalopram and its metabolite desmethylescitalopram into breastmilk. British Journal of Clinical Pharmacology, 62: 316–322.

Rampono J, Kristensen JH, Ilett KF, et al (2007) Quetiapine and breast feeding. Annals of Pharmacotherapy, 41: 711–714.

Rampono J, Teoh S, Hackett LP, et al (2011) Estimation of desvenlafaxine transfer into milk and infant exposure during its use in lactating women with postnatal depression. Archives of Women's Mental Health, 14: 49–53.

Ritz S (2005) Quetiapine monotherapy in post-partum onset bipolar disorder with a mixed affective state. European Neuropsychopharmacology, 15 (Suppl 3): S407.

Schäfer MR, Klier CM, Lenz G, et al (2005) St. John's Wort (hypericum perforatum) and breastfeeding: concentrations of hyperforin in nursing infants and breast milk. Pharmacopsychiatry, 38: 38.

Schlotterbeck P, Leube D, Kircher T, et al (2007) Aripiprazole in human milk. International Journal of Neuropsychopharmacology, 10: 433.

Schlotterbeck P, Saur F, Heimke C, et al (2009) Low concentration of ziprasidone in human milk: a case report. International Journal of Neuropsychopharmacology, 12: 437–438.

Schmidt K, Olesen OV, Jensen PN (2000) Citalopram and breast-feeding: serum concentration and side effects in the infant. Biological Psychiatry, 47: 164–165.

Schou M, Amdisen A (1973) Lithium and pregnancy 3: lithium ingestion by children breast-fed by women on lithium treatment. BMJ, 2: 138.

Skausig OB, Schou M (1977) Breastfeeding during lithium therapy. Ugeskr Laeger, 139: 400–401.

Spigset O, Carleborg L, Öhman R, et al (1997) Excretion of citalopram in breast milk. British Journal of Clinical Pharmacology, 44: 295–298.

Stahl MM, Neiderud J, Vinge E (1997) Thrombocytopenic purpura and anemia in a breast-fed infant whose mother was treated with valproic acid. Journal of Pediatrics, 130: 1001–1003.

Stein A, Pearson RM, Goodman S, et al (2014) Effects of perinatal mental health disorders on the fetus and child. Lancet, 384: 1800–1819.

Stowe ZN, Owens MJ, Landry JC, et al (1997) Sertraline and desmethylsertraline in human breast milk and nursing infants. American Journal of Psychiatry, 154: 1255–1260.

Stowe ZN, Hostetter AL, Owens MJ, et al (2003) The pharmacokinetics of sertraline excretion into human breast milk: determinants of infant serum concentrations. Journal of Clinical Psychiatry, 64: 73–80.

Stowe ZN Cohen LS, Hostetter A, et al (2000) Paroxetine in human breast milk and nursing infants. American Journal of Psychiatry, 157: 185–189.

Suri R, Stowe ZN, Hendrick V, et al (2002) Estimates of nursing infant daily dose of fluoxetine through breast milk. Biological Psychiatry, 52: 446–451.

Sykes PA, Quarrie J, Alexander FW (1976) Lithium carbonate and breast–feeding. BMJ, 2: 1299.

Taddio A, Ito S, Koren G (1996) Excretion of fluoxetine and its metabolite norfluoxetine in human breast milk. Pediatrics, 36: 42–47.

Tomson T, Öhman I, Vitols S (1997) Lamotrigine in pregnancy and lactation: a case report. Epilepsia, 38: 1039–1041.

Tonn P, Reuter SC, Hiemke C, et al (2009) High mirtazapine plasma levels in infant after breast feeding: case report and review of the literature. Journal of Clinical Psychopharmacology, 29: 191–192.

Trixler M, Tényi T (1997) Antipsychotic use in pregnancy. What are the best treatment options? Drug Safety, 16: 403–410.

Tunnessen WW, Hertz CG (1972) Toxic effects of lithium in newborn infants: a commentary. Journal of Pediatrics, 81: 804–807.

Verbeeck RK, Ross SG, McKenna EA (1986) Excretion of trazodone in breast milk. *British Journal of Clinical Pharmacology*, **22**: 367–370.

Viguera AC, Newport DJ, Ritchie J, *et al* (2007) Lithium in breast milk and nursing infants: clinical implications. *American Journal of Psychiatry*, **164**: 342–345.

Whalley LJ, Blain PG, Prime JK (1981) Haloperidol secreted in breast milk. *BMJ*, **282**: 1746–1747.

Wisner KL, Perel JM (1991) Serum nortriptyline levels in nursing mothers and their infants. *American Journal of Psychiatry*, **148**: 1234–1236.

Wisner KL, Perel JM (1998) Serum levels of valproate and carbamazepine in breastfeeding mother–infant pairs. *Journal of Clinical Psychopharmacology*, **18**: 167–169.

Wright S, Dawling S, Ashford D (1991) Excretion of fluvoxamine in breast milk. *British Journal of Clinical Pharmacology*, **31**: 209.

Yapp P, Ilett KF, Kristensen JH, *et al* (2000) Drowsiness and poor feeding in a breast-fed infant: association with nefazodone and its metabolites. *Annals of Pharmacotherapy*, **34**: 1269–1272.

Yoshida K, Kumar R (1996) Breast feeding and psychotropic drugs. *International Review of Psychiatry*, **8**: 117–124.

Yoshida K, Smith B, Craggs M, *et al* (1997a) Investigation of pharmacokinetics and of possible adverse effects in infants exposed to tricyclic antidepressants in breast–milk. *Journal of Affective Disorders*, **43**: 225-237.

Yoshida K, Smith B, Kumar RC (1997b) Fluvoxamine in breast milk and infant development. *British Journal of Clinical Pharmacology*, **44**: 210–211.

Yoshida K, Smith B, Craggs M, *et al* (1998a) Fluoxetine in breast-milk and developments outcome of breast-fed infants. *British Journal of Psychiatry*, **172**: 175–179.

Yoshida K, Smith B, Craggs M, *et al* (1998b) Neuroleptic drugs in breast-milk: a study of pharmacokinetics and of possible adverse effects in breast-fed infants. *Psychological Medicine*, **28**: 81–91.

# Further reading

American Academy of Pediatrics and American College of Obstetricians and Gynecologists (2014) *Breastfeeding Handbook for Physicians* (2nd edn). American Academy of Pediatrics.

## Drugs and Lactation Database (LactMed)

A US peer-reviewed and fully referenced database, including maternal and infant levels of drugs, possible effects on infants, and alternatives. There is a free app (www.toxnet.nlm.nih.gov/newtoxnet/lactmed.htm).

## The Specialist Pharmacy Service (SPS)

The website (www.sps.nhs.uk) includes information on the safety of drugs in lactation.

# CHAPTER 10

# Service provision

Service provision in the UK remains patchy and inadequate (Bauer *et al*, 2014). Although the National Institute for Health and Care Excellence (NICE, 2014) guideline on antenatal and postnatal mental health stated that there should be a multidisciplinary perinatal service in each locality, access to specialist expert advice, clear referral and management protocols, there remain many areas of the UK where there is no service at all and others where only some elements of a comprehensive service exist.

A recent report by the Centre for Mental Health (Bauer *et al*, 2014) estimates that half the women in the UK have no access to specialist perinatal mental health services. NICE estimates that there is a shortfall of around 60–80 beds in mother and baby units. Nearly all of the recent maternal deaths from psychiatric causes were women being cared for by non-specialist mental health teams (Centre for Maternal and Child Enquiries, 2011). The Maternal Mental Health Alliance Map of specialist community services and mother and baby units can be found on their website (http://everyonesbusiness.org.uk/?page_id=349).

Regional clinical networks can help to develop more equitable services, but in some areas these have only recently been established. The Royal College of Psychiatrists' Perinatal Quality Network (www.rcpsych.ac.uk/researchandtrainingunit/centreforqualityimprovement/perinatalqualitynetwork.aspx) should ensure that mother and baby unit and community teams' standards are uniform.

Services must take account of the fact that perinatal psychiatric disorders include new, chronic and recurrent illness in relation to pregnancy and childbirth across the whole range (and range of severity) of psychiatric disorders. Adjustment disorders and distress, anxiety and depressive disorders of a severity below that requiring referral to secondary care should be appropriately managed in primary care. More severe and complex cases – such as women with comorbidity and severe and enduring mental illness – will require assessment and/or management by a specialist team.

The service provision for any defined area or population must relate to the epidemiology. This has been clearly defined and is based on the birth rate rather than the total population (Royal College of Psychiatrists, 2001; Joint Commissioning Panel for Mental Health, 2012). Care should be taken to note any factors that could lead to an increase in the population of reproductive age in an area, such as a new factory opening and attracting a young workforce to the area, or the arrival of migrant workers, refugees or asylum seekers who may be concentrated in a particular town or city. Such groups can elevate the birth rate in an area and might have specific needs that must be addressed.

Although services may be targeted at mothers, many of their partners will also be experiencing mental health problems (Ballard *et al*, 1994; Glangeaud-Freudenthal *et al*, 2004), and a mechanism of assessing and meeting their needs should be considered. Closer relationships and joint working with child and adolescent services are essential because of the well-established links between parental mental illness and associated emotional and behavioural problems in children and teenagers. Maternal depression, for example, is associated not only with an increase in behavioural problems in children, but also with a poorer response to treatment directed at the behaviour disorder (Rishel *et al*, 2006). Young people moving from child and adolescent services to adult mental healthcare should be managed according to Department of Health Guidance (http://webarchive. nationalarchives.gov.uk/20130107105354/http://www.dh.gov.uk/en/ Publicationsandstatistics/Publications/PublicationsPolicyAndGuidance/ DH_4132145).

## Primary care

The role of primary care services is to detect and treat mild and moderate mental health problems in relation to pregnancy and childbearing and to detect and refer individuals with more severe problems or at risk of more serious problems to secondary or tertiary services. When referring women with a history of mental health problems to maternity care, information regarding the psychiatric history must be included in the referral. This is less likely to happen now that pregnant women can directly access midwifery care.

Health visitors can be trained in both non-directive counselling and elements of cognitive–behavioural therapy, termed 'cognitive behavioural counselling'. Such additional skills can lead to more assessments of women's mental health being carried out, and better recording of contacts, but also more referrals to mental health services (Appleby *et al*, 2003). Women suffering from depression treated by health visitors trained in either a cognitive–behavioural or a person-centred approach have better outcomes at 6 months than those treated with usual health visitor care (Morrell *et al*, 2009, 2011), and these interventions have proved cost-effective. However, some women, particularly those who are younger and of lower educational status, exclude themselves from healthcare (Murray *et al*,

2003), and primary care professionals must consider what additional input might be required to engage these vulnerable women whose infants have poorer outcomes. Educating women about perinatal depression using a case vignette enabled better recognition of depression and a better assessment of their own mental state (Buist *et al*, 2007); this is strategy that could be employed by the primary care team.

Training is available (see Appendix 3) both for individual professionals and for those wishing to train others. However, trainers who had attended one course reported several barriers to implementing training in their own trust, including only recently having been trained themselves, lack of time allocated to training, lack of referral systems and health visitors declining training (Elliott *et al*, 2003). There has been recent investment in training 5000 more midwives and 4200 more health visitors, and in increasing the training for them and for doctors in perinatal mental health (Department of Health, 2014).

Some Sure Start Children's Centres (www.childrenscentres.info), have projects in perinatal mental health, e.g. specific groups for adolescent mothers. Services such as Home-Start (www.home-start.org.uk), although not focused on perinatal mental health, work with many women with perinatal mental illness. There are many support and information services provided by the voluntary sector, some of which are outlined in Chapter 2.

# Secondary care

## *Maternity services*

In England, National Health Service (NHS) trusts consist of service provider organisations within secondary care, and clinical commissioning groups, which provide primary care and commission services from secondary care. All trusts providing maternity care should have guidelines for the management of women at risk of a relapse or recurrence of severe mental illness following delivery. Women with substance misuse should be managed according to national guidelines (see Chapter 5).

Midwives must make a systematic enquiry about current and past mental health and substance misuse at antenatal booking; however, this should not be implemented until appropriate training has taken place and there is a mechanism in place for regular updating.

Psychiatric disorders must be identified as specific syndromes and the abbreviation 'PND' should not be used. Women with serious mental illness or problem drug and/or alcohol histories have high-risk pregnancies and should have their management supervised by an obstetrician. Obstetricians and midwives must be aware of the law in relation to child and vulnerable adult protection, and when and to whom to refer if concerns arise.

Trusts should ensure that self-medication on maternity units is controlled by using secure lockers for storage to reduce the risk of overdose.

## Mental health services

Psychiatric services must share information and management plans with maternity services, social services and other agencies involved in a woman's care. They must assess women at risk of puerperal illness, even if they are well during pregnancy, and must consider contraception in childbearing women, particularly if the woman is known not to attend primary care services for this. Referral can be made to the local family planning service.

Psychiatric health professionals must consider the possibility of serious physical illness in recently delivered women suffering from unusual symptoms and must not automatically attribute these to a psychiatric disorder. Deaths continue to occur when physical symptoms are misattributed to psychiatric disorder, resulting in a delay in diagnosis and effective treatment (Centre for Maternal and Child Enquiries, 2011).

## Specialist perinatal psychiatric services

These are justified by:

- the special needs of perinatal women and their infants
- the specialist knowledge, skills and understanding required of staff, especially the assessment and management of the mother–infant relationship, including the diagnosis and treatment of severe mother–infant relationship disorders
- the critical mass of patients required to afford adequate experience in developing and maintaining staff skills and to justify the material and human resources
- the difficulty for general services of maintaining skills and understanding and prioritising the needs of this group of patients in the face of competing demands.

### Functions of a specialist service

- To assess and manage those suffering from puerperal psychosis and other severe postnatal mental illnesses.
- To provide a range of facilities, including an in-patient mother and baby unit (or access to one), out-patient clinics, alternatives to admission (intensive home nursing and/or day hospital) and community treatment.
- To advise on, and manage where necessary, patients with continuing psychiatric disorder who become pregnant while under the care of other adult psychiatrists, and to work closely with child and adolescent and intellectual disability services, jointly managing cases where necessary.
- To liaise with primary healthcare professionals to assist in the management of less serious psychiatric conditions.

- To provide an obstetric liaison service, assessing mental health problems associated with pregnancy and the postpartum period, and deal with emergencies.
- To provide preconceptual counselling and high-risk management for women at risk of developing an illness postpartum owing to previous major mental illness.
- To undertake the assessment of women with severe chronic mental illness in respect of their ability to parent their child and provide expert medico-legal advice.

A multidisciplinary specialist perinatal mental health service will also be in a position to take a lead role in the development of services at all levels of healthcare provision, to contribute to the education and training of other healthcare professionals and will function at different levels, relating to primary care and providing specialist advice and management.

### Community services: day care and home treatment

Oates (1988) developed a community-based treatment for puerperal psychosis which allowed some women to be entirely treated at home and reduced the length of stay for others. This might be achieved today with community-based specialist perinatal mental health staff working alongside home treatment teams. Home treatment teams are unlikely to have the skills and expertise to manage these women and their infants without such collaboration.

Day units may be situated alongside mother and baby units and share staff or be sited in the community. The Parent and Baby Day Unit in Stoke-on-Trent, England, has been well described in the literature and shown to be cost-effective compared with routine primary care of women with postnatal depression (Boath *et al*, 2003). It continues to offer care delivered by a multidisciplinary team who provide individual and group psychological and social interventions, nursery nurse support, and psychiatric medical review and treatment.

Howard *et al* (2006) describe a mother and baby day hospital programme in the USA, which offers various individual and group interventions. Most of the care is offered on a short-term basis (mean duration 5 days, range 1–22). The majority of patients are suffering from major depressive disorder and around three-quarters receive medication (Battle *et al*, 2006).

### In-patient units

The first recorded admission of a mother and baby to a psychiatric hospital is credited to Main (1948) and was arranged to avoid any detrimental effect on the baby or reduction in maternal confidence if they were separated. Since then – in the UK, France, Germany, Belgium, Australia and New Zealand in particular – several specialised mother and baby units have been established. Units in Geneva (Alberque *et al*, 2006) and Jerusalem (Maizel *et al*, 2005) have also been described. However, in many other parts of the world, there are none or very few.

**271**

Despite admission to a specialist mother and baby unit being recommended in the UK for all women requiring in-patient psychiatric care who have an infant under the age of 12 months (Scottish Intercollegiate Guidelines Network, 2012; NICE, 2014; Royal College of Psychiatrists, 2015), there remain an insufficient number of beds. The beds are not uniformly distributed throughout the country in relation to population centres but are concentrated in some regions, with none at all in others (Bauer et al, 2014). The Maternal Mental Health Alliance have mapped service provision across the UK (http://everyonesbusiness. org.uk/?page_id=349).

The mean duration of admission in a more recent series of 100 consecutive admissions in the UK was 2 months (Kumar et al, 1995). Almost half of the patients were admitted under the Mental Health Act. Most had become ill within 2 weeks of delivery and admitted acutely. An Australian unit reported the mean duration of admission as 21.7 days; the majority of their patients suffered from schizophrenia, other psychoses or major depression (Milgrom et al, 1998). Salmon et al (2004) audited data from 1217 UK admissions between 1996 and 2002. The most common primary diagnoses were depressive illness (43%), schizophrenia (21%) and bipolar disorder (14%). The only predictor of self-harm was depressed mood and behavioural disturbance; self-harm and the age of the mother (16–25 years) were found to predict harm to the child. Mothers with schizophrenia were three times more likely to experience a poor outcome and more likely to be separated from their infant on discharge. In a similar audit in France and Belgium of a smaller number of mother–baby admissions (176), schizophrenia was the most common diagnosis and the majority (65%) of admissions resulted in a symptom-free or considerably improved maternal mental state (Glangeaud-Freudenthal et al, 2004). Problems relating to risk of harm to the infant or poor emotional response were more common in mothers with schizophrenia, delusional disorders, personality disorder or intellectual disability than in mothers with bipolar disorder or bouffée délirante. A larger study of 869 admissions to units in France (Glangeaud-Freudenthal et al, 2011) reported very similar findings.

There are naturalistic follow-up studies of women who have been admitted to mother and baby units and general wards, as well as case reports and service descriptions, many dating from the 1960s and 1970s. These are comprehensively described in the final chapter of Brockington (1996). Only one controlled trial compares outcomes in mothers admitted with their infant and those admitted without their baby, although they were not randomised (Baker et al, 1961). All of the 20 mothers admitted to the mother and baby unit were able to care for their infant on discharge home, whereas 13 of the 20 admitted alone were not. The average duration of admission was 10 weeks in the mother and baby unit and 16 weeks on the general ward.

Specialist in-patient units should have between 6 and 12 beds, and should be staffed by specialist professionals who are able to care for acutely ill mothers and also their infants. Hence, there should be nursery nurses on the staff, nursery and play areas, and a milk preparation area, in addition to rooms for mothers, sitting and dining areas, offices and interview rooms. The units should offer a range of therapeutic services and be closely linked to maternity, general medical, mental health and community services.

Initial nursing and psychiatric assessment should consider the needs and safety of the infant. The observation level required should take this into account, with infants sleeping in the nursery if the mother is too disturbed or any risk is posed. This should be reviewed regularly and observation levels may be reduced if the mother poses no risk and is able to engage in infant care with support. Treatment is likely to include medication, psychological therapy, mothering skills interventions, perhaps family or couple work, and there may be social needs such as housing and financial issues. Discharge planning should involve community services closely and include contraceptive advice, as well as advice regarding the risk of recurrence of the illness after any future pregnancies.

Women admitted to mother and baby units appear to be satisfied with the care they receive and prefer the units to general acute psychiatric wards (Neil *et al*, 2006). It is recommended that women who require acute psychiatric admission following childbirth are admitted to a specialist mother and baby unit (Centre for Maternal and Child Enquiries, 2011; SIGN 2012; NICE, 2014).

## Obstetric liaison

This involves not only assessing pregnant or postpartum women referred by maternity services, but also being available for consultation and advice on specific problems. Psychiatrists providing obstetric liaison should ensure that screening at booking for antenatal care is carried out, and should educate midwifery and obstetric staff when required. Establishing good working relationships with local maternity services is essential. An understanding of the normal and abnormal pregnancy, delivery and postpartum period, in addition to embryology, fetal and infant development, not only aids communication with other professionals but enables the psychiatrist to detect problems and know when to refer for specialist opinion.

## Child protection

In England and Wales, the Children Act 2004 (2007) (www.legislation. gov.uk/ukpga/2004/31/contents) and the most recent guidance *Working Together to Safeguard Children* (HM Government, 2015) provide a framework for established local safeguarding children's boards and actual or virtual 'Children's Trusts' under the auspices of local authorities. They also clarify the duty of all agencies to make arrangements to safeguard and promote the welfare of children (a child is defined as anyone who has not yet reached their 18th birthday (16 in Scotland)). Section 11 of the Children Act 2004 (2007) places a duty on strategic health authorities, special hospitals, commissioners, NHS trusts and foundation trusts to ensure that they have regard to the need to safeguard and promote the welfare of children.

### Links with other agencies

Clinical networks already exist in some UK areas, and more should follow as the NICE (2014) guideline is implemented. Each network should be managed by a coordinating board of health professionals, commissioners, managers, patients and carers. They should provide a multidisciplinary perinatal service in each locality that can provide the following functions:

- direct services, consultation and advice to maternity, mental health and community services, both urgent and routine
- specialist expert advice on the risks and benefits of psychotropic medication during pregnancy and while breastfeeding
- clear referral and management protocols at all levels of care
- clear pathways of care for patients
- designated specialist in-patient services.

## What skills do perinatal psychiatrists need?

Perinatal psychiatrists require knowledge and skill in managing mental disorders at all levels of severity and complexity in pregnant and postpartum women. Therefore, in addition to general psychiatric skills they must have knowledge and awareness of normal pregnancy and postpartum psychological and physiological changes, embryology, fetal and infant development, and the organisation of maternity care in the UK. They should be aware of the pharmacodynamic and pharmacokinetic changes of pregnancy and the postpartum and have knowledge of psychopharmacology in relation to this (see Chapters 8 & 9).

Joan Raphael-Leff (1991) explored the issues relating to psychotherapy with pregnant women and highlighted the countertransference reactions in different types of therapists. These include envy in some male or childless female therapists, repressed elements from a non-pregnant therapist's own past pregnancies, and 'powerful transference implants' from the patient, which may induce the therapist to enact the parental role. She described maternal therapists who may feel anxious about the patient, and the difficulties that might surround a pregnant therapist whose own vulnerability and introspection may have increased.

Perinatal psychiatrists must be able to consult and liaise with psychiatric, maternity and obstetric staff and primary care, and should have skills in multi-agency working, particularly with child social services. They should ensure that they make themselves fully aware of local services for mothers in their area. They should be familiar with policies and guidelines relating to perinatal mental health, both national and those of any devolved part of the UK they are working in.

Skills in the assessment of parenting may be required and are discussed in Chapter 4. For up-to-date information regarding specialist training in perinatal psychiatry in the UK, please see the Royal College of Psychiatrists' website (www.rcpsych.ac.uk/workinpsychiatry/faculties/perinatal/training/highertraining.aspx).

### Medico-legal expertise

Perinatal psychiatrists should have knowledge of the legislation and guidance in relation to child protection. They will be asked for reports by numerous bodies, including social services, Mental Health Act Review Tribunals and the courts. It is essential to develop skills in producing reports that will withstand the scrutiny of these agencies and cross-examination at tribunals and in court. Psychiatrists may be asked about parenting capacity, but should not give expert opinion on this unless they are skilled in assessing it. Such assessment cannot be made on the basis of psychiatric interview and perusal of records alone and must involve direct observation of parent–child interaction and interview of any others involved in child care, e.g. foster parents or other family members (Bass & Adshead, 2007).

# Conclusion

It is to be hoped that service provision in the UK will improve to ensure that a more equitable and comprehensive service is available to every woman who needs it, and that more collaborative working between services and agencies will improve the care available to families and hence their well-being.

# References

Alberque C, Robert V, Eytan A (2006) A peripartum inpatient psychiatric program for mothers and infants. *Psychiatric Services*, **57**: 721.

Appleby L, Hirst E, Marshall S, *et al* (2003) The treatment of postnatal depression by health visitors: impact of brief training on skills and clinical practice. *Journal of Affective Disorders*, **77**: 261–266.

Baker AA, Morison M, Game JA, *et al* (1961) Admitting schizophrenic mothers with their babies. *Lancet*, **ii**: 237–239.

Ballard CG, Davis R, Cullen PC, *et al* (1994) Prevalence of postnatal psychiatric morbidity in mothers and fathers. *British Journal of Psychiatry*, **164**: 782–788.

Bass C, Adshead G (2007) Fabrication and induction of illness in children: the psychopathology of abuse. *Advances in Psychiatric Treatment*, **13**: 169–177.

Battle CL, Zlotnick C, Miller IW, *et al* (2006) Clinical characteristic of perinatal psychiatric patients: a chart review study. *Journal of Nervous and Mental Disease*, **194**: 369–377.

Bauer A, Parsonage M, Knapp M, *et al* (2014) *The Costs of Perinatal Mental Illness*. Centre for Mental Health and London School of Economics.

Boath E, Major K, Cox J (2003) When the cradle falls II: the cost-effectiveness of treating postnatal depression in a psychiatric day hospital compared with routine primary care. *Journal of Affective Disorders*, **74**: 159–166.

Brockington I (1996) *Motherhood and Mental Health*. Oxford University Press.

Buist A, Speelman C, Hayes B, *et al* (2007) Impact of education on women with perinatal depression. *Journal of Psychosomatic Obstetrics and Gynaecology*, **28**: 49–54.

Centre for Maternal and Child Enquiries (2011) Saving Mothers' Lives: reviewing maternal deaths to make motherhood safer: 2006–2008. *British Journal of Obstetrics and Gynaecology*, **118** (Suppl 1): 134–144.

Department of Health (2014) *Closing the Gap: Priorities for Essential Change in Mental Health*. Department of Health.

Elliott SA, Ashton C, Gerrard J, *et al* (2003) Is trainer training an effective method for disseminating evidence-based practice for postnatal depression? *Journal of Reproductive and Infant Psychology*, **21**: 219–228.

Glangeaud-Freudenthal NM-C, MBU-SMF Working Group (2004) Mother-Baby psychiatric units (MBUs): national data collection in France and Belgium (1999-2000). *Archives of Women's Mental Health*, **7, 59-64.**

Glangeaud-Freudenthal NM-C, Sutter A-L, Thieulin A-C, *et al* (2011) Inpatient mother-and-child postpartum psychiatric care: factors associated with improvement in maternal mental health. *European Psychiatry*, **26**: 215-223.

HM Government (2015) *Working Together to Safeguard Children: a guide to inter-agency working to safeguard and promote the welfare of children*. HM Government.

Howard M, Battle CL, Pearlstein T, *et al* (2006) A psychiatric mother-baby day hospital for pregnant and postpartum women. *Archives of Women's Mental Health*, 9: 213–218.

Joint Commissioning Panel for Mental Health (2012) *Guidance for Commissioners of Perinatal Mental Health Services*. JCPMH.

Kumar R, Marks M, Platz C, et al (1995) Clinical survey of a psychiatric mother and baby unit: characteristics of 100 consecutive admissions. *Journal of Affective Disorders*, **33**: 11–22.

Main TF (1948) Mothers with children in a psychiatric hospital. *Lancet*, **272**: 845–847.

Maizel S, Kandel Katzenelson S, Fainstein V (2005) The Jerusalem psychiatric mother-baby unit. *Archives of Women's Mental Health*, **8**: 200–202.

Milgrom J, Burrows GD, Snellen M, *et al* (1998) Psychiatric illness in women: a review of the function of a specialist mother-baby unit. *Australian and New Zealand Journal of Psychiatry*, **32**: 680–686.

Morrell CJ, Warner R, Slade P, *et al* (2009) Psychological interventions for postnatal depression: cluster randomised trial and economic evaluation. The PoNDER trial. *Health Technology Assessment*, **13**: 1–153.

Morrell CJ, Ricketts T, Tudor T, *et al* (2011) Training health visitors in cognitive behavioural and person-centred approaches for depression in postnatal women as part of a cluster randomised trial and economic evaluation in primary care: the PoNDER trial. *Primary Health Care Research and Development,* **12**: 11–20.

Murray L, Woolgar M, Murray J, *et al* (2003) Self-exclusion from healthcare in women at risk for postnatal depression. *Public Health Medicine*, **25**: 131–137.

National Institute for Health and Care Excellence (2014) *Antenatal and Postnatal Mental Health: Clinical Management and Service Guidance*. NICE.

Neil S, Sanderson H, Wieck A (2006) A satisfaction survey of women admitted to a psychiatric mother and baby unit in the northwest of England. *Archives of Women's Mental Health*, **9**: 109.

Oates M (1988) The development of an integrated community-orientated service for severe postnatal mental illness. In *Motherhood and Mental Illness: Causes and consequences* (eds R Kumar, IF Brockington). Wright.

Raphael-Leff J (1991) Psychotherapy with pregnant women. In *Psychological Processes of Childbearing* (pp. 91–116). Chapman & Hall.

Rishel CW, Greeno CG, Marcus SC, *et al* (2006) Effect of maternal mental health problems on child treatment response in community-based services. *Psychiatric Services*, **57**: 716.

Royal College of Psychiatrists (2001) *Perinatal Mental Health Services: Recommendations for Provision of Services for Childbearing Women*. RCPsych.

Royal College of Psychiatrists (2015) *Perinatal Mental Health Services: Recommendations for the Provision of Services for Childbearing Women (CR197)*. RCPsych.

Salmon MP, Abel K, Webb R, *et al* (2004) A national audit of joint mother and baby admissions to UK psychiatric hospitals: an overview of findings. *Archives of Women's Mental Health*, **7**: 65–70.

Scottish Intercollegiate Guidelines Network (2012) *Management of Perinatal Mood Disorders*. SIGN.

# CHAPTER 11

# Perinatal psychiatry
# in multi-ethnic societies

'In no known culture was pregnancy found to be ignored or treated with indifference, instead it elicited a gamut of emotions and feelings including responsibility and accountability by the parents as well as solicitude by social groups' (Mead & Newton, 1967).

Childbirth in traditional societies has been regarded by anthropologists as a rite of passage with three linked phases of adjustment. The first was the rite of separation, followed by a liminal period during which the mother was confined for the birth and was in 'limbo', and finally the third phase of incorporation when she re-entered society with a new status. In modern secular societies, this transition is often incomplete or non-existent. Kinship bonds and family rituals are changing in many societies because of rapid economic development, competitive market economies and increased voluntary migration, as well as forced migration of refugees and asylum seekers.

Parenting is a process intimately linked to cultural values and beliefs (Bernstein, 2013). The free movement of labour in the European Union has resulted in increased numbers of migrants coming to the UK to work and to better the opportunities for their families. Other changes in UK society over recent decades include an increased proportion of absent fathers, more serial marriages, increased divorce rates, same-sex marriage, shorter stays in the maternity unit, a decline in institutional religion, and an expectation of prompt return to work with no defined period of postpartum rest. The status of the childbearing woman has become more ambiguous in Western Europe. Childbirth may elicit condolences from friends and family members, and questions about who will look after the baby. A journalist writing in the *Guardian* newspaper has drawn attention to the fall in birth rate with the headline 'Behind the baby gap lies a culture of contempt for parenthood' (Bunting, 2006). She suggested that present-day culture values consumption, choice and independence, which may be incompatible with the inherent demands of parenthood.

A sociocultural approach to understanding the current stresses of childbirth in society is necessary for a comprehensive grasp of the causes and management of perinatal mental disorders. Health professionals' familiarity with local values and culture (including language and religion), and how these change over time, is particularly important when developing a perinatal service for a multicultural society. Transcultural psychiatry begins 'at home', where the values of post-modern families may include, for example, excessive deference to biomedicine (Littlewood, 1992). This sociocultural approach to perinatal psychiatry is, in our experience, central to any working model for a perinatal service (Cox, 1999). Furthermore, it is within this broad social context that advances in the neuroscience or genetics of puerperal psychosis (Chapter 3) are best understood. The biopsychosocial model (Engel, 1980), which has guided much research, may no longer be an adequate framework to investigate the mother's personal narrative, her attachment to the baby and the 'ghosts in the nursery' (Fraiberg et al, 1987). For these reasons, a different paradigm could be considered, such as a body–mind–spirit paradigm, which incorporates meaning and purpose (spirit) as well as the valences of relationships. Perinatal psychiatry is, at its core, a relationship-based specialty, and may also be a key to liberate medical practice from excessive biomedical and managerial reductionism.

## Low- and middle-income countries

In Africa, Collomb et al (1972) described Senegalese childbearing women as entering a world of worries and fears, and noticed that quite often anxiety 'wins out over veneration and contentment'. In many other low-income countries, childbirth and the associated mental disorders represent great risk to the well-being and longevity of the mother and her infant. It is estimated that 1 in 16 mothers in some low- and middle-income countries die in childbirth (World Health Organization, 2005), and in the UN Millennium Development Goals (MDGs) this staggering statistic has at last become an international public health priority and led to a call for action. Empowering women and improving maternal mental health are the third and fifth development goal targets.

## Social support

Stern and Kruckman (1983) described the sociocultural components that provided social support in traditional societies, and suggest that the extent of this support may 'cushion or prevent the experience of post partum depression'. The components they considered include:

- structuring of a distinctive postpartum time period
- protective measures and rituals reflecting the vulnerability of the mother
- social exclusion

- mandated rest
- assistance from relatives or a midwife
- social recognition (through rituals, gifts, etc.) of the new social status of the mother.

They pointed out that postnatal depression was, at the time, infrequently described in traditional societies compared with Europe or the USA, and attributed this to the possibility that social support and higher status protected against maternal mental disorder. Their observation spurred on subsequent perinatal community studies in low- and middle-income countries, which in general found that depressive symptoms were readily identified in traditional societies, but that their impact and duration may be different from those found in high-income countries.

## Transcultural study of postnatal depression

An international study (Marks *et al*, 2004) brought together research groups in Europe (France, UK, Sweden, Portugal, Italy, Switzerland and Austria) as well as Japan, the USA and Uganda, to develop, harmonise and validate culturally sensitive research instruments for use in the perinatal field. Each research centre used qualitative research methods (focus groups and key informant interviews) to explore whether or not 'postnatal depression' was a recognised condition (see Oates *et al*, 2004). A morbid state of unhappiness postpartum was found in most of the cultures and countries studied, with symptoms similar to those commonly identified in 'postnatal depression'; however, these symptoms were not universally regarded as a medical condition that requires treatment by health professionals. In Uganda, there was no folk disorder similar to postnatal depression that was familiar to local informants – although there was a traditional illness, amakiro, which included symptoms found in the puerperal psychoses (Cox, 1979). The functional disability of many mothers with non-psychotic perinatal depression was nevertheless found to be considerable and included difficulty with household tasks (digging and carrying water) as well as problems with childcare.

In a study from Malta by Felice *et al* (2006), low rates of depression postpartum were reported in a cohesive Catholic island community. In an ongoing study from the Faroe Islands, led by Anna Sofia Fjällheim and using the Faroese version of the Edinburgh Postnatal Depression Rating Scale (EPDS), it is hypothesised that the prevalence of perinatal mental disorder may be similarly reduced. Likewise in Japan, where sex roles are more traditionally determined, and in Uganda, where the status and social support from co-wives and tradition were clearly evident (Cox 1983), the rates of depression in stable rural villages was less than that reported in urban areas of many high-income countries.

It is likely that the social support available to mothers during pregnancy and in the year postpartum is an important variable that determines the duration of depression during pregnancy and postpartum, as well as its severity. Knowledge of sociology (role change, gender tasks, family structure), psychology (personality traits, dependency, self-esteem) and social anthropology (values, meaning of symptoms and childbirth rituals) is important if a full understanding of the maintaining factors for perinatal mental health is to be achieved. Psychoanalysts (such as Joan Raphael-Leff, 2001) have also contributed much to this field and describe the unconscious identification between the mother and her baby, and with the mother's own mother, as well as the problems that occur and if the mother had herself an unhappy childhood.

The mother–infant relationship is thus the vehicle through which most knowledge and culture are passed between generations. Breaks in 'women's knowledge' (Fitzgerald, 1998) – interruptions in the transmission of birth experience across generations – which may occur in modern societies because of increased mobility, globalisation and more short-term relationships can cause difficulty with parenting owing to a lack of knowledge about childcare and access to supportive postnatal customs. The benefits of health visitor 'listening visits' and of structured counselling postpartum are best explained by an understanding that these intergenerational psychological processes are a component of any professional relationship. The community perinatal health worker provides advice, validation of status and specific practical knowledge about feeding and infant development that might have been given in traditional societies by the mother's own mother.

The anthropologist Lewis (1976) said that if a mother does not know how to bring up her children, then the cultural heritage is in jeopardy. There are present-day attempts to diminish subsequent challenging behaviour in adolescent boys and so help vulnerable families to attempt to compensate for these 'breaks in women's knowledge'. If successful, they could enhance the neurodevelopmental processes of the infant and facilitate more secure attachment to the parents.

## Public health considerations

Perinatal mental health problems are increasingly prominent in public health planning throughout the world. They affect the viability of young families and influence the extent to which the next generation of parents fulfil their responsibilities and maintain good enough mental health. There is also evidence that perinatal mental disorders can adversely affect attachment and cognitive development, particularly of boys in Western societies (see Chapter 6). In the developing world, the result can be weight loss in the infant and failure to thrive (Patel *et al*, 2005). A community study from Stoke-on-Trent (O'Brien *et al*, 2004) found a twofold increase in the likelihood of clinical depression in mothers whose babies had non-organic failure to thrive. Explanations for this finding included feeding difficulties caused by an irritable or crying baby, as well as the depressed mother having difficulty in persisting with feeding or having insufficient breast milk.

The preferred gender of the infant is has marked cultural assumptions. The birth of a girl was associated with maternal postnatal depression in the Sikh community in Wolverhampton (Clifford et al, 1997), as well as in studies from India (Chandran et al, 2002), Nigeria (Abiodun, 2006) and China (Xie et al, 2007). In Western Europe, 11-year-old boys whose mothers were depressed following their birth were more likely than girls to show behavioural disturbances, and to have elevated morning cortisol (Hay et al, 2001).

## Grandparents

Transcultural research shows that, in many societies, grandparents still provide much support in the immediate postpartum months. However, in almost all the centres in an international study of perinatal mental disorder (Marks et al, 2004), mothers-in-law were a possible source of unhappiness.

In modern Japan, the custom 'Satogaeri bunben', in which a mother goes to her own mother's house for the delivery and remains there for the first 40 days, is still practised, but it does not necessarily protect against postnatal depression (Yoshida et al, 2001). In China, doing the month, when the mother should not go outside or be blown by the wind, should not have sex with her husband, should eat chicken and should be supported by her mother, is still customary. These proscriptions can be helpful to clarify the responsibilities for the new mother, and the expected practical and emotional support from the family. In Hong Kong, however, Lee et al (2004) found that this practice was not always helpful and could heighten conflict between filial respect for the woman's own mother and the wish for autonomy. In Uganda, before the AIDS pandemic, support for a new mother who was married was available from co-wives or neighbours – and older children might help with household tasks. The naming ceremony and baptism were important, and the name was traditionally chosen by a grandparent. A single mother was often ostracised, as the baby would have no name – and therefore no family.

A qualitative study of same-sex parents identified lack of support from their families of origin, challenges in negotiating parenting roles, and legal and policy barriers as stressors (Ross, 2005). Eberhard-Gran et al (2010) have suggested that many of the postnatal customs that were common before 1950 may no longer exist as modern societies are changing in their attitudes to childbirth.

## Refugees and asylum seekers

Mothers are particularly vulnerable to the stresses of migration and cultural change. Those who have become parents in a new, and alien, country are particularly at risk of becoming depressed after childbirth. Studies of immigrants from Cambodia and Vietnam to Australia (Matthey et al, 1997) found that such women were particularly vulnerable to postnatal depression. In the Beyond Blue programme in Australia, a country where over 45% of the population were born overseas or had parents born overseas, familiarity with these cultural issues was regarded as of fundamental importance. This understanding was of special relevance to the Aboriginal peoples and the Torres Strait Islanders (www.beyondblue.org.au/resources/for-me/aboriginal-and-torres-strait-islander-people/risk-factors).

In some immigrant communities, the father may be working away from home and is absorbing the new culture and language, while the mother is less exposed to these influences and becomes more isolated. Other difficulties for migrants include the conflict of values as the mother and baby socialise with local women who have different attitudes towards childcare and different religious traditions.

It is estimated that in parts of the UK 20% of births occur in refugee families, who are often exposed to distinctive stressors. Asylum seekers have often experienced severe stresses and trauma outside normal experience. It may be difficult to distinguish post-traumatic stress disorder from depression or anxiety. The refugee parents may have experienced a 'sequential traumatisation' and, as a consequence, may have an increased risk of mental health problems. The stresses these refugees may experience include:

- events back home, including violence, torture and rape
- the journey here, not knowing where they were going
- living here, unfamiliar language, food and culture, poverty/fiscal trauma
- pregnancy and motherhood, other major stressors
- isolation
- racism, stigmatisation
- moves, of house, school and city
- the asylum claim and legal issues.

Other community healthcare workers (Teng et al, 2007) identify a healing relationship, safety, remembrance and mourning, and re-connection as important components of the refugees' recovery. They describe the stresses for the health professionals working with these vulnerable refugees, and the difficulties of overcoming language and cultural barriers, as well as the intrusion of their own feelings. Drennan & Joseph (2005) have described the issues relevant to professional practice, and the need to prioritise the mother's basic needs, as well as the needs of the infant. The practical barriers and culturally determined barriers to care, such as limited access to services and language difficulties, as well as stigma, were other factors to consider (Teng et al, 2007).

The health professional working with immigrant groups may fear being de-skilled by cultural uncertainty and language problems, as well as having inadequate assessment tools. Midwives working in London with Somali refugees, for example, need to be aware of the effects of female genital mutilation (FGM) on birth, which include depression and anxiety, as well as reproductive and obstetric difficulties (Straus *et al*, 2009). FGM is illegal in the UK and the health worker must therefore be vigilant of the law as well as being sensitive to cultural practices (www.england.nhs.uk/2014/12/08/fgm-prevention/).

## Edinburgh Postnatal Depression Scale: cultural issues

The EPDS (Cox *et al*, 1987) was developed and validated in Scotland and has been translated into over 50 languages and validated on all continents (Henshaw & Elliott, 2005; Cox *et al*, 2014). The process of translating the scale and using it in a non-English-speaking community brings the clinician face to face with the cultural components of perinatal mental disorders and their satisfactory management. The issues of translation are fully discussed by Flaherty *et al* (1988). These include the need to establish semantic validity, content validity, technical equivalence and construct validity.

## Management issues

It is apparent from the issues discussed in this chapter that the development of a perinatal mental health service, with appropriate referral pathways, can only be established if there is a full awareness of the sociocultural dimensions. Clinicians and managers are required to be culturally competent and fully aware of their own cultural assumptions. It is also necessary to have hands-on experience of the assessment and the psychology of refugees and their particular experience of stress. The provision of readily available trained interpreters, advocates and culture brokers is crucial in the contemporary world.

Awareness of the impact of changes in family structure on social support, familiarity with naming customs in ethnic minorities, and understanding the values and beliefs of patients, as well as the pitfalls of superficial translation, are other examples of the required core skills and competencies.

## References

Abiodun OA (2006) Postnatal depression in primary care populations in Nigeria. *General Hospital Psychiatry*, **28**: 133–136.

Bernstein MH (2013) Parenting and child mental health: a cross cultural perspective. *World Psychiatry*, **12**: 258–265.

Bunting M (2006) Behind the baby gap lies a culture of contempt for parenthood. *The Guardian*, Tuesday 7 March.

Chandran M, Tharyan P, Muliyil J, *et al* (2002) Post-partum depression in a cohort of women from a rural area of Tamil Nadu, India: incidence and risk factors. *British Journal of Psychiatry*, 181: 499–504.

Clifford C, Day A, Cox J (1997) Women's health after birth. Developing the use of EPDS in a Punjabi-speaking community. *British Journal of Midwifery*, 5: 616–619.

Collomb H, Guena R, Diop B (1972) Psychological and social factors in the pathology of childbearing. *Foreign Psychiatry*, 1: 77–89.

Cox JL (1979) Amakiro: a Ugandan puerperal psychosis? *Social Psychiatry*, 14: 49–52.

Cox JL (1983) Postnatal depression: a comparison of African and Scottish women. *Social Psychiatry*, 18: 25–28.

Cox JL (1999) Perinatal mood disorder in a changing culture: a trans-cultural European and African perspective. *International Review of Psychiatry*, 11: 103–110.

Cox JL, Holden JM, Sagovsky R (1987) Detection of postnatal depression. Development of the 10-item Edinburgh Postnatal Depression Scale. *British Journal of Psychiatry*, 150: 782–786.

Cox JL, Holden J, Henshaw C (2014) *Perinatal Mental Health: the Edinburgh Postnatal Depression Scale Manual (2nd edn)*. Royal College of Psychiatrists.

Drennan VM, Joseph J (2005) Health visiting and refugee families: Issues in professional practice. *Journal of Advanced Nursing*, 49:155–163.

Eberhard-Gran M, Garthus–Nagel S, Garthus–Nagel K, *et al* (2010) Post natal care: cross-cultural and historical perspective. *Archives of Women's Mental Health*, 13: 459–466.

Engel G (1980) The clinical application of the Bio-psycho-social model. *American Journal of Psychiatry*, 137: 534–554.

Felice E, Saliba J, Grech V, *et al* (2006) Validation of the Maltese version of the Edinburgh Postnatal Depression Scale. *Archives of Women's Mental Health*, 9: 75–80.

Fitzgerald MH (1998) Hear our Voices: Trauma, Birthing and Mental Health among Cambodian Women. *Sydney Transcultural Mental Health Centre.*

Flaherty JA, Gaviria FM, Pathak D, *et al* (1988) Developing instruments for transcultural psychiatric research. *Journal of Nervous and Mental Disease*, 176: 257–264.

Fraiberg S, Adelson E, Shapiro V (1987) Ghosts in the nursery: a psychoanalytic approach to the problems of impaired infant-mother relationships. In *Selected Writings of Selma Fraiberg* (ed L. Fraiberg; pp. 100–136). Ohio State University Press.

Hay DF, Pawlby S, Sharp D, *et al* (2001) Intellectual problems shown by 11 year old children, whose mothers had postnatal depression. *Journal of Child Psychology and Psychiatry*, 42: 871–889

Henshaw C, Elliott S (2005) Bibliography of translations and validation studies. In *Screening for Perinatal Depression* (pp. 205–211). Jessica Kingsley.

Lee DTS, Alexander SK, Tony YS, *et al* (2004) Ethnoepidemiology of postnatal depression: Prospective multivariate study of socio-cultural risk factors in a Chinese population in Hong Kong. *British Journal of Psychiatry*, 184: 36–40.

Lewis IM (1976) *Social Anthropology in Perspective*. Penguin Books.

Littlewood R (1992) Russian dolls and Chinese boxes: an anthropological approach to the implicit models of comparative psychiatry. In *Transcultural Psychiatry* (ed JL Cox). Croom Helm.

Marks M, O'Hara M, Glangeaud-Freudenthal N, *et al* (2004) Transcultural study of postnatal depression: development of harmonised research methods. *British Journal of Psychiatry*, 184 (Suppl 46).

Matthey S, Barnett BE, Elliott A (1997) Vietnamese and Arabic women's responses to the Diagnostic Interview Schedule (depression) and self-report questionnaires: cause for concern. *Australian and New Zealand Journal of Psychiatry*, 31: 360–369.

Mead M, Newton N (1967) Cultural patterning of perinatal behavior. In *Childbearing: Its Social and Psychological Aspects* (eds SA Richardson, AF Guttmacher). Williams & Wilkins.

Oates M, Cox JL, Neema S, *et al* (2004) Postnatal depression across countries and cultures. *British Journal of Psychiatry*, 84: 10–16.

O'Brien IM, Haycock L, Hanna P, et al (2004) Postnatal depression and faltering growth: a community study. *Paediatrics*, **11**: 1242–1247.

Patel V, Desouza N, Rodrigues M (2005) Postnatal depression and infant growth and development in low-income countries: a short study from Goa, India. *Archives of Diseases of the Child*, **88**: 34–37.

Raphael-Leff J (2001) *Psychological Processes of Childbearing*. Psychoanalytic Publication Series, University of Essex.

Ross LE (2005) Perinatal mental health in lesbian mothers: a review of potential risk and protective factors. *Women & Health*, **41**: 113–128.

Stern C, Kruckman L (1983) Multi-disciplinary perspectives on post partum depression; an anthropological critique. *Social Science and Medicine*, **17**: 1027–1041.

Straus L, McEwen A, Hussein FM (2009) Somali women's experience of childbirth in the UK: perspectives from Somali health workers. *Midwifery*, **25**: 181–186

Teng L, Robertson Blackmore E, Stewart DE (2007) Healthcare workers' perceptions of barriers to care by immigrant women with postpartum depression: an exploratory qualitative study. *Archives of Women's Mental Health*, **10**: 93–101.

World Health Organization (2005) *The World Health Report 2005: Make Every Mother and Child Count*. WHO.

Xie R, He G, Liu A, et al (2007) Foetal gender and postpartum depression in a cohort of Chinese women. *Social Science and Medicine*, **65**: 680–684.

Yoshida K, Yamashita H, Ueda M, et al (2001) Postnatal depression in Japanese mothers and the reconsideration of 'Satogeri-bunben'. *Paediatrics International*, **43**: 189–193.

# Further reading

Ingleby D (2004) *Forced Migration and Mental Health: Rethinking the Care of Refugees and Displaced Persons*. Springer-Verlag.

Wilson JP, Drožek B (2004) *Broken Spirits: The Treatment of Traumatized Asylum Seekers, Refugees, War and Torture Victims*. Routledge.

# Appendix I
# Organisations offering support and information

| Source | Contact information | What's there |
|---|---|---|
| Action on Puerperal Psychosis FREEPOST RTEX-YBCH-CGJR Hadyn Ellis Building Maindy Road Cardiff CF24 4HQ | Tel: 020 3322 9900 Web: www.app-network.org | Provide advice, resources, signposting to help and support, and an online forum for support via the website |
| Association for Post-Natal Illness 145 Dawes Road Fulham London SW6 7EB | Helpline: 020 7386 0868 Email: info@apni.org Web: www.apni.org | Support and information for women with postnatal illness |
| Cry-sis BM Cry-sis London WC1N 3XX | Helpline: 08451 228 669 Email: info@cry-sis.org.uk Web: www.cry-sis.org.uk | Support, help, advice and information for parents with a crying baby |
| Home-Start UK 2 Salisbury Road Leicester LE1 7QR | Tel: 0116 233 9955 Email: info@home-start.org.uk Web: www.home-start.org.uk | Volunteers offer support, friendship and practical help in their own home to families with at least one child under 5 who are having difficulties |
| Meet-a-Mum Association (MAMA) 7 Southcourt Road Linslade Leighton Buzzard Bedfordshire LU7 2QFR | Enquiries: 0845 120 6162 Helpline: 0845 120 3746 Web: www.mama.co.uk | Support and help for women with postnatal depressive illness, or who feel tired or isolated after having a baby or are simply in need of a friend |
| National Childbirth Trust 30 Euston Square London NW1 2FB | Helpline: 0300 330 0700 Web: www.nct.org.uk | Information and support for expectant and new parents including antenatal classes, breastfeeding counselling and postnatal support groups |
| Netmums 124 Mildred Avenue Watford WD18 7DX | Web: www.netmums.com | Support and information – a network of local websites, chat rooms and blogs |

| | | |
|---|---|---|
| Perinatal Illness UK<br>PO Box 49769<br>London WC1H 9WH | Enquiries: 01530 560645<br>Helpline: 01654 713833<br>Web: www.pni-uk.com | Support and information<br>Message board, chat room<br>and email support |
| Postpartum Support<br>International<br>6706 SW 54th<br>Avenue<br>Portland, Oregon<br>92719<br>USA | Tel: +1 503 894 9453<br>Helpline: +1 800 944 400D<br>(4773)[a]<br>Web: www.postpartum.net | Provide information and<br>advice via their website,<br>run support groups and are<br>a network of professionals<br>who can provide training<br>and run an annual<br>conference; most members<br>are based in the USA |

a. The toll-free number only works in the USA.

There are other charities and organisations that work in specific areas – ask your health visitor or at your nearest Children's Centre for information about local services.

# Appendix II
# Edinburgh Postnatal Depression Scale

## The Edinburgh Postnatal Depression Scale

Name...........................................

Today's date..............................

Please UNDERLINE the answer which comes closest to how you have felt IN THE PAST WEEK, <u>not just how you feel today</u>.

IN THE PAST WEEK

I have been able to laugh and see the funny side of things:

| | |
|---|---|
| As much as I always could | 0 |
| Not quite so much now | 1 |
| Definitely not so much now | 2 |
| Not at all | 3 |

I have looked forward with enjoyment to things:

| | |
|---|---|
| As much as I ever did | 0 |
| Rather less than I used to | 1 |
| Definitely less than I used to | 2 |
| .Hardly at all | 3 |

I have blamed myself unnecessarily when things went wrong:

| | |
|---|---|
| Yes, most of the time | 3 |
| Yes, some of the time | 2 |
| Not very often | 1 |
| No, never | 0 |

I have been anxious or worried for no good reason:

| | |
|---|---|
| No, not at all | 0 |
| Hardly ever | 1 |
| Yes, sometimes | 2 |
| Yes, very often | 3 |

I have felt scared or panicky for no very good reason:

|  |  |
|---|---|
| Yes, quite a lot | 3 |
| Yes, sometimes | 2 |
| No, not much | 1 |
| No, not at all | 0 |

Things have been getting on top of me:

|  |  |
|---|---|
| Yes, most of the time I haven't been able to cope at all | 3 |
| Yes, sometimes I haven't been coping as well as usual | 2 |
| No, most of the time I have coped quite well | 1 |
| No, I have been coping as well as ever | 0 |

I have been so unhappy that I have had difficulty sleeping:

|  |  |
|---|---|
| Yes, most of the time | 3 |
| Yes, sometimes | 2 |
| No, not very often | 1 |
| No, not at all | 0 |

I have felt sad or miserable:

|  |  |
|---|---|
| Yes, most of the time | 3 |
| Yes, sometimes | 2 |
| No, not very often | 1 |
| No, not at all | 0 |

I have been so unhappy that I have been crying:

|  |  |
|---|---|
| Yes, most of the time | 3 |
| Yes, quite often | 2 |
| Only occasionally | 1 |
| No, not at all | 0 |

The thought of harming myself has occurred to me:

|  |  |
|---|---|
| Yes, quite often | 3 |
| Sometimes | 2 |
| Hardly ever | 1 |
| Never | 0 |

# Appendix III
# Resources

## For professionals

### Antenatal Psychosocial Health Assessment (ALPHA)
This form is available from the Department of Family and Community Medicine, University of Toronto (http://ocfp.on.ca/docs/default-source/cme/alpha-guidead64b74ce3a6.pdf?sfvrsn=0).

### Postnatal Depression Training
One- and two-day courses are offered, either at their venue near Swansea or at the client's base.

### Postpartum Depression Screening Scale (PDSS)
This scale is published and distributed by Western Psychological Services (www.wpspublish.com).

### The Royal College of Psychiatrists
The RCPsych has a number of online training modules, including 'Psychiatric aspects of perinatal loss', 'Psychotropic medication in breastfeeding' and 'Practical child protection'. It also has others under development: 'Adoption and fostering', 'Infanticide', 'Safeguarding children in perinatal mental health' and 'The assessment and management of postnatal depression'. (www.psychiatrycpd.org/learningmodules.aspx).

### Beating Bipolar
Has an online training module for midwives (www.beatingbipolar.org/perinataltraining).

### Maternal Mental Health Alliance
Is campaigning for improvements in services. Their website (www.everyonesbusiness.org.uk) has information for professionals including commissioners and directories of support organisations.

# For patients and carers

See Appendix I for organisations that can offer help, advice and support.

### Mind

Has information on postnatal depression, including a leaflet that you can download. It also has information on a wider range of mental disorders. www.mind.org.uk

### The Royal College of Psychiatrists

Has information leaflets on a wide range of disorders and treatments, free to download. www.rcpsych.ac.uk/expertadvice.aspx

# Index

Compiled by Linda English

abortion 30, 95, 204
abuse, of mothers 23, 73, 86, 93–94, 117, 122–123, 143
acupuncture 39, 40
adjustment and transition 27–28
admission, of mothers 98
adolescents
    fathers 157–158
    mothers 13, 73, 157–158, 176
    services 268
Adult Attachment Interview 160
agomelatine 214, 253
Ainsworth, Mary 145
alcohol misuse 86, 108, 115–121, 122, 143, 157, 201
    binge drinking 116–117, 118
    breastfeeding 119
    child outcome 110–111, 115–116, 118, 151–152
    detoxification 121
    dose–response association 118
    infant withdrawal 123–124
    interventions 120–121
    screening and detection 119–120
alcohol-related neurodevelopmental disorder 115
alprazolam 254–255
amakiro 3, 280
amisulpride 221
amitriptyline 247
amniotic fluid, drugs transfer through 199–200
amphetamines 124, 125, 126
anorexia nervosa 95–98, 151
Antenatal Psychosocial Health Assessment (ALPHA) 181
Antenatal Risk Questionnaire 181
anticholinergics 222–223
anticoagulant therapy 76–77
anticonvulsants 92, 224–226, 256–257

antidepressants 37–38, 76, 92, 93, 186
    breastfeeding 246–254
    pregnancy 38, 196–214
    women's opinion about 43, 44
antipsychotics 76, 77, 87, 88
    atypical 38, 86, 92, 215, 218–222, 258–260
    breastfeeding 257–260
    pregnancy 215–222, 227
    typical 216–217, 258
anxiety disorders 7, 23–31
    in postnatal depression 11, 13, 15, 18, 20, 21
    pre-existing 92–94
    pregnancy 23, 30–31, 40–41, 42, 92–94, 147, 151, 154–155, 229–230
    screening 177, 178, 180, 183
anxiolytics 196, 214–215
Apgar scores 92, 202, 206, 208
aripiprazole 221, 260
aromatherapy 229–230
assessment
    admission of mothers 98
    child outcome 160–161
    in non-psychotic disorder 31–32
    parenting capacity 99–100, 271, 275
    puerperal psychosis 75–76
    residential 100
    risk–benefit in bipolar disorder 91
    substance misuse 109, 119, 127
assisted reproductive technologies (ART) 17
atomoxetine 214, 253
attachment 18, 144–150
    anxious 145
    anxious avoidant 18, 145
    assessment 160
    disorders of 146
    disorganised 28, 145
    impact of parental mental illness 146–148
    parental 148–150
    prenatal 141–142
    secure 145, 146

**293**

attention-deficit hyperactivity disorder
   (ADHD) 110, 118, 144, 208–209, 214,
   227
AUDIT-C instrument 119, 120
AUDIT instrument 119, 120
autism spectrum disorder (ASD) 208–209
Avon Longitudinal Study of Pregnancy and
   Childhood (ALSPAC) 122

baby massage 161
Bayley Scales of Infant Development 160
Beck Depression Inventory (BDI) 178
benzodiazepine receptor agonists 215
benzodiazepines 126, 196, 214–215, 227,
   254–255
Bethlem Mother–Infant Interaction Scale 75
Beyond Blue programme 283
binge drinking 116–117, 118
binge-eating disorder 95, 151
biological factors, in postnatal
depression 13, 19–21
biopsychosociocultural model 15, 279
bipolar disorder 1, 7, 15, 84, 85, 89–92
   abortion 30
   drugs during pregnancy 38, 226–227
   in-patient units 272
   management 91–92
   obstetric complications 151
   postpartum recurrence 64, 89, 91–92
   prevention 91, 188
   and puerperal psychosis 63, 66, 68, 69,
      70, 71
   screening 182, 188
birth weight, low see low-birth weight babies
blues, postpartum 15, 181, 183
body–mind–spirit paradigm 279
borderline personality disorder (BPD) 147
Bowlby, John 144–145
breastfeeding 31
   alcohol misuse 119
   eating disorders 96
   physical treatments 245–266
      anticonvulsants 256–257
      antidepressants 246–255
      antipsychotics 257–260
      benzodiazepines and hypnotics 254–
         255
      factors influencing infant
         exposure 245–246
      general guidelines 246
      mood stabilisers 255–257
      non-drug interventions 260
      same drug used during pregnancy 246

   puerperal psychosis 76, 188
   sleep disturbance 187
   substance misuse 119, 124, 129
bright light therapy
   breastfeeding 260
   pregnancy 229
British Association for
   Psychopharmacology 230
Bromley Postnatal Depression Scale 175,
   177
bromocriptine 70
bulimia nervosa 95–98
Bumps website 230
buprenorphine 128–129
bupropion 37, 113, 211–212, 253
buspirone 215
butyrophenones 217

Caesarean section 17, 25, 30, 35, 41, 65, 87,
   96, 110
CAGE questionnaire 119, 120, 122
calcium carbonate 187
calcium channel blockers 226–227
cannabis 109, 110–111, 122, 126, 127,
   152–153, 157
carbamazepine 92, 224, 256
cardiac malformations 86, 204–205, 209,
   211–212, 220, 223
care plan 88
catatonic symptoms 65, 68, 228
CHARGE syndrome 220
child abuse and neglect 16–17, 87, 148,
   149, 155–156
   see also child sexual abuse
Child Behaviour Checklist 1.5-5 161
childbirth
   'fear of childbirth teams' 41
   fear of (tokophobia) 25–26, 35, 41
   rite of passage in traditional societies 278
   sociocultural approach 278–279
child health settings, screening in 184
child homicide 86, 155
childhood acute myeloid leukaemia 118
child mental health services, and adult
   services 163, 164, 268
child protection 98, 100, 155–156, 269,
   273–274, 275
children 139–173, 197–198
   alcohol misuse in mothers 110–111,
      115–116, 118, 151–152
   antenatal mental illness 150–152
   assessment 160–161
   development 152–154

emotional and behavioural problems 150,
153, 154–155, 157, 160–161, 162, 268,
282
gender 154, 281
interventions and 159–163
mental health problems 154–155, 156
outcome 150–154, 159, 160, 281
physical health 152
resilience 139–140, 149–150
schizophrenia in mothers 86–87
separation from 84, 87, 98, 146, 163
substance misuse in mothers 110–111,
118, 126
Children Act 2004 (2007) 273–274
child sexual abuse (CSA) 16, 22, 155
chlorpromazine 207, 216–217, 258
cholestasis 202, 205
cholesterol 20
churching, of mothers 2
citalopram 198, 199, 203, 205, 249, 250
classification 2–8
cleft lip and palate 214, 221, 224
clinical networks 267, 274
clomipramine 42, 201–202
clonazepam 254–255, 259
clozapine 88, 218, 219, 221–222, 257
club foot 204
cocaine 122, 125, 126, 152, 153
cognitive–behavioural counselling
(CBC) 33, 268
cognitive–behavioural therapy (CBT) 32,
34, 40–41, 42, 87, 121
cognitive deficits
in children 118, 125, 154
puerperal psychosis 65
command hallucinations 74, 75
community services, specialist 267
comorbidity 23, 26, 267
complementary therapies 40, 201
congenital malformations 41, 112, 125, 230
drugs in pregnancy 200
antidepressants 203–205, 209, 210–212
antipsychotics 216, 217, 218–219,
220–222
anxiolytics and hypnotics 214, 215
mood stabilisers 223, 224–226, 227
electroconvulsive therapy in
pregnancy 228
schizophrenia 86
see also cardiac malformations; neural tube
defects
contraception 78, 84, 92, 129, 147–148,
226, 270
Coroners and Justice Act 2009 74

cortico-limbic networks 149
corticotrophin-releasing hormone
(CRH) 19, 20, 21–22, 180
cortisol 19, 93, 144, 208, 282
Cotard's syndrome 68
counselling 32, 33, 112, 184, 201, 268, 281
countertransference 274
Couvade syndrome 88
culture
classification 2, 8
perinatal psychiatry in multi-ethnic
societies 278–286
cycloid psychosis 63, 68

day care 271
delirium 63–64
delusional misidentification 65
delusions 65, 68, 74, 75, 87, 156, 272
depot medication 88, 197, 216–217
depression 84, 174, 269
fathers 157
interventions 32–42
major 7, 10, 63, 182, 272
pregnancy 10, 15, 20–21, 22–23, 30–31,
114, 141–142, 146–147, 151, 180,
227–229
pregnancy loss 28
prevalence 10, 11, 22
psychotic 63, 67, 73
subsyndromal or subthreshold 7
see also antidepressants; postnatal
depression
desipramine 42
desvenlafaxine 251–252
detoxification
alcohol 121
substance misuse 128
diazepam 121, 126
diphenylbutylpiperidines 217
distress, after delivery 24
diuretics 97
domestic violence 13, 16, 22, 93–94, 108,
143, 155, 180
Doop Chaon instrument 178
dopamine receptors 20, 70
dothiepin 202, 247
doxepin 247
drug misuse see substance misuse
Drugs and Lactation Database
(LactMed) 266
DSM-IV 2–3, 5
DSM-V 2, 3–4, 5, 7
duloxetine 199, 213, 251

eating disorders 95–98
  child outcome 151, 153
  consequences 95–97
  management 97–98
Ebstein's anomaly 223
eclampsia 68, 126, 129
Edinburgh Postnatal Depression Scale
  (EPDS) 160, 175–177, 178, 179, 180,
  183, 185, 284, 289–290 Appendix
electroconvulsive therapy (ECT) 77, 92,
  161, 227–228, 260
emotional and behavioural problems,
  in children 150, 153, 154–155, 157,
  160–161, 162, 268, 282
emotional reciprocity 145
Emson, Daksha 3
encephalitis 64, 68
encephalopathy 64, 65
epidural anaesthesia 17, 30
escitalopram 203, 206, 250–251
ethnic minorities 109–110, 176, 178, 179,
  196
  see also multi-ethnic societies
euphoria 15, 64–65
exercise 35–36
explanatory models 2, 8
expressed emotion 150
extrapyramidal side effects 197, 222–223, 258
eye movement desensitisation and
  reprocessing treatment 41–42

factitious disorder by proxy 74
failure to thrive 152, 153, 281–282
family, parental mental illness and 158
fathers 151
  adolescent 157–158
  assessment of parenting capacity 99
  attachment 145
  cannabis 126
  Couvade syndrome 88
  infant homicide 156
  mental illness 156–157
  obsessive–compulsive disorder 27, 42
  pregnancy loss 28
  relationship with 13, 18
  services for 268
fatigue, postnatal depression and 18–19
fatty acids 20–21, 22, 39, 187, 229
female genital mutilation (FGM) 283–284
fertility 84–85, 117–118
fetal alcohol spectrum disorder (FASD) 115,
  151–152
fetal alcohol syndrome 115, 126

fetal cardiogram 223
fetus
  abuse 142–143
  activity 144, 151
  experiences 143–144
  growth retardation 111, 151, 200, 213,
    230
  intrauterine death 200
  pain perception 143
  risks of drug exposure 200
  routes of drug exposure 198–200
  teratogenicity 198, 200, 224, 226
  see also congenital malformations
filicide 156
floppy infant syndrome 215, 222, 227
fluoxetine 42, 198, 203–205, 206, 207, 208,
  248–249
fluphenazine decanoate 216–217
fluvoxamine 42, 199, 250, 251
folate 40, 222, 225
folic acid 85, 86
Framework for Assessing Children in Need and
  their Families 99–100
Fregoli syndrome 65

gabapentin 92, 226, 257
gamma-hydroxybutyrate (GBH) 127
gay couples 159
gender, of infant 13, 154, 282
General Health Questionnaire
  (GHQ-30) 177, 178
generalised anxiety disorder (GAD) 23–24,
  147
Generalised Anxiety Disorder Scale 178
General Medical Council guidelines, on
  prescribing 197
general practitioners (GPs) 44, 109, 114,
  182
genetic factors 2, 150
  postnatal depression 21–22
  puerperal psychosis 69–70, 279
gestational age
  large for (LGA) 151, 218, 219
  small for (SGA) 96, 118, 123, 124, 126,
    209, 216
gestational diabetes 96, 110, 205, 215–216,
  218, 222
gonadal steroid hormones 19–20, 70
grandparents 145, 158
Greek physicians 2
group interventions 32, 34–36
growth hormone responses, to
  apomorphine 20, 70

growth retardation, fetal 111, 151, 200, 213, 230
Gruen therapy 36

hair analysis 127
hallucinations 65, 68, 74, 75, 76
hallucinogens 125
haloperidol 217, 218, 258
Hamilton Rating Scale for Depression (HRSD) 177, 180
harm to infant 24, 26–27, 31, 42, 64, 75, 147, 272
health visitors 32–33, 44, 184, 185–186, 268–269, 281
herbal medicines 40, 201, 213–214, 254
heroin 123–124
historical perspectives 1–2
HIV infection 126, 129
home-based intervention 100, 162, 186, 271
HOME Inventory 160
homelessness 123
Home-Start 269
hormones 2, 19–20, 38–39, 186–187, 188
Hospital Anxiety and Depression Scale (HADS) 178
*How Are You Feeling?* booklet 178
hyperemesis 94, 95–96, 98, 210, 215
hyperprolactinaemia 87
hyperventilation 228
hypnosis 40, 187
hypnotics 214–215, 254–255
hypoglycaemia 202
hypothalamic–pituitary–adrenal (HPA) axis 19, 20, 93, 118, 143, 144, 151, 208

ICD-9 2
ICD-10 2–3, 4–5
ICD-11 3–4, 7
'Identify, Screen, Intervene, Support' programme 180
imipramine 202, 247
immune system dysregulation, in puerperal psychosis 70–71
infanticide 156, 182
  obsessions of 24
  puerperal psychosis 73–75
Infanticide Act 1938 74
Infanticide Act (Northern Ireland) 1939 74
infants
  assessment 160–161
  death 66
  factors in postnatal depression 19

harm to 24, 26–27, 31, 42, 64, 75, 147, 272
substance misuse in mothers 110, 111, 123–129
temperament 144, 149–150, 154
Infant Toddler Symptom Checklist 161
infective psychoses 63–64
inflammation mediators 21
information and education 36, 41, 78, 269, 287–288 Appendix
in-laws, relationship with 13, 18
in-patient care 76, 271–273
intellectual disability 73, 74, 272
  parenting 147–148
  screening 176, 178
international classifications 2–5
internet interventions 36–37
internet screening 179
interpersonal therapy (IPT) 32, 33–35, 44, 186
intimate partner violence (IPV) 13, 143, 155
IQ, parental 148

Kempe, Margery 2
ketamine 127

lactation *see* breastfeeding
'lactational psychosis' 1
lamotrigine 92, 225–226, 256–257
laxatives 97
LBW *see* low-birth weight babies
lesbian mothers 159
life events
  birth of child as 140
  depression during pregnancy 22
  postnatal depression 16–17
'listening visits' 32, 33, 184, 281
lithium 92, 188, 216, 223–224, 255
lofepramine 247
looked after children 146
lorazepam 93, 214, 254–255
low-birth weight babies (LBW) 142, 143
  anorexia nervosa 96
  depression in pregnancy 30–31, 151
  postnatal depression 19
  psychotropics in pregnancy 202, 206, 216, 217, 219
  schizophrenia 86
  self-harm 73
  substance misuse 112, 115, 118, 121, 123, 124, 125, 126

low- and middle-income countries 13, 35, 64, 66, 279, 280–281
lurasidone 221, 260
lysergic acid diethylamide (LSD) 125

mania 63, 64–65, 67, 71, 92, 187–188
Marcé, Louis Victor 1
Marcé Society 1
marital relationship, postnatal depression and 18
massage 39, 40, 161, 229–230
maternal deaths 71–72, 108, 143, 267, 270, 279
Maternal Mental Health Alliance Map 267, 272
maternity, delusions of 87
maternity services 269
MedEdPPD 36–37, 62
Medicines and Healthcare Products Regulatory Agency 208, 225, 230
medico-legal expertise 275
Mellow Bumps 161
meningioma 64
menstrual cycle 70
mental disorders
    maternal services 269
    misattribution of physical symptoms to 32, 270
    pre-existing 84–107
Mental Health Act 1983 Code of Practice 98
Mental Health Care and Treatment Act (Scotland) 76
mental health services 268, 270
mephedrone 127
methadone 123–124, 127, 129
methamphetamine 122, 152
methylenedioxymethamphetamine (MDMA; ecstasy) 124
methylphenidate 227
midwives 114–115, 182–183, 268, 269, 283–284
migrants 12, 268, 278, 282–284
Minding the Baby programme 162
mirtazapine 210–211, 252
miscarriage 28, 69, 177
    anorexia nervosa 96
    obsessive–compulsive disorder 95
    post-traumatic stress disorder 29, 94
    psychotropics during pregnancy 200, 202, 203, 209, 210
    substance misuse 110, 116, 117–118
moclobemide 213

monoamine oxidase inhibitors (MAOIs) 213, 252
monocytes 70, 71
mood stabilisers 76, 89–91, 188, 223–227, 255–257
mother and baby units 76, 99, 222, 267, 270, 271–273
mother–infant bonding disorders 179
mother–infant relationship 2, 4, 35, 75, 88, 154, 161–162, 179, 270, 281
Motherisk website 230, 255
Mother to Baby website 230
motivation interviewing 121
multi-ethnic societies 278–286

nefazodone 37, 211, 253
neonatal abstinence syndrome (NAS) 123–124, 128, 129, 152, 161
neonatal adaptation syndrome 161
neonatal intensive care unit (NICU) admission 198, 218, 219
neonates
    complications and psychotropics 202–203, 205–208, 214–227
    death 28–29, 124, 143, 151, 228
    pulmonary hypertension 206
    withdrawal symptoms 123–124, 128, 129, 161, 200, 201, 214–215, 250, 251
neonaticide 73–74, 142
neural tube defects (NTD) 85, 86, 91, 222, 224, 225
neuroleptic malignant syndrome (NMS) 76
neurotransmitters 19–20, 70, 151
NHS trusts 269
NICE (National Institute for Health and Care Excellence)
    breastfeeding and drugs 255, 256
    child outcomes 140, 159
    pregnancy and drugs 198, 215, 225
    rapid tranquillisation in pregnancy 227
    screening 175, 178
    service provision 267, 274
    substance misuse 113, 115, 116–117, 120
nicotine 109–115, 151–152, 154
nicotine replacement therapy (NRT) 112–113, 114
nitrazepam 73
norfluoxetine 203
nortriptyline 186, 202, 247

obesity 222
object relations theory 145

obsessional thoughts 24, 31, 38, 147
obsessive–compulsive disorder (OCD) 26–27, 259
  attachment 147
  interventions 42
  postpartum depression and 23–24
  pre-existing 95
obstetric complications
  antidepressants 202–203, 205–208
  schizophrenia 86
obstetric factors
  postnatal depression 17–18
  puerperal psychosis 71
obstetricians 182–183, 269
obstetric liaison 270–271, 273, 274
oestradiol/oestrogens
  postnatal depression 19–20, 39, 77, 187–188
  puerperal psychosis 69–70
olanzapine 91, 188, 218–219, 258
omega-3 fatty acids 22, 39, 187, 229
omphalocele 204
opiates 122, 123–124, 126, 128–129, 152, 153
organic pseudo-pregnancy 88
organic psychosis 63–64, 65
organisations 37, 287–288 Appendix
overdose 72, 73, 247, 269
oxytocin 21, 149

pain, fetal perception 143
paliperidone 221, 260
panic disorder 23–24, 26, 32, 92, 93, 259
Parental Bonding Instrument 160
parent and baby day unit (PBDU) 44, 271
Parent–Child Early Relational
    Assessment 160
parent–child psychotherapy 162
parent–child relationships 140, 141,
    144–145, 149, 152, 159, 161, 162
parenting
  assessment of capacity 99–100, 271, 275
  culture 278, 281
  intellectual disability 147–148
  interventions 100, 161–162
  parents' childhood experience of 16–17,
    141, 160
'Parenting and Mental Illness Group'
    programme 100
Parenting Stress Index 160
parent management training (PMT) 162
parents
  guilt 163
  mental illness and problems in
    children 268

parental attachment 148–150
  psychological adjustment 140–142
paroxetine 198, 203, 204–206, 207, 208,
    209, 249, 250
Patient Health Questionnaire (PHQ-9) 178
Perinatal Anxiety Screening Scale
    (PASS) 178
perinatal mental disorders
  alternative diagnoses 32, 270
  biopsychosociocultural model 15
  characteristics of 6–7
  children and family 139–173
  continuum from mild to severe 7
perinatal psychiatrists, skills needed 274–275
peripartum onset specifier 5, 7, 8
personality disorder 74, 99, 118, 147, 272
personality, postnatal depression and 18
pharmacokinetics, in pregnancy 198, 203
phenothiazines 216–217
phobic anxiety 25–26
physical illness 63–64, 66, 75–76, 78, 270
physical treatments
  breastfeeding 245–266
  pregnancy 196–244
pimozide 217
placenta
  drug transfer through 198–199, 218,
    256–257
  substance abuse 111, 118, 125
'PND' abbreviation 269
polypharmacy 197, 205, 218, 226
poor neonatal adaptation syndrome
    (PNAS) 207–208, 209
postnatal depression 4, 10–22, 23–24, 62, 93
  adjustment 27–28
  adolescent mothers 157
  adversity 16–17
  biological factors 13, 19–21, 180
  child outcome 153–155, 160–161, 268,
    281–282
  classification 4, 7
  eating disorders 96, 98
  epidemiology 12
  genetic factors 21–22
  infant factors 19
  interventions 32–44, 186–187, 268, 271
  life events 16–17
  marital relationship 18
  mood during pregnancy and early
    puerperium 15–17
  obstetric factors 17–18
  past psychiatric history 15–17
  personality 18

predictors 12–22
prevention 186–187
protective factors 13
public health problem 10
recurrence 11–12
screening 174–181, 183, 184, 185
self-harm 73
sleep deprivation and fatigue 18–19
social support 16–17, 18, 279–281
sociodemographic factors 17
specificity as concept 11–12
transcultural study 13, 280–283
Postpartum Bonding Instrument 179
Postpartum Depression Predictors Inventory
(PDPI-R) 181
Postpartum Depression Screening Scale
(PDSS) 175, 176, 179
post-traumatic stress disorder (PTSD) 23–
25, 180
attachment 147
interventions 41–42, 43
management 94
neonaticide 74
pre-existing 93–94
pregnancy loss 25, 28–29
refugees and asylum seekers 283
poverty 12, 13, 17, 86, 157
pre-eclampsia 17–18, 30, 94, 111, 151, 202,
224
pregnancy
advice against 85
anxiety disorders 23, 30–31, 40–41, 42,
92–94, 147, 151, 154–155, 229–230
bipolar disorder 89–91
child outcome of mental illness
during 150–152, 153, 154–155
concealment of 73–74, 142
culture 278
delusions of 87–88
denial of 87, 142–143
depression 10, 15, 20–21, 22–23, 30–31,
114, 141–142, 146–147, 151, 180,
227–229
eating disorders 95–96
ectopic 94
fear of future 17–18
fetal abuse 142–143
fetal experiences 143–144
intimate partner violence 143
loss 28–29, 41–42, 85, 141
obsessive–compulsive disorder 95
obstetric outcomes and anxiety/
depression during 30–31
organic pseudo-pregnancy 88

parental psychological adjustment 140–
142
physical treatments 196–244
anticholinergics 222–223
antidepressants 38, 196–214
antipsychotics 215–222
anxiolytics and hypnotics 214–215
discontinuing antidepressants 38, 197,
200
electroconvulsive therapy 161, 227–228
first-trimester exposure to drugs 201–
202, 203–204, 209
general principles 197–198
long-term neurodevelopmental
outcomes 203, 208–209
mood stabilisers 223–227
non-drug interventions 39–42, 227–230
pharmacokinetics 198, 203
rapid tranquillisation 227
risk–benefit analysis 196–197
risks to fetus 200
routes of fetal exposure 198–200
women's perceptions of drugs 200–201
postnatal depression and 15, 16
pre-birth planning 100
prenatal attachment 141–142, 146–147
pseudocyesis 87
'psychological' 140–141
psychosis 68–69, 142, 147, 228
psychotherapy 274
resources 230
screening 176, 177, 178, 180–183
self-harm 72–73
simulated 87
smoking 109–115, 154
stress 154
substance misuse 109–129, 154, 181
suicide 73
termination 30, 41, 69
unplanned 143, 151, 200
unwanted 142
Pregnancy Risk Questionnaire (PRQ) 181
premenstrual dysphoric disorder
(PMDD) 15
preterm birth 19, 73, 141, 142, 143
anxiety and depression in
pregnancy 30–31, 151
breastfeeding 246, 249, 253
electroconvulsive therapy in
pregnancy 228
pre-existing mental disorders 85, 86, 92,
94, 96
psychotropics in pregnancy 202, 206, 210,
216, 217, 218, 226

substance misuse 111, 112, 118, 120, 123, 124, 125, 126
prevention 186–188
primary care 267, 268–269
primiparity 65, 66, 71
progesterone 19–20, 38, 77, 186–187, 188
progestogens 38, 186–187
promethazine 215
Protecting the Next Pregnancy project 121
pseudocyesis 87
psychoanalytic theory 141, 145, 281
psychological/psychosocial therapies 162, 274
  depression and anxiety 32–36, 40–41, 186
  puerperal psychosis 78
  schizophrenia 88
psychosis 30, 86, 110, 272
  acute mixed atypical 7
  attachment 147
  cycloid 63, 68
  depressive 63, 67, 73
  fertility 84–85
  infective 63–64
  'lactational' 1
  organic 63–64, 65
  in pregnancy 68–69, 142, 147, 228
  unspecified functional 63
  see also bipolar disorder; puerperal psychosis; schizophrenia
public health 10, 281–282
puerperal psychosis 1, 63–83, 280
  aetiology 69–71
  assessment 75–76
  classification 3, 4, 5, 7, 8
  contraception 78
  dopamine 70
  drug treatment 76–77
  electroconvulsive therapy 77
  epidemiology 65–66
  genetics 69–70, 279
  immune system dysregulation 70–71
  infanticide 73–75
  in-patient care 76
  management 75–78
  obstetric factors 71
  onset, course and prognosis 66–68
  organic psychosis 63–64, 65
  phenomena 64–65
  prevention 187–188
  psychological treatment 78
  relationship to bipolar disorder 69
  screening 182, 183, 187–188
  self-harm 72–73
  services 270, 271

  suicide 71–72, 73, 74, 75, 76
  thyroid function 70
  women's experiences 71
Punjabi Postnatal Depression Scale 178

querulant (complaining) disorder 25
quetiapine 42, 218, 219–220, 259

rapid tranquillisation, in pregnancy 227
reboxetine 213, 253
refugees and asylum seekers 268, 278, 282–284
relaxation therapy 41
resilience, in children 139–140, 149–150
resources 195, 230, 291–292 Appendix
risperidone 218, 219, 220–221, 259
Romanian institutions 146
Royal College of Psychiatrists 3–4, 267, 275

S-adenosylmethionine 40
safeguarding issues 87, 152, 155–156, 273–274
St John's wort (hypericum) 40, 213–214, 254
Saving Mothers' Lives 72, 85
schizophrenia 63, 85–88, 110, 183, 259
  attachment 147
  child outcome 151, 156
  course 67, 68
  fertility 84
  mother and baby units 272
  parenting capacity 99
  pregnancy 216, 218, 222, 227–228
screening 3
  acceptability 179
  alcohol misuse 119–120
  case finding 174
  definition 174–175
  disclosure 179, 184, 185
  instruments 175–179
  internet-based 179
  and intervention 184–185, 186–187
  location 183–184
  postpartum 183
  pregnancy 180–183
  and prevention 186–188
  puerperal psychosis 182, 183, 187–188
  resources 195
  role of midwives and obstetricians 182–183
  women's opinions 185–186

secondary care 269–275
selective serotonin reuptake inhibitors
    (SSRIs) 37
  bipolar disorder 92
  breastfeeding 248–251
  obsessive–compulsive disorder 38, 42
  postnatal depression 38
  pregnancy 196, 197, 198–200, 203–209
  serotonergic syndrome in infant 161
selenium 187
self-harm 72–73, 151, 272
Self-Rating Depression Scale 178
separation, from children 84, 87, 98, 146,
    163, 272
serotonergic syndrome, in infants 161
serotonin levels, in depression 180
serotonin–noradrenaline reuptake inhibitors
    (SNRIs) 161, 214
serotonin transporter 20, 21–22, 69–70,
    248
sertraline 186, 198, 199, 203, 204, 205,
    249–250
service provision 267–277
  birth rate 267–268
  maternity services 269
  mental health services 270
  multi-ethnic societies 284
  primary care 268–269
  secondary care 269–275
  specialist perinatal psychiatric
services 270–275
sexual abuse
  of child 16, 22, 155
  of mother 26, 122–123
SGA (small for gestational age) 96, 118,
    123, 124, 126, 209, 216
siblings 158
sleep problems
  breastfeeding 246, 260
  infant 19
  intervention 40, 187
  postnatal depression 18–19, 40, 187
  pregnancy 215
  puerperal psychosis 187–188
  smoking 111–112
smoking 85, 108, 109–115, 122, 125, 143
  alcohol 117, 120
  cessation interventions 112–115
  child behavioural problems 154
  depression in pregnancy 22–23
  pharmacological interventions 112–113
  providers of interventions 114–115
  relapse prevention 112
  reluctance to engage in cessation 113–115

social factors
  adolescent mothers 157
  postnatal depression 12, 17
  substance misuse 122–123, 181
social services
  children 98, 156
  supervision on discharge 99, 147
social support
  depression during pregnancy 22
  group treatment 35
  postnatal depression 16–17, 18, 279–281
  smoking cessation 112
sodium valproate 91, 224–225, 256
sound, fetal experiences of 143
specialist community services 267
specialist perinatal psychiatric services 3,
    267, 270–275
  child protection 273–274
  community services 271
  functions 270–271
  in-patient units 271–273
  links with other agencies 274
  obstetric liaison 273
  psychiatrists' skills 274–275
Specialist Pharmacy Service (SPS) 266
status, of mother 278, 280
stillbirth 25, 28–29, 86, 118, 151, 200
stimulants 124–125, 227
Strengths and Difficulties
  Questionnaire 160
stress, maternal 16–17, 22, 23–31, 144, 151,
    153, 154
stressors, for refugees and asylum
  seekers 282–284
subdural haematoma 64, 75–76
substance misuse 85, 108–138, 143, 161, 198
  attachment 141–142, 146
  child outcome 151–152
  definitions 108
  dependence syndrome (addiction) 108
  depression in pregnancy 22–23
  detoxification 128
  harmful use 108
  infanticide 74
  management during pregnancy 127–129
  polydrug use 122
  postnatal care 129
  post-traumatic stress disorder 94
  in pregnancy, and infant outcomes 123–
    129
  pregnancy loss 28
  prevalence 122–123
  residential treatment programmes 162
  schizophrenia 86

screening and detection 109, 127, 181
self-harm 73
substitution and maintenance 128–129
*see also* alcohol misuse; smoking
sudden infant death syndrome 22, 24, 86,
111–112, 118, 126
suicide/suicidality 150–151
antidepressants in pregnancy 38, 196
depression in pregnancy 20–21, 22
filicide 156
harm to infant 31
puerperal psychosis 71–72, 73, 74, 75, 76
screening 180, 182
substance misuse 108
Sure Start Children's Centres 269


T-ACE questionnaire 119–120
taste, fetal experiences of 143
T cell levels 70–71
telephone interventions 36–37, 112
temazepam 255
temperament, of infant 144, 149–150, 154
teratogenicity 198, 200–201, 224, 226, 230
thrombocytopenia 125, 128
thyroid dysfunction
lithium via breastfeeding 255
postnatal depression 21, 187
puerperal psychosis 70
tokophobia 25–26
toluene 122, 126
topiramate 92
toxicity 198, 200, 203, 255
training 183, 184, 185, 268, 269, 275
transcranial magnetic stimulation
breastfeeding 260
pregnancy 228–229
transcultural psychiatry 279
trazodone 212, 252
tricyclic antidepressants (TCAs) 197,
201–203, 247
trifluoperazine 258
tryptophan hydroxylase gene
polymorphisms 21
TWEAK instrument 119, 120


Uganda 3, 280
UK National Screening Committee
(NSC) 174–175

ultrasound scans 94, 142, 214, 223
umbilical artery resistance 111
UN Millennium Development Goals 279
urine analysis 127
uterine artery resistance 93, 111


vagus nerve stimulation, in pregnancy 229
valproate 91, 92, 224–225, 226, 256
varenicline 113
venlafaxine 37, 42, 198–200, 203, 205,
209–210, 249, 251–252
venous thromboembolism 76–77, 86, 187,
215–216
verapamil 227, 257
Victoria Climbié inquiry report 87
vitamins 85, 121
B12 86
D 21
K 224
volatile substance misuse ('glue
sniffing') 122, 126–127


Watching, Waiting and Wondering
programme 162
*What to do if you're worried a child is being
abused* 87
*Why Mothers Die* 71–72
withdrawal symptoms, in neonate 123–124,
128, 129, 161, 200, 250, 251
women's opinions
drugs in pregnancy 200–201
puerperal psychosis 71
screening 185–186
treatment 42–44
*Working Together to Safeguard Children* 87, 273
World Health Organization's Self-Reporting
Questionnaire 176
World Psychiatric Association, International
Guidelines for Diagnostic Assessment 4


zaleplon 215
ziprasidone 221, 260
zolpidem 37, 215, 255
zopiclone 215
zotepine 221, 260

Printed in the United States
By Bookmasters